# Ayurvedic Perspectives on Selected Pathologies

# Other Books by Vasant D. Lad

Ayurveda: The Science of Self-Healing. 1985

Secrets of the Pulse: The Ancient Art
of Ayurvedic Pulse Diagnosis. 1996

The Complete Book of Ayurvedic Home Remedies. 1998

The Textbook of Ayurveda: Fundamental Principles,
Volume One. 2002

Strands of Eternity: A Compilation of
Mystical Poetry and Discourses. 2004

The Textbook of Ayurveda: A Complete Guide
to Clinical Assessment, Volume Two. 2006

The Textbook of Ayurveda: General Principles
of Management and Treatment, Volume Three. 2012

The Yoga of Herbs: An Ayurvedic Guide to Herbal Medicine. 1986
by Vasant Lad and David Frawley

Ayurvedic Cooking for Self-Healing. 2nd ed., 1997
by Usha and Vasant Lad

Marma Points of Ayurveda: The Energy Pathways
for Healing Body, Mind and Consciousness with a
Comparison to Traditional Chinese Medicine. 2008
by Vasant Lad and Anisha Durve

# Ayurvedic Perspectives on Selected Pathologies

*An Anthology of Essential Reading
from* Ayurveda Today
*Second Edition*

by
## Vasant D. Lad, B.A.M.&S., M.A.Sc.

Anthology Compiled by Vasant D. Lad
First Edition Compiled by Glen Crowther

The
Ayurvedic
Press

Albuquerque, New Mexico

Although the information contained in this book is based on Ayurvedic principles practiced for thousands of years, it should not be taken or construed as standard medical diagnosis or treatment. For any medical condition, always consult with a qualified physician.

Traditional Ayurvedic medicine may contain botanicals (herbs), minerals, animal substances or any combination of them. The remedies in this book follow the traditional Ayurvedic pharmacopoeia and may contain substances that modern science and conventional medicine do not consider to be safe or effective. Consult with a qualified physician before using any of the formulations listed in this book.

This book is printed on acid-free paper.

Cover design by Michael Quanci.
Project management and layout by Laura Humphreys.

First Edition 2005
Second Edition 2012, revised and expanded
ISBN 978-1-883725-16-7
Printed in the United States of America

---

**Library of Congress Cataloging-in-Publication Data**

Lad, Vasant, 1943-
   Ayurvedic perspectives on selected pathologies : an anthology of essential reading from ayurveda today / by Vasant Lad ; anthology compiled by Vasant Lad. -- 2nd ed.
      p. cm.
   Includes bibliographical references.
   ISBN 978-1-883725-16-7 (alk. paper)
   1. Medicine, Ayurvedic. I. Title.
   R605.L25 2012
   615.5'38--dc23
                          2012007966

---

Published by **The Ayurvedic Press** • P.O. Box 23445 • Albuquerque, NM 87192-1445
*For more information on Ayurveda, contact:*
The Ayurvedic Institute • 11311 Menaul Blvd. NE • Albuquerque, NM 87112
(505) 291-9698 • Fax 505.294.7572 • www.ayurveda.com

# Table of Contents

# Editor's Preface

IN THIS EDITION, Dr. Lad selected the additional titles for the book from the numerous articles that he has written in the ensuing seven years' publication of *Ayurveda Today*. Dr. Lad has grouped the articles according to srotamsi, the bodily channels, and this is noted in the Table of Contents. Primarily oriented to the practitioner, these articles give in-depth descriptions of pathologies from an Ayurvedic understanding along with detailed recommendations to correct these imbalances.

There are more than 200 substances used for healing mentioned in this text. The appendix has a comprehensive table providing details about each of these substances. Additionally, there are illustrations in the appendix for the marma therapy protocols recommended within the text.

Meditation is an important part of health for body, mind, and spirit. Dr. Lad suggests several meditation techniques in the text. Instructions for Empty Bowl and So'hum Meditation are available on our website at http://www.ayurveda.com/online_resource/index.html. He also mentions pranayama (breathing exercises) as a form of self-healing. These can be learned from qualified yoga instructors. Also available is a DVD, *Pranayama for Self-Healing,* with full instructions by Dr. Lad in the Products Section of our website. He talks about beneficial yoga postures many times in the text, most often with their English names. See Table 10, "Yogāsana Used in this Book," on page 247 for the Sanskrit and English names of the poses.

***Sanskrit.*** Knowledge of Ayurveda originates in the Sanskrit language. Sanskrit is a precise phonetic language that uses a set of written symbols not familiar to most Westerners. The phonetic representation of Sanskrit words using the English alphabet is called transliteration. We can transliterate Sanskrit to English characters, but not every sound translates directly. There are quite a few sounds that do not exist in the English language, requiring special characters to represent them accurately.

One example is वात ,which translates to vāta. The first 'a' in vāta is a 'long a,' as in "father"; it is held for two beats. The second 'a' is a 'short a,' as in "what." Another example is a sound somewhere between an 'i,' a 'u' and an 'r' that occurs in the word प्रकृति. This word is transliterated as prakṛti. The 'ṛ' is pronounced as the 'ri' in the English spelling of the word Krishna. To make things even more complicated, among those who use Sanskrit the 'ṛ' is pronounced in northern India as the 'i' in "it" and in southern India as the 'u' sound in "root." Because of the regional variations in pronunciation, in this book both ru and ri are found in place of the technically correct 'ṛ'.

Another consideration is that the trailing 'a' in Sanskrit words is sometimes omitted because of the influence of the Hindi language. It is included in many of the words in this book. The trailing 'a' is also subject to grammatical changes depending on the letters that follow it and, for simplicity's sake, we generally ignore these rules. For example, the word *meda* (fat) can be transliterated as *medo, medas,* and meda depending on the word following it. Ordinarily, we use the most common form, meda, so that you, the reader, will have to learn only the one word. Of course, it would be wonderful if all our readers began the study of Sanskrit, inspired by the knowledge available in these ancient texts, but it is not our purpose here to teach that language.

In *Ayurvedic Perspectives*, we have chosen to use transliteration characters only for long vowels, denoted by an overscore or macron character, and for the 'nya' sound denoted by 'ñ'. The pronunciations of the vowels are:

a as in about; ā as in father

i as in ink; ī as in fee

u as in put; ū as in food

e as in pay; ai as in I

o as in corn; au as in loud

In all of our texts, we have elected to italicize the first occurrence of the Ayurvedic terms used in the text,[1] since they are used repeatedly throughout the text.

## Acknowledgements

The idea for the first edition of this book originated with Glen Crowther, Dr. Lad's long time editor and student. He selected the articles and edited them to fit within the publication, with Dr. Lad's input, of course. He brings creativity, precision, and a deep knowledge of Ayurveda to his work. We are grateful to him for his long association with The Ayurvedic Press and Dr. Lad.

Photos listed here are © iStockphoto.com/ page 20, 235, red_frog; page 169, 236, 237, izusek; page 235, LindaMarieB; page 236, janulla; page 75, Eraxion. Front cover photos are © iStockphoto.com/ AgnieszkaS (stomach), MedicalArtInc (knee), pukrufus (brain, lungs), and mladn61 (microscope).

All other illustrations are by Vasant D. Lad, BAM&S, MASc, © copyright 2012. Photos page 181, © copyright The Ayurvedic Institute.

---

1. *The Chicago Manual of Style,* 15th ed. (Chicago: University of Chicago Press, 2003), 292.

# Chapter 1

# Causative Factors of Āma

Fall 1999, Volume 12, Number 2

उष्मणोऽल्प बलत्वेन धातुमाद्यमपाचितम् ।
दुष्टमामशयगतं रसमामं प्रचक्षते
वाग सु १३ढ२५

Ushmano 'lpa balatvena dhātum ādyama pāchitam
Dushṭam āmashaya gatam rasam āmam prachakshate

*The first dhātu (rasa) which by the weakness of the (digestive) fire remaining uncooked and becoming vitiated accumulates in the stomach and small intestine is known as āma.*

Vāg. Su. 13.25

THESE SUTRAS DESCRIBE the formation of *āma* in the body and mind. You should learn this first *sūtra* by heart. The first line of the sūtra means: because of the low, inner fire, *āhāra rasa*—the food precursors of all subsequent *dhātus*—remains *apachita,* remains undigested, unprocessed and raw.

In the second line of the sūtra, the raw, unprocessed ahāra rasa, which is disturbed by āma, goes into the *āmāshaya,* the stomach. The drawing on the next page illustrates the lesser curvature of the stomach and its blood vessels as well as the greater curvature and its many blood vessels. Also shown are *jāthara agni* and the thoracic duct or chyle duct which contains *ādyām apachitam rasam,* the undigested food precursors. Ādyām apachita rasa refluxes back into the stomach through the blood vessels because of low agni. This means that āma formation takes place when the end product of previously eaten food contains materials that have not been fully digested. This end product, whether fully digested or not, is the food precursor for the dhātus. This food precursor is the *ādyāhāra rasa* which is not digested completely or processed properly because of low jāthara agni. Because it is

> *ushmano:* ushma means heat referring to inner heat, fire, agni
> *'lpa:* 'lpa means low, little, scanty
> *balatvena:* by the strength
> *dhātum:* the tissue
> *ādyāma:* the first; first dhātu, the rasa
> *pachitam:* undigested, unprocessed, unassimilated
> *gata:* to go
> *rasam:* it goes to the rasa dhātu
> *āmāshaya:* stomach
> *chaksa:* to look
> *prachaksa:* means not only looking but knowing

1

undigested, it is called āma which is *dushtam*—disturbed—by quality. Translating the entire sūtra: *Because of the low inner fire, the first food precursors of the dhātus remain unprocessed. Those disturbed, unprocessed, raw food precursors then enter the stomach instead of going to feed the dhātus, at which point they are called āma.*

Āma formation due to low agni causes unprocessed micro-chyle to regurgitate back into the stomach.

This first sūtra is one of the beautiful definitions of āma. It puts emphasis on jāthara agni, the gastric fire. Because of the low strength of inner fire, agni, the first āhāra rasa remains undigested and disturbed. That undigested and disturbed āhāra rasa enters back into the stomach for further digestion because the tissue does not accept and cannot process anything raw. This is the intelligence of the body. This is the reason a person's tongue looks coated. Before eating look at your tongue in the mirror. If the tongue is coated because of āma, that means undigested, unprocessed *rasa* is regurgitating back into the stomach. You should not eat if your tongue is coated. That is going against the intelligence of the body. Modern medicine does not give any importance to a white coating; they say do not worry, it is there. However, Ayurveda says this is the root cause of all disease; that disease is born out of āma. That is why disease is called *āmaya*. It means that which is born out of āma.

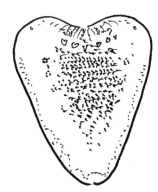

A white coating on the tongue indicates āma in the gastrointestinal tract.

आमं अन्नरसं केचित् केदित्तु मल संचयं ।
प्रथम दोष दुष्टिं च केचित् आमं प्रचक्षते ॥

अनाम

Āmam annarasam kechit kedittu mala sanchayam
Prathama doṣa dushṭim cha kechit āmam pracakshate

*According to some, accumulated wastes are āma but, according to others, undigested ahara rasa is āma and according to others the previously disturbed dosha is called āma.*

Anon.

The second definition is more complete. This sūtra is not in the classical texts; it is from an enlightened master, *kechit*. Kechit can even be translated as "someone" or "some authority." *Amam* is āma and *anna rasam* means undigested food juice. Therefore, according to an authority, āma is undigested food juice. That is the whole meaning of this first phrase, *amam annarasam kechit*. The second phrase, *kedittu mala sanchayam*, means that when a person does not sweat properly, then this unexpressed sweat will make the body impure. If a person does not urinate for three days then non-eliminated urine will make the body impure. It is the same if a person does not defecate for four or five days, those constipated feces make the body impure. When the *malas* stay in the body for too long they make the body impure. Mala means the impurities of the body, which are urine, sweat, and feces. These are the three malas.

According to this sage, āma is simply accumulated impurities, malas. Meaning that when a person has constipation, scanty urination or no perspiration, then those impurities become āma. This is a very beautiful definition. This sūtra also says āma is undigested food juice and that āma is due to previously disturbed dosha. This is a very complete definition.

In the first sūtra, āma is defined as undigested āhāra rasa because of low agni. According to the next sūtra, āma is accumulated, stagnated impurities or malas because of improper elimination of urine, feces or sweat. This sūtra also says that āma is nothing but previously disturbed *dosha*. These sūtras are good explanations of the sources of āma. They give us a complete, three-dimensional picture of the formation of āma in the body.

*amam*: Ām
*annarasam*: the food juice, the end product of digested food juic
*kechit*: according to someone, according to some authority; the repeated reference, *kedit*, means according to another authority
*tu*: but
*mala*: the three *mala* — urine, feces and sweat; that which makes the body impure if it is accumulated
*samchayam*: accumulation, stagnation
*pratamama*: previous, the first, the one before
*dosha*: vāta, pitta, kapha
*dushtim*: disturbed
*cha*: and
*prachakshate*: is called

स्रोतोरोध बल भ्रंश गौरवानिल मूढताः ।
आलस्यापक्ति निष्ठिव मलसङ्गारुचि क्लमाः ॥

अष्ट हृ सु १३ २३

Sroto rodha bala bhramsha gauravānila mūḍatāḥ
Ālasyāpakti nishtiva malasaṅgāruchi klamāḥ

*The signs and symptoms of āma are clogging of channels, sense of heaviness, low energy, restlessness, lethargy, indigestion, kaphatype congestion (expectoration), accumulation of the three malas (wastes), loss of taste and sexual debility.*

Aṣṭ Hṛd. Su. 30.23

This third sūtra is important and supplements the previous two. The first word is *sroto rodha*. Sroto rodha is blocking the channels. In this sūtra, they are using this very beautiful, specific phrase: Whenever āma is formed in the system, it creates clogging of the channels. These blocked channels can mean many things: coronary occlusion, pulmonary embolism, stagnation, venous engorgement or lymphatic obstruction. For all these, they are using just one phrase: sroto rodha which is due to āma in the system.

*Bala bhramsha* refers to having low energy or strength. This can manifest as someone having chronic fatigue syndrome which is due to too much āma in the liver. If you feel tired and weak, drink agni tea. It will burn āma and you will get energy. This first phrase, sroto rodha bala bhramsha, refers to low energy, fatigue and tiredness. *Gaurava* is a sense of heaviness. The person feels heavy subjectively—heaviness in the body, hands, belly or head. Whenever you feel heaviness anywhere, it is due to āma.

*Anila mūdhatā* means the *vāta* channels are blocked. Vāta starts moving about seeking an open channel and, in its constant movement, gains momentum due to the pressure created by the blockage. These efforts to find its own way around that blockage cause vāta to become restless. This restlessness of vāta creates breathlessness, tingling and numb-

srotas: channels
rodha: blocked, blockage, blocking
   the channels
balā: strength, energy
bhramsha: low, lack of energy,
   fatigue
gaurva: sense of heaviness
anila: vāyu
mūdhatā: restlessness and confusion
   of vāta dosha
ālasya: lethargy, malaise
apakti: indecision. Pakti means
   decision; apakti no decision
malasanga: accumulation of
   impurities
aruchi: lack of taste
klamaha: means sexual debility, or
   sexual weakness

ness, burping, flatulence, and hyper-peristalsis. Mental confusion and restless or excessive thinking are signs of blocked vāta. Anila mūdhatā is as if a heavy storm has happened in the body because of āma, creating ringing in the ear, insomnia, "ungroundedness," confusion, constipation, vague intestinal pain, increased peristalsis, tremors, ticks, or spasms.

It is as if vāta becomes hyperactive because of being blocked by āma. Another meaning of the phrase anila mūdhatā refers to mental confusion, lack of clarity, and poor perception. This restlessness and confusion cause the mind to become foggy resulting in mental āma.

In the second sentence, the person has no enthusiasm to do anything because of *ālasya* and the inability to decide whether to take an action, caused by *apakti*. *Nishthiva* has a very significant meaning. A meaning of the word *nishtha* is faith, but because of āma, it becomes nishthiva, which means faithlessness. One hidden meaning of the word nishthiva is lack of mental faith. The disciple who has a lot of āma in his or her mind loses faith, because faith is trust, clarity and love. When there is mental āma the person does not trust, so nishthiva means doubt or delusion. That is one meaning of nishthiva.

Another meaning of nishthiva is to spit out or expectorate *kapha. Kapha nishthivanam* means pulmonary congestion. When veins are clogged with kapha that is also āma. Āma and kapha are very similar in quality. They are both heavy, oily, sticky and cloudy. Āma creates nishthiva, congestion, adhesions and fibrocystic changes in the breasts. Even when you do oil massage, if there is too much āma the person's body will ache. In a case like this, have them take trikatu and ginger tea to burn that āma and the pain will go away.

*Malasanga* is the accumulation of malas—urine, feces, sweat—but can also mean the accumulation of mental mala—conclusion, judgment, criticism. When the suppression of unresolved anger, fear or frustration accumulates in the mind, it becomes polluted and that is another form of malasanga or mental āma. *Aruchi,* which means a lack of taste or flavor, can also mean a lack of interest or enthusiasm. *Klamaha* means sexual debility or weakness. The accumulation of malas is a sroto rodha and it leads to a lack of enthusiasm and sexual debility, which is the result of āma.

A modern definition of āma could include high cholesterol, high triglycerides, high sugar and increased white blood cells—leukocytosis—or decreased white blood cells—leukocytopenia. Āma also is indicated by an accumulation of antibodies, increased blood urea, increased platelet count and increased red blood cell count—called polycythemia, which is āma resulting from aggravated *pitta.* Stagnant bile in the gallbladder is āma, which can create gallstones. Increased liver enzymes (SGOT, SGPT) are indications of āma in the liver, leading to chronic fatigue syndrome. Āma in the eye increases intraocular pressure creating glaucoma. According to the definition of āma in the second sūtra, even the accumulation of bacteria leading to bacterial infection is pittagenic āma. These examples help us to understand the role āma plays in terms of modern science and in Ayurveda.

We can see from these sūtras that āma can be classified according to the doshic disturbance, to improper digestion of the āhāra rasa and to the blockage of the *srotas* or channels of the body. There can also be mental āma. It is interesting that āma creates mūdhatā, restlessness because restlessness also creates āma. The cause becomes the effect and the effect then becomes a cause.

I would like to add one more. According to my observations, āma is also formed from unresolved emotion. If you have unexpressed anger, emotions or fears, it will create mental āma. So, I can add one more sūtra and say: According to a kechit or an authority who lives in Albuquerque, āma could be formed by unresolved, unexpressed emotions.

To be one with the present moment is clarity, but we live in the past or we live in the future. Because of its sticky, gluey qualities, āma creates attachment to the past and, because of its liquid, slimy qualities, it causes us to skate or slide into the future. It is the past and the future that gives meaning to life. The present moment is deeply connected to the past and when you stay with the present moment, you can see the past clearly.

Mental āma is formed from unresolved emotions.

To be in the present moment is to be with agni and agni is clarity, love, digestion. When we are stuck with the past, our emotion never gets digested or processed into love or intelligence. So, be in the present moment! In the present moment, when an unresolved emotion or thought from the past comes up and you are in the present moment, you are looking at it with clarity, with love. Then you can act from that clarity, call your friend or loved one and ask for forgiveness. By remaining in the present moment, you can heal your past. Getting stuck with the past is mūdhatā. It is apakti when you remain with the past; then there is no digestion of the past hurt and you blame yourself. Do not blame yourself. Love yourself and forgive yourself. Forgiving happens in the present moment.

In the present moment, you can see the beauty of the blue sky, the lonely shadow of a tree, marvel at the beautiful face of a child, or the innocent face of your wife or husband. When you are here, be here, at this moment. Buddha taught this meditation: eating mindfully, sitting mindfully, sleeping mindfully. If you really practice mindfulness, you live in the present moment. This awareness brings perfect digestion of our moment-to-moment experiences. By practicing this art of being one with this present moment, we can easily burn mental āma. Practicing mindfulness burns āma.

Thank God, we are given one moment at a time, not two, not three! One moment at a time, but even so we cannot live that moment completely. We are either stuck with past grief, sadness and emotions, or we are worried about the divine future. If I live fully, completely this moment, this moment will make my future. Therefore, instead of saying, "make my day" you can say, "make my moment." Meditation is the simplest thing to do, there is nothing as simple as breathing, there is nothing as simple as paying attention to this very moment. So, when you live in the present moment, a tremendous energy comes to you, you become the central focus of the entire universe. If you stay in the present moment, the Universe is blessing you, showering a benediction upon you from all directions. This moment is called *pakti*. Pakti means digestion. In the present moment there is no āma. The present moment is poetry, the present moment is art, and it is ecstasy and joy. So, my dear friend, let us learn this art of living mindfully every moment, not to judge, not to criticize, but to be one with this moment.

# Chapter 2

# Shat Kriyā Kāla: Vāta
## Management of the Six Stages of Samprāpti for Vāta

Spring 2010, Volume 22, Number 4

THE FIVE CLINICAL barometers used in Ayurvedic medicine in order to study a disease are called *nidāna pañchakam*. These are *nidāna,* etiology, *pūrva rūpa,* prodromal signs and symptoms, *rūpa,* the cardinal signs and symptoms, *upashaya,* therapeutic trial and *samprāpti,* pathogenesis.

We have discussed this topic numerous times and most students are very familiar with the six stages of samprāpti. In this article, we will see how the *shat kriyā kāla,* the six important stages of samprāpti, can be effectively managed when we pay complete, undivided attention to the signs and symptoms of the patient.

Each individual has his or her unique *prakruti,* personal genetic code, which maintains his or her unique psycho-physiological balance. This balance can be disturbed by environmental changes, seasonal changes, change within a relationship and the moment-to-moment changes of emotions. Due to the influence of these factors, the doshas undergo qualitative and quantitative changes. The *gunas* (qualities, attributes) related to each stage of samprāpti, beautifully explained in volume two of the *Textbook of Ayurveda* series, are shown in the table below.

**Table 1: Gunas (Qualities) Relating to Each Stage of Samprāpti**

| Stage | Vāta | Pitta | Kapha |
|---|---|---|---|
| Sañchaya (accumulation) | Cold | Liquid, Sour | Heavy, Cool |
| Prakopa (provocation) | + Dry, Light | + Hot, Pungent | + Liquid, Slow, Dull |
| Prasara (spread) | + Mobile | + Spreading, Oily | + Oily |
| Sthāna Samshraya (deposition) | + Subtle | + Sharp | +Sticky, Slimy |
| Vyakti (manifestation) | + Rough | + Light | + Cloudy, Soft |
| Bheda (complication) | + Clear | + Fleshy smell | +Hard, Dense, Static, Gross |

If we look closely at these qualitative expressions of the doshas in the stages of samprāpti then one can see that it is beneficial to use the opposite quality to oppose the aggravation by using the table of the pairs of opposites.

## Vāta Management and the Stages of Samprāpti

In this article, we will attempt to cover the management of vāta in the various stages of samprāpti.

In the *sañchaya* stage, the cold quality accumulates in the anal canal and the rectum producing constipation, lower abdominal distention and gas. In this case, we can apply our theory of using the opposite quality to oppose or balance the aggravated quality by placing a hot castor oil heavy compress on the abdomen or a hot water bottle followed by a warm sesame oil *basti*.

In the *prakopa* stage, the cold, dry and light qualities cause vāta to become aggravated in the colon. These will require more space and produce fullness in the flanks, increased peristalsis and pressure under the diaphragm accompanied by difficulty in breathing. To compensate for this, a warm dashamūla tea basti can be used. Prepare this by boiling 1 Tbs. of dashamūla powder in 1 pint of water. Then strain and allow to cool. While it is still warm, add ½ cup of sesame oil then administer the basti. This type of basti will conquer vāta in its second stage. To prevent further prakopa, use triphalā guggulu 300 mg in capsules three times a day (TID) or gandharva harītakī, 1 tsp. at bedtime with warm water as necessary.

| |
|---|
| T.I.D. = from the Latin means *ter in diem,* three times a day |
| B.I.D. = from the Latin means *bis in diem,* two times a day |

With the *prasara* stage, the mobile quality helps vāta to leave the gastrointestinal (GI) tract. Any dosha entering circulation comes into contact with the heart, the capillary layer, *rakta dhātu* and the topmost layer of the skin, *rasa dhātu*. During this stage, vāta creates dry skin, goose bumps, poor circulation, cold hands and feet, palpitations, ringing in the ears, and abnormal pulsations in the veins. This stage requires *abhyanga* (massage) or *snehana* (self-massage with oil) and *svedana* (sudation) to stabilize vāta. The vāta types can use sesame oil, pitta can use sunflower oil and kapha can use olive oil. This should be followed by svedana. For vāta types a few drops of nirgundī oil can added to the steam box; a couple of drops of sandalwood oil for pitta types and three to five drops of eucalyptus oil can be added for the kapha types. For the palpitations that occur during this stage, take a dashamūla tea with ½ tsp. of arjuna. For the ringing in the ears, *karna pūrana* is well indicated.

As for the abnormal pulsation in the veins, a formula consisting of equal parts of manjishthā, rakta chandana, and jatamāmsi can be taken ½ tsp. TID with warm water until the symptom subsides.

### Sthāna Samshraya and the Dhātus

In *sthāna samshraya,* the addition of the subtle quality of vāta in the process of samprāpti allows vāta to enter any weakened dhātu (tissue) or to impair the agni (meta-bolic fire) of the dhātu. If all *dhātu agnis* are healthy then vāta is not able to enter into any dhātu and will return to the colon This is a state called *prashama avastha,* in which all dhātu agnis are healthy and there is no *khavaigunya* (defective space). However, it is very rare for this to happen. It is far more usual for vāta to enter the tissues or to skip one dhātu and move to the subsequent one, wherever the agni is impaired.

**The 20 Paired Opposite Gunas**

| Heavy | Light |
|---|---|
| Slow / Dull | Sharp |
| Cold | Hot |
| Oily | Dry |
| Slimy / Smooth | Rough |
| Dense | Liquid |
| Soft | Hard |
| Static (stable) | Mobile |
| Subtle | Gross |
| Clear | Sticky / Cloudy |

*Rasa Dhātu.* When *rasa dhātu agni* is low, vāta enters this tissue creating fever with chills, dry dark skin, malaise, fatigue, general body ache, acne, palpitations, goose bumps and dehydration. This is the textbook picture of *vāta jvara* (fever) and is best treated by using a formula with dashamūla 500 mg, tribhuvan kirti 200 mg, or sudarshan gana vati 200 mg with tulsi tea.[1] In the west, we can use dashamūla 500 mg, tagara 200 mg, and mahāsudarshan 200 mg with ginger, cinnamon, and basil tea. The person should be wrapped in a warm blanket and, to correct dehydration, given a homemade dextro-saline solution made by adding 5 tsp. of sugar, ½ tsp. of salt, and the juice of ½ lime to a pint of water.

*Rakta Dhātu.* If the mobile and subtle qualities of vāta encounter a strong rasa dhātu agni and are warded off, then vāta attempts to enter rakta dhātu. If rakta dhātu is low, then *rakta gata vāta* occurs.[2] In this case, there will be poor circulation and cold hands and feet. This vāta condition will create very small red blood cells (microcytic anemia), blood clots, varicose veins, craving for meat, and aneurism.

For the poor circulation, massage briskly, creating friction, with mahānārāyana oil to improve circulation. Afterwards, soak in a bath containing  cup each of ginger powder and baking soda for at least 5-10 minutes. This can be done daily until the condition subsides.

In the case of microcytic anemia, one should use 1 tsp. of mahatikta ghrita before each meal, take 4 Tbs. of kumārī āsava with equal amounts of water after lunch and dinner, or take loha āsava in the same way. Additionally, add supplements such as vitamin $B_{12}$, 500 mg per day, and folic acid, 60 mg per day.

In the case of blood clots, Ayurveda recommends the use of kaishore guggulu, 200 mg TID, or trikatu in the same dosage. This regimen would be very similar to the use of 85 mg of aspirin to prevent clotting.

The craving for protein can be met by having chicken broth, liver soup, fried rabbit blood, or blood sausage sautéed with ghee. Alternatively, a vegetarian could consume beet juice, carrot juice, barley greens, blue green algae, spinach, or red cabbage, which are also sources of the iron that the body is craving.

Varicose veins can be aided by taking ½ tsp. TID of a formula containing kaishore guggulu 200 mg, trikatu 200 mg, and pushkaramūla 200 mg. Foods like garlic, onions, turmeric, and ginger will help the blood fluidity. Apply mahānārāyana oil to the varicose

---

1. Vati are tablets, usually flattened.
2. Gata means 'gone;' in this context, entering into.

veins, then keep the legs elevated or in the *viparīta karanī* (legs up the wall) yogic posture at least once daily.

***Māmsa Dhātu.*** In the case that both the rasa and the rakta dhātu agnis are functioning properly and not allowing vāta to enter the dosha, then *māmsa dhātu* will be the next to be affected, if its agni is not strong. When vāta enters this tissue, it creates *māmsa gata vāta,* which will manifest as muscle spasm, muscle pain, tics and tremors, muscle wasting, and low muscle power, tone and coordination, which can lead to paralysis, foot drop, restless leg syndrome, or even dancing chorea (involuntary dancing).

For the muscle pain, simply do abhyanga or snehana with mahānārāyana oil, followed by a svedana with nirgundī oil. Furthermore, it would be beneficial to take internally ½ tsp. TID a formula containing equal proportions of yogarāja guggulu, mustā, and tagara with warm water.

In case of emaciation, a formula containing ashvagandhā 500 mg, balā 400 mg and vidārī 300 mg can be given with milk in the dosage of ½ tsp. TID. Additionally, increasing the consumption of cashews, almonds or almond milk, protein intake, and/or eating meat will generally reverse muscle wasting.

To enhance power and coordination, use a formula containing sarasvatī 500 mg, brahmī 300 mg, and jatamāmsi 300 mg. Take ½ tsp. of this TID with either dashamūla arishta, ashvagandhā arishta, or balā arishta. These are Ayurvedic herbal wine preparations that kindle *māmsa dhātu agni.* If not available, use warm water as the *anupāna.*

For cases of paralysis, paraplegia or foot drop in India, highly potentized compounds are given such as mahāyogaraja guggulu 200 mg TID or mahā vāta vidvamsa 200 mg tablets TID. Another option is to administer a *madhu tailam basti* (honey and oil basti). For this, mix ½ cup of honey and ½ cup of warm sesame oil and retain the mixture to strengthen the muscles. Nutritive foods such as quinoa, amaranth, milk, tofu, almond milk, goat cheese, and medicated ghee such as balā ghrita (ghee) or shatāvarī ghrita should be favored.

The mobile quality of vāta creates abnormal muscular movements resembling dance (dancing chorea). Use a formula of dashamūla 500 mg, ashvagandhā 400 mg, balā 300 mg, vidārī 200 mg, yogarāja guggulu 200 mg, and sarasvatī 200 mg. Take ½ tsp. TID with almond milk. Additionally, the person should do self-massage, applying balā tailam or ashvagandhā oil as the massage oil, and use vacha-medicated nasya oil.

***Meda Dhātu.*** If all the dhātu agnis prior to *meda dhātu agni* are strong and meda dhātu agni is impaired, vāta will enter this tissue instead, creating *meda gata vāta.* Lack of lubrication, lack of sweat, dry skin, lumbago, displacement of organs such as descending kidneys or spleen, osteopenia, and dislocation of the joints are some of the signs and symptoms of vāta entering *meda dhātu.* When this occurs, the first line of treatment is plenty of deep oil massages using oils like ashvagandhā tailam, dashamūla oil, dhanvantari tailam (an oil preparation with balā in it), or balā tailam. Internally to support meda dhātu, medicated ghees are given such as shatāvarī ghee, balā ghrita, vidārī ghee, or yashthi madhu ghrita in a dosage of 1 tsp. TID before food.

Additionally take ½ tsp. TID after meals of a formula containing dashamūla 500 mg, ashvagandhā 400 mg, balā 300 mg, and vidārī 300 mg with shatāvarī ghee. A special soup, called *mahasneha* soup, is recommended as well. It contains ghee, animal fat and bone marrow. Use an oil enema or make a tea of dashamūla and ashvagandhā vidārī and combine with oil for a tea and oil enema.

In the case of organ displacement, the classic formulas use ½ tsp. of a mixture of ashvagandhā, vidārī, balā, kākolī, and kshirakākolī in milk TID. It is also recommended to bandage the organ site to support the ligaments. A similar protocol is used in the case of dislocation of the joints.

As for osteopenia, Ayurveda uses a mixture of herbs and bhāsmas, so the typical formula would contain dashamūla 500 mg, pravāl pañchāmrit 200 mg, moti bhāsma 200 mg, and kaishore guggulu 200 mg; ½ tsp. of this mixture TID with goat's milk.

*Asthi Dhātu.* Cracking and popping of the joints, osteoporosis, spinal misalignment, scoliosis, lower back ache, neck ache, splitting hair ends, receding gums, hair loss, thyroid dysfunction, and ringing in the ear are all signs that vāta has entered *asthi dhātu.*

Mahānārāyana oil is widely used topically for local lubrication in this case. Internally, for osteoporosis, a formula containing dashamūla 500 mg, yogarāja guggulu 300 mg, and pravāl pañchāmrit 200 mg is used in the dosage of ½ tsp. TID with milk. For spinal misalignment, the internal formula is dashamūla 500 mg, ashvagandhā 400 mg, and balā 300 mg. In India, this formula would be supplemented with a bone supporting tablet called asthi poshaka vati, which contains egg shell ash, coral ash, and calcium from antlers, among other ingredients.

For lower backache, application of mahānārāyana oil in a *kati basti* (pooling of oil on the lower back) is indicated as well as massage with mahānārāyana oil. Dashamūla tea basti is also commonly advised. Internally, take a formula containing ashvagandhā 400 mg, yogarāja guggulu 200 mg, tagara 200 mg, and pravāl pañchāmrit 200 mg, ½ tsp. TID with warm water.

In the case of receding gums, chew sesame seeds in the early morning and massage the gums. *Gandūsha,* filling the mouth with oil, swishing it, and retaining it before spitting it out, is also very useful.

With irregular thyroid function, there is a deficient calcium metabolism, so the person looks chubby but the bones are weak. To support the system, classic Ayurveda recommends the use of kaishore guggulu and pravāl pañchāmrit and, in modern Ayurveda, kelp is also recommended. *Bhrāmarī prāṇāyāma* and *ujjāyi prāṇāyāma* are very good tools as well and can be added to the protocols used in the vāta sañchaya and prokopa stage.

*Majjā Dhātu.* When vāta enters *majjā dhātu,* there is tingling and numbness in the extremities. *Majjā gata vāta* creates habitual ticks, spasms, muscle tremors, and gradual muscle wasting. As majjā dhātu includes the brain, spinal cord, eyeball, and articular surface of the joint, majjā gata vāta can create cluster headaches, spinal pain (pain along vertebra), nystagmus (involuntary eye movement), and stiffness in the joints. As vāta runs along the tract of the nerve, it can then cause classic conditions such as neuralgia, trigeminal neuralgia, and sciatica. According to the Ayurvedic system of medicine, majjā dhātu is the substratum of consciousness, thoughts, feelings, and emotions. Due to high vāta in majjā, there can be rushing of thoughts, mood swings, poor memory, forgetfulness, anxiety, fear, and insomnia.

In general, for *majjā gata vāta samprāpti* the herbal protocol is dashamūla 500 mg, sarasvatī 300 mg, brahmī 200 mg, shankha pushpī 200 mg, and tagara 200 mg, ½ tsp. TID with warm water. For *virechana* (purgation), 1 tsp. of plain harītakī at night in hot water is recommended. For nasya in the morning, use 5 drops per nostril of brahmī ghee, vacha tailam, or anu tailam. *Shirodhāra* three times a week is beneficial and rub brahmī or bhringarāja oil on the skull at night before bed. Karna pūrana (filling of the ear with warm oil) with a medicated vacha oil can also calm vāta in majjā. Dashamūla basti should be administered daily in the vāta time of day until symptomatic relief has been achieved.

In the case of trigeminal neuralgia, mahā yogarāja guggulu should be added to the above general herbal protocol and a local application of mahānārāyana oil with massage to the area would be ideal.

With majjā gata vāta in the eye, *netra basti* with plain ghee is advised in addition to the recommendations above.

For muscle tremors and wasting, the formula changes to dashamūla 500 mg, ashvagandhā 400 mg, vidārī 300 mg, and balā 200 mg. Take ½ tsp. TID with warm milk. For abhyanga or snehana, use ashvagandhā or balā tailam.

For neuro-psychiatric disorders such as anxiety, fear, memory loss, etc., the formula is dashamūla 500 mg, brahmī 200 mg, jatamāmsi 200 mg, and sarasvatī 200 mg, ½ tsp. taken TID with brahmī ghee.

Unfortunately, long lingering majjā gata vāta can lead to Parkinson's and Alzheimer's. In these cases, add 200 mg of ātma guptā to the general majjā gata vāta neuro-psychiatric herbal protocol.

***Shukra Dhātu.*** Vāta in *shukra dhātu* can produce oligospermia (scanty formation of semen), temporary or permanent deficiency of spermatozoa in seminal fluid, erectile dysfunction, premature ejaculation, dyspareunia (painful coitus), sexual impotency, lower back ache, fear associated with sex, or even deformed sperm leading to cleft palate, spina bifida, talipes equinovarus (club feet), depleted ojas, difficulty in conception, multiple miscarriages that affect the offspring and partner.

For general management, the herbal protocol requires dashamūla 500 mg, ashvagandhā 400 mg, vidārī 300 mg, ātma guptā 200 mg, and tagara 200 mg; take ½ tsp. TID with milk. Additionally, a dashamūla, ashvagandhā, balā, or madhu tailam basti can be done every day to protect *ojas*. Take ashvagandhā ghee, ashvagandhā arishta, or dashamūla arishta TID. Topical application to the glans penis of ashvagandhā or balā oil or a vidārī and nutmeg ointment are encouraged. Foods to favor include goat testicle soup, bone marrow soup, or chicken soup, accompanied by red wine.

***Ārtava Dhātu.*** Vāta in *ārtava dhātu* gives rise to infertility, sterility, amenorrhea, irregular menses, pain during ovulation, constriction of the cervix, cervical dysplasia, dryness in the vagina, dyspareunia, irregular menstruation, vaginal and uterine prolapse, retroverted uterus, and/or premature orgasm. These conditions can be alleviated by a general herbal protocol of dashamūla 300 mg, shatāvarī or ashvagandhā 300 mg, tagara 300 mg, and ashoka 300 mg. Take ½ tsp. internally TID with warm water. Traditionally a *pichu* (vaginal tampon) using shatāvarī ghee or dashamūla ghee is inserted at least twice a week. Also, take ashokarishta or kumārī āsava twice a day before each meal, 4 Tbs. with an equal amount of water. To lessen vāta in ārtava, perform a kati basti with sesame oil, a warm massage to the lower back, or apply a warm oil compress to the abdomen.

### Vyakti Stage

In the vyakti stage the rough qualities of vāta will create the full manifestation of the disease, *vyādhi darshana,* and basically the treatment protocols are the same as those provided in the sthāna samshraya stage.

### Bheda Stage

In the *bheda* stage of samprāpti where the clear quality of vāta manifests, there are more complications. Bheda stage in rasa dhātu creates severe dehydration; in rakta dhātu, it generates severe anemia; in māmsa, muscle wasting, emaciation, and atrophy occur; in meda, the depletion of normal, healthy fatty tissue leads to degenerative changes; in asthi, osteoporosis, spontaneous fractures, deposition of calcium in soft tissue, and reduction of height manifest. Vāta in bheda stage penetrating the majjā dhātu creates a loss of function of cerebral activity, epileptic convulsions, severe Parkinson's, Alzheimer's with total memory loss, loss of consciousness, and coma. If instead the vāta in bheda stage moves to the shukra or ārtava dhātu, there is total loss of libido, total reproductive dysfunction, and loss of secondary sexual characteristics.

## Management in Bheda Stage

Critical care is needed at this stage and, in most incidences, hospitalization is required. The following guidelines are given for each tissue so that you can prevent additional aggravation of the dosha and dhātu.

For rasa dhātu, maintain water electrolyte balance and avoid dehydrating herbs like punarnavā, gokshura, or triphalā. Cleansing therapies and even mild virechana should not be administered. For rakta dhātu, blood-building foods can be eaten such as beets, red cabbage, black raisins, currants, and blueberries. In India, loha āsava is recommended. For māmsa dhātu, give a gentle yet deep massage with ashvagandhā and balā medicated oils, followed by svedana, daily for three to four weeks. In terms of food guidelines, meat soup, chicken broth, almond milk, and milk with ashvagandhā are favored.

For meda dhātu, this is the time when Ayurveda recommends fatty fried food and internal consumption of shatāvarī ghee, balā ghee, or licorice ghee, all preceded by a pinch of rock salt or trikatu to aid the digestion. For asthi dhātu, calcium, magnesium, and zinc supplementation may be needed. In India, a typical medicine is asthi poshaka vati, which in essence is very similar to coral calcium. Gentle weight-bearing exercises and yoga are also advised.

For majjā dhātu, shirodhāra and shirobasti are the therapies that bring the most benefit. Nasya with vacha tailam and *prāṇāyāma* are helpful as well.

For shukra, in India, strong *rasāyanas* are used such as mākaradvāja 200 mg twice a day, kapikacchū vati 300 mg TID, or ashvagandhā vati 300 mg TID. For ārtava, licorice tea *uttara basti* is recommended daily, then weekly. For both shukra and ārtava, yogic postures like *vajrāsana* (thunderbolt pose), *utthita padmāsana* (elevated lotus pose), *halāsana* (plow pose), *bhujangāsana* (cobra pose) and *balāsana* (child's pose) are very beneficial at this stage. Beneficial *mudras* are *vāyu mudrā* and *agni mudrā,* and y*oni mudrā* for women.

# Chapter 3

# Ṣhat Kriyā Kāla: Pitta
## Management of the Six Stages of Samprāpti for Pitta

Summer 2010, Volume 23, Number 1

AS PROMISED IN the previous chapter, in this article we will cover the management of *pitta dosha* in the various stages of samprāti.

In the sañchaya stage, the liquid and sour qualities (see Table 1 on page 7) cause umbilical pain, intense hunger, and yellow discoloration of urine and sclera. In this condition, we can use one teaspoon at night of āmalakī, to counteract the increased liquid quality, with aloe vera juice, to counteract the sour or in India,[3] they would use shanka vati, a *bhasma* of calcinated shell.

In the prakopa stage, the hot and pungent qualities mingle with the liquid and sour qualities that were already present and give rise to acid indigestion, hyperacidity, heartburn, nausea, and gastric pain. In this condition, use a mixture of shatāvarī or gudūchī 500 milligrams (mg), gulvel sattva 200 mg, shanka bhasma 200 mg, and kāma dudhā 200 mg, ½ teaspoon three times a day (TID) before meals with cup of milk.

Up to this stage, the doshas are excited, overwhelmed, and filling their organs completely. Vāta inflates the colon, pitta overwhelms the small intestines, and kapha is ready to overflow the stomach. Now is the crucial time for proper management because, if not handled with treatment, the dosha will leave its site and start traveling throughout the body. It will start by trying to enter rasa and rakta dhātu in the prasara stage. In the prasara stage, the qualities of pitta are spreading and oily, which precipitates pitta aggravation and leads it to sthāna samshraya. These two qualities actually help the entry of pitta into the dhātus. As long as the doshas are in the gastrointestinal (GI) tract, it is fairly easy to remove them from the system. However, once they enter the *bāhya mārga*, then management and removal becomes more complicated as it progresses to the sthāna samshraya stage. (see Vyādhi Mārga Illustration page 16)

---

3. There are herbs, compounds, and bhasmas that are available only in India or are no longer made. Lad includes these to give a complete picture of the recommended remedies in the ancient texts.

## Sthāna Samshraya

***Rasa Dhātu.*** If sthāna samshraya occurs in the rasa dhātu—the plasma tissue (serum, white blood cells, lymphatic system)—the individual gets repeated hives, rash, urticaria, hyper-pyrexia (high fever), acne on the face or on the body, dermatitis, eczema, and psoriasis. Even melanin cells under the skin become irritated, leading to red spots under the skin that can turn into multiple moles. A person with *sthāna samshraya pitta* in the rasa dhātu may become subject to skin cancer or malignant melanoma, a highly metastasizing cancer, and for that reason entry of pitta into the rasa dhātu should not be taken lightly.

The protocols for sthāna samshraya pitta in the rasa dhātu vary according to the condition. For high fever, one can use ½ teaspoon TID of an herbal compound containing mahāsudarshan 300 mg, gulvel sattva 200 mg, kāma dudhā 200 mg, and pravāl pañchāmrit[4] 200 mg with either lemongrass tea or cinnamon, ginger, sandalwood, and mustā tea where the ingredients are combined in equal proportion. Also, one should sponge the forehead with a tepid mixture of rose and camphor water TID and away from food. Should the person in question be a child, the caregiver should grate one onion. Take half of the grated onion, wrap in a cotton cloth and apply it to the forehead; wrap the other half and apply it to the belly button. This type of *lepa,* application of paste, is also quite common in cases of febrile convulsions. Externally onion is cooling and can have an immediate effect on body temperature.

One should never undergo virechana, purgation, during high fever and the person should stay hydrated to avoid dehydration. In India, they use sutshekhar pills 200 mg TID

4. A compound of coral, conch, oyster, pearls and cowrie shells processed in aloe vera and rose water.

and 4 Tbs. of mahāsudarshan qwath (an alcoholic preparation of mahāsudarshan) with equal amounts of water, two times daily (BID).

T.I.D. = from the Latin means *ter in diem*, three times a day

B.I.D. = from the Latin means *bis in diem*, two times a day

For hives and rashes, a lepa consisting of equal proportions of sandalwood, rose, and manjishthā and prepared with milk can be applied topically at night or early morning. Allow the lepa to dry then rinse off. Juice fresh cilantro and drink this TID. You can then use the pulp residue as an additional topical application. Should the rash be an allergic reaction due to contact, for example, with poison oak or ivy, then tikta ghrita can be applied on the rash. Internally take ½ tsp. TID of an herbal mixture consisting of equal proportions of gudūchī, manjishthā, and turmeric.

For urticaria, active dermatitis, take ½ tsp. TID of a bitter herbal combination comprising shatāvarī 500 mg, kutki 200 mg, manjishthā 200 mg, and neem 200 mg. The anupāna (vehicle) can be pomegranate juice or even milk.

For chronic, long-lingering pitta, sthāna samshraya of pitta in the rasa dhātu can create eczema and psoriasis. In these conditions there is burning, itching, red lesions of inflammatory changes, and there can also be bleeding in spots. In India for this type of condition, one is given ārogya vardhini capsules of 200 mg and capsules of sutshekhar 200 mg and kāma dudhā with moti 200 mg. Since these medicines are not available here in the United States, we use a mixture of shatāvarī 500 mg, gudūchī 200 mg, manjishthā 300 mg, neem 200 mg, and turmeric 200 mg. Use this combination ½ tsp. TID with aloe vera gel. Aloe vera gel has a sustained action versus the short acting juice.

Acne, a common problem in teenage boys and girls who are arriving at the pitta time of life, may be due to hormonal changes. Young boys have excess testosterone in their blood stream and girls have excess estrogen; as a result, they break out in the form of acne. In pitta-predominant prakruti and *vikruti,* stress can also trigger sthāna samshraya pitta in the rasa dhātu, which may manifest as acne.

In India, the internal treatment protocol is very similar to that prescribed for eczema and psoriasis. In the west we can differentiate and for the female use a mixture of shatāvarī 200 mg, gudūchī 300 mg, manjishthā 200 mg, neem 200 mg, and harītakī 200 mg, taken ½ tsp TID with aloe vera juice. For males, the mixture would consist of ashvagandhā 500 mg, vidārī 400 mg, gudūchī 300 mg, manjishthā 200 mg, neem 200 mg, and harītakī 200 mg, taken ½ tsp TID with milk.

For external treatment, wash the affected area with neem soap or sandalwood soap to remove all the oil and then apply a simple turmeric-sandalwood paste, an almond-nutmeg-milk paste, or a multani mitti-sandalwood-manjishthā-rose paste for skin healing. Allow to dry and then rinse to remove. In some serious cases of acne, the best recommendation is *rakta moksha,* blood letting, which can be done easily by donating blood to the blood bank. This method can clear acne within one week.

Generally, pitta prakruti/vikruti individuals tend to get multiple moles on the skin. As a rule, they should avoid long exposure to sun light. Usually when the mole has clear-cut margins, is round or oval in shape, the boundaries are cleanly distinguished, and surface is smooth, it is a benign mole. You can apply a mixture of coconut oil and castor oil, half and half, to the mole area. However, if mole looks puckered, the margins have merged into the peripheral tissue, the mole has discoloration spots or brownish areas, and/or the surface looks granular, then this type of mole can create more itching and slight bleeding. Additionally, it may be malignant. You should immediately go to the dermatologist for an expert opinion and biopsy. If they want to remove the mole, let them do so.

***Rakta Dhātu.*** If rasa dhātu agni is strong and healthy then pitta has no chance to deposit into the rasa dhātu, red blood cells. Such angry and irritated pitta will then go to the rakta and, if the rakta dhātu agni is weak and impaired, pitta will enter the rakta dhātu. Pitta and rakta…they have very similar qualities. Pitta is *ushna* (hot), rakta is ushna. Pitta is *tīkshna* (sharp), rakta is tīkshna. Pitta is *sūkshma* (subtle), rakta is sūkshma. Pitta is *sara* (spreading), rakta is spreading. The condition of sthāna samshraya of pitta in the rakta is called *rakta pitta.*

Pitta gives its hot, sharp, sour qualities to rakta; and rakta gives its red fleshy smell and spreading quality to pitta. This condition creates bleeding disorders. Due to the hot and sharp qualities of pitta and rakta, the platelet count diminishes. When platelet count diminishes, the prothrombin[5] and thrombin[6] clotting factors are affected and the blood becomes thinner, easily rupturing the peripheral capillaries or blood vessels and creating bleeding disorders.

If rakta pitta is pushed upward by *udāna vāyu* then the person gets bleeding from the upper pathways, i.e., the nose, gums, eyes, and ears. If rakta pitta is pushed downward by *apāna vāyu* then the individual can get bleeding from the lower pathways, i.e, the urethra, vagina, and rectum. If rakta pitta is pushed inward or outward by *samāna vāyu* or *vyāna vāyu,* the person can get petechial hemorrhage or hemophilia purpura. Charaka states a very important sūtra in the *Chikitsā Sthāna* that says, *pratimārgam cha haranam cha rakta pittam vidhiyate,* meaning that bleeding disorders are treated with herbs that encourage the opposite flow of direction of the disorder. Hence, with an upward flow of blood to the nose, gums, or teeth, we use a sweet, mild virechana like āmalakī that will give an opposite downward pull to the dosha. For the downward flow of bleeding, we have to induce a mild emetic, which creates an upward pull on the dosha, using licorice, neem, or madana phala with either pomegranate juice or milk. In both cases, virechana and *vamana* are not expected; we want only to change the vector.

When samāna pushes rakta pitta creating petechial hemorrhage, one can use gulvel satva, kāma dudhā, manjishthā, lodhra, and sandalwood in equal proportions, ½ tsp TID with aloe vera juice. Then give a mild virechana of bhumi āmalakī. Externally apply sandalwood-rose paste or sandalwood-rose-camphor paste. Camphor is cooling. You can use mustā in place of sandalwood, in case sandalwood is too expensive.

If there is severe bleeding with sputum, then use iced water, sip by sip. This will also stop bleeding. In general, ice is not nice but here ice is nice because it helps to clot the blood. It is observed that if there is bleeding and you put ice on it, it will freeze the blood,

---

5. A coagulation (clotting) factor that is needed for the normal clotting of blood.
6. A key clot promoter, thrombin is an enzyme that presides over the conversion of a substance called fibrinogen to fibrin, creating the right conditions for a clot.

acting as a hemostatic; conversely, when you apply heat, it will increase the bleeding. So bleeding time increases by application of heat and bleeding time reduces by application of cold.

Another condition of pitta sthāna samshraya in the rakta is inflammatory arthritis such as gout, where high uric acid levels create crystals, which go into the joint and irritate the synovial membrane, creating inflammation, deformity, and pain in the interphalangeal joint. In this case, vāta is pushing pitta in the *rakta vaha srotas* and rakta dhātu, creating gout. This condition is called *vāta rakta* in Ayurvedic literature. The treatment protocol is a mixture of kaishore guggulu 200 mg, amrita guggulu 200 mg, kāma dudhā 200 mg, and pravāl pañchāmrit 200 mg. Take ½ tsp. TID with aloe vera juice. Use a topical application of an anti-inflammatory paste of red sandalwood and turmeric.

For any kind of bleeding disorder, use *pitta-rakta* soothing and pacifying herbs. They are shatāvarī, gulvel sattva, manjishthā, neem, turmeric mixed with neem, rose, red sandalwood, white sandalwood, lodhra, and mocha rasa. These herbs will separate pitta from rakta and act as a hemostatic, acting to arrest bleeding or hemorrhaging.

The next condition of sthāna samshraya pitta in the rakta is hot flashes. This condition occurs as a woman enters perimenopausal and menopausal stages. Lack of estrogen hormone may push pitta in the hematopoietic system. The treatment protocol for hot flashes is a mixture of shatāvarī 500 mg, kāma dudhā 200 mg, gulvel sattva 200 mg, and moti bhasma 200 mg. Take ½ tsp. TID with aloe vera juice, which is also a source of estrogen. To further maintain estrogen balance, use evening primrose oil 500 mg, one capsule after dinner for 15 days on, 15 days off.

Sthāna samshraya of pitta in the rakta dhātu may create weeping eczema. Use a topical paste of equal proportions of catechu, neem, manjishthā, and sandalwood, twice daily. Internally take a mixture of shatāvarī 200 mg, gudūchī 200 mg, neem 200 mg, manjishthā 200 mg, and kāma dudhā 200 mg, ½ tsp. TID with aloe vera gel.

*Māmsa Dhātu.* If the rakta dhātu agni is strong, it will never allow pitta to enter its territory. One could say this disappoints pitta, since pitta thought that rakta was a brother and yet was sent away. Pitta then travels to māmsa dhātu and, if māmsa dhātu agni is low, enters the muscle tissue where it can create fibromyalgia or fibromyositis. In fibromyalgia, there are nine bilateral trigger points (18 points in all, see page 20) that are exceptionally sensitive to the touch; they feel like sensitive *marmāni*. Generally, 11 points must be sensitive for three months before one can diagnose fibromyalgia. The treatment protocol is a mixture of ashvagandhā 500 mg, as a vehicle to carry the medicine to the māmsa dhātu, shatāvarī 400 mg, as *pitta pratyanika,* specific to the dosha, then gudūchī 300 mg, kaishore guggulu 200 mg, both as anti-inflammatory, mustā 200 mg, a muscle relaxant and analgesic, and tagara 200 mg, analgesic. Take ½ tsp. TID with warm water. Topically one can apply mahānārāyana oil to the troubled area. For fibromyositis, the treatment protocol is the same as for fibromyalgia.

Another condition of sthāna samshraya pitta in the māmsa is bursitis, an inflammation of the bursa around the joints and ligaments. The treatment protocol for this is a mixture of ashvagandhā 500 mg, kaishore guggulu 200 mg, mustā 300 mg, and tagara 200 mg taken orally ½ tsp. TID with warm water. Topically apply mahānārāyana tailam for any inflammatory muscle disorder.

## The Bilateral Trigger Points of Fibromyalgia

*Māmsa gata pitta,*[7] another name for sthāna samshraya pitta in the māmsa, can create bleeding and spongy gums like scurvy. For that, Ayurveda recommends a triphalā tea gargle with a pinch of alum or a neem oil *kavala gandūsha.* Kavala gandūsha is to fill the mouth with oil, swishing it for several minutes, and retain it before spitting it out. One tsp. of āmalakī at night is good source of Vitamin C.

Long lingering pitta in the sthāna samshraya stage of māmsa dhātu can cause multiple boils and abscesses. In my experience, when a patient comes with multiple boils and abscesses, we must first rule out diabetes.

The abscess and boil is an inflammatory condition called *pacāmana avasthā,* which is a stage of inflammation. The next stage is the ripe stage or *pakvāsthā,* which is suppuration with pus formation. For a boil, we can apply local heat like ginger, black pepper, or piper longum as a paste. This will help should the boil still need to ripen and it will increase the suppuration. Once ripe, the pus will come out easily. Internally one can give a natural, herbal antibiotic like sūkshma triphalā, available in India. Here in the west, we can use gulvel sattva 200 mg, neem 200 mg, turmeric 200 mg, echinacea 200 mg, osha 200 mg, and goldenseal 200 mg as an antibacterial mixture. Take this ½ tsp. TID until the infection comes under control or for a maximum two weeks.

For māmsa gata pitta creating myositis, local inflammation, one can take internally ½ tsp. TID of a mixture containing kaishore guggulu 200 mg, ashvagandhā 500 mg, and mustā 300 mg with water.

---

7. Gata means 'gone;' in this context, entering into.

*Meda Dhātu.* *Meda gata pitta* is the term given to pitta sthāna samshraya in meda dhātu, adipose tissue or fat. If māmsa dhātu agni is strong, not allowing pitta to enter the dhātu, then pitta will turn away and possibly penetrate meda's door. Meda gata pitta will create profuse sweating and excess thirst. Excess kleda is eliminated through human sweat as well as through the urinary tract so pitta will have access to the urinary tract and create repeated cystitis. Then high excess pitta in the meda dhātu effects fat metabolism, creating fatty degenerative changes in the liver and impairing fat metabolism in the liver, therefore the person will get fatty diarrhea and undigested fat will pass through the urine or to the stool. Furthermore, there is a connection between meda dhātu and the adrenal glands as well as meda dhātu and the thyroid gland. High pitta in the meda dhātu creates low adrenals and can produce the autoimmune thyroid disorder known as Hashimoto's thyroiditis.

For profuse perspiration, dusting therapy called *uddhūlanam* will help. Use a superfine powder of calamus, sandalwood, and jatamāmsi or chickpea flour or oatmeal powder and then gentle brushing to help minimize sweating. Internally give shatāvarī 500 mg, gudūchī 300 mg, kāma dudhā 200 mg, and kutki 200 mg, ½ tsp. TID with cool water.

For cystitis the herbal protocol calls for a mixture of punarnavā 500 mg, gokshura 400 mg, mustā 300 mg, kāma dudhā 200 mg, and fennel 200 mg. Take ½ tsp. TID with aloe vera juice or gel. As in cystitis, there is a tendency for the urine to become acidic. It is customary in India to have ushīrāsava, a self-generating alcoholic preparation whose main ingredient is ushīra. Alternatively, one can drink a tea made out of sandalwood, ushīra, and coriander in equal proportions.

For fatty liver, in India we use ārogya vardhini 200 mg TID. However, here we use a mixture of shatāvarī 500 mg, gulvel sattva 400 mg, katukā 300 mg, neem 200 mg, and shilājit 200 mg. Take ½ tsp. TID with aloe vera gel. In addition, prānāyāma can help this condition. Recommended practices are shītalī, shītkāri, and kapāla bhāti.

For low adrenals where there may be postural hypotension, fatigue, exhaustion, or development of dark circles around the eyes, we can use a compound of ashvagandhā 500 mg, vidārī 300 mg, yashthi madhu 200 mg, and ātma guptā 200 mg. Take ½ tsp. TID with either milk or warm water.

For the thyroid dysfunction of Hashimoto's disease, one can use a formula of kaishore guggulu 200 mg, gudūchī 300 mg, kāma dudhā 200 mg, and pravāl pañchāmrit 200 mg. Take ½ tsp. TID with pomegranate juice. If thyroid function is low then we can use a mixture of punarnavā 500 mg, kutki 200 mg, chitrak 200 mg, shilājit 200 mg, and kāma dudhā 200 mg. Have ½ tsp. TID with warm water.

*Asthi Dhātu.* If meda dhātu agni is strong then pitta cannot access the tissue during the prasara stage and will move to the next tissue, asthi dhātu, bone and cartilage tissue. Pitta sthāna samshraya in asthi will create inflammatory changes either in the periosteum or within the matrix of asthi dhātu. As a result, the *upadhātu* of asthi, *danta* (teeth), and the *mala, kesha* (hair) and *nakha* (nails), will be affected. Long lingering pitta in the asthi dhātu can enter into the articular surface of the joint, which will affect the synovial membrane, leading to inflammatory arthritis of the joints, with heat, swelling, and generalized inflammation. During the journey from superficial to deep in the asthi dhātu, pitta dosha by its ushna (hot) and tīkshna (sharp) qualities can create periostitis.[8] Pitta dosha can also cause alopecia by affecting the root of hair and creating gingivitis, tooth abscess, bleeding gums and yellowing of teeth by affecting the root of teeth.

*Asthi dhara kalā*—the periosteum, the membranous structure covering the bone, is intimately connected with calcium metabolism and indirectly governed by the thyroid gland. The glandular system is a bridge between asthi dhātu and majjā dhātu. Therefore, pitta in the asthi dhātu has access to disturbed thyroid function and hyperthyroidism, leading to generalized heat in the body, increased perspiration, and impairment of calcium metabolism.

To deal with pitta in asthi dhātu, the treatment protocol is to use shatāvarī 500 mg as *dosha pratyanika,* kaishore guggulu, or amrita guggulu 300 mg as anti-inflammatory and pravāl pañchāmrit 200 mg and kāma dudhā 200 mg also as anti-inflammatory. This mixture is to be taken ½ tsp. TID with two tablespoons of aloe vera gel. Topically one can apply bhringarāja, brahmī, or coconut oil on the joint.

The asthi dhara kalā contains specialized osteo plasma,[9] which is rich in calcium, magnesium, and zinc, and produces and nourishes asthi dhātu. In my clinical practice of the last 40 years, I have found a connection between ulcerative colitis, osteo arthritis, and osteoporosis. To treat these conditions I have had success with a dashamūla and gudūchī tea basti and an internal herbal mixture consisting of dashamūla 500 mg, kāma dudhā 200 mg, pravāl pañchāmrit 200 mg, and swayambhu guggulu 200 mg, ½ tsp. TID with warm milk after meals.

To make the dashamūla-gudūchī basti, take 1 pint of water and add 1 tablespoon of dashamūla and one tablespoon of gudūchī. Bring to a boil and simmer for 3 minutes; allow to cool. Strain the tea before administering the basti.

For the treatment of alopecia, one must first rule out other serious illnesses such as severe depression, stress, dermatitis, exposure to radiation, an iatrogenic condition, or the process of aging. In India, one can use ārogya vardhini 200 mg, kaishore guggulu 200 mg, and brahmī 200 mg. Apply topically neem, brahmī, or bhringarāja oil, any combination of these three.

For tooth abscess and dental disorders, Ayurveda recommends brushing the teeth with neem and gargling with ½ cup of aloe vera juice. If there is infection or gingivitis, internally take a mixture of mahāsudarshan 300 mg, neem 200 mg, manjishthā 200 mg, echinacea 200 mg, and goldenseal 200 mg, ½ tsp. TID with aloe vera juice.

For the treatment of pitta in asthi dhātu with hyperactive thyroid and excess heat we can use a mixture of shatāvarī 500 mg, gulvel sattva 200 mg, kāma dudhā 200 mg, and kaishore guggulu 200 mg, ½ tsp. TID with aloe vera gel.

In general, it is a good practice of a person suffering with *asthi gata pitta* to have shatāvarī milk, brahmī milk, or dashamūla milk at bedtime to help both bones and pitta.

---

8. Inflammation of the periosteum, a layer of connective tissue that surrounds bone.
9. Bone tissue has pathways through the cells for nutrients and waste, so even though bone is hard, there is plasma in it.

*Majjā Dhātu.* When the *asthi dhātu agni* is strong and healthy, pitta will not be allowed to enter its territory, and pitta then tries to enter majjā dhātu, the marrow, nerve, and connective tissue. As pitta is hot, sharp, penetrating, and spreading, it will create first burning sensations, burning hands and feet, burning in the eyes, then insomnia, dizziness, nausea, and vomiting leading to pitta-type fever and, if long lingering, syncope, coma, and even death. On a psychological level, pitta may create a chemical form of depression, even suicidal depression. Pitta in majjā can also create demyelinating disorders, multiple sclerosis (MS), migraine headaches, meningitis, or encephalitis. Therefore, *majjā gata pitta* is a very serious condition.

Since the upadhātu of majjā is lacrimal secretions and *akshi vitta sneha,* the oily secretions of feces and eyes, majjā gata pitta will cause the person to wake up with sticky eyes and have mucousy yellow stool, with yellow discoloration of the sclera and photosensitivity, which may lead to ophthalmic migraine.

For burning sensation of the hands and the feet, rub coconut or castor oil on the soles of the feet and palms of the hands. Internally take TID a mixture of brahmī, bhringarāja, and gudūchī, 300 mg each.

For burning sensation in the eyes one can use a goat milk compress, a triphalā tea eyewash, netra basti with plain ghee or *netra bindu,* which are eye drops available in India that contain rose, camphor, and alum.

For dizziness, nausea, and vomiting, one can take internally shatāvarī 500 mg, brahmī 200 mg, and sarasvatī 200 mg, ½ tsp. TID with aloe vera juice.

For fever and migraines, one can take gudūchī 300 mg, mahāsudarshan 300 mg, and brahmī 200 mg, TID with water.

When pitta enters majjā and leads to suicidal thoughts, violence, aggression, and possible chemical depression, the situation should not be taken lightly and one should seek proper counseling. It may be necessary at some point to call for emergency care (911).

For demyelinating disorders leading to MS, *pañchakarma,* abhyanga, svedana, basti, and nasya can be quite helpful. The herbal protocol for this uses a mixture of shatāvarī 500 mg, dashamūla 400 mg, kaishore guggulu 200 mg, brahmī 200 mg, and ātma guptā 200 mg, ½ tsp. TID with tikta ghrita or brahmī prash (an alcoholic preparation of brahmī).

Meningitis and encephalitis are very serious conditions that require hospitalization.

*Shukra /Ārtava Dhātus.* When majjā dhātu agni is strong and pitta could not penetrate the tissue the next tissue in the pathway is shukra or ārtava dhātu, male or female reproductive tissue. Shukra and ārtava dhātu occupy the whole body. Though the top most layer of the skin represents rasa, the seventh layer is shukra/ārtava and it comes to the surface of the body at the mucocutaneous[10] junction of the lips, then at the nipple and areola, and on the skin of the penis and clitoris. These areas are very sensitive as are the throat, heart, belly button, and *linea alba.*[11] The *kama kalā nādī* (an energetic pathway) passes through these

---

10. A mucocutaneous zone is a region of the body in which mucosa transitions to skin.
11. "White line;" a fibrous band that runs vertically along the center of the anterior abdominal wall and receives the attachments of the oblique and transverse abdominal muscles.

areas and kissing or touching these areas yields an intense desire to make love, as mentioned in the *Kama Sūtra,* the book on the secret science of erotic pleasure.

When pitta enters shukra/ārtava dhātu, the person will become oversensitive to touch and have irritability, anger, and even repulsion towards their sexual partner. The lips become too sensitive to kiss, the areola and nipples are tender and painful and even intercourse is painful (*sakastha maithuna*).

Depending on how deep the pitta has gone into the shukra/ārtava dhātu, the signs and symptoms vary accordingly. In men, it will manifest as urethritis, orchitis, epididymitis, excess pitta in sperm and semen, leading to burning in the spermatic cord, urethra, and prostate. There can also be premature ejaculation. During these conditions all sexual acts are painful, irritating, and may create, as complications, outbreaks of herpes, gonorrhea, or syphilis. In women, the ovaries become sore and painful; there is pain along the fallopian tubes and repeated endometritis. There will be pitta-type pre-menstrual syndrome. The woman will suffer from tenderness in the breasts, irritability, and anger pre-menstrually and have profuse menstrual bleeding.

The pure essence of shukra/ārtava is ojas and *pitta ojo vyāpat*[12] may develop or may manifest in both individuals, where tejas is burning ojas and may lead to autoimmune disorder.

For generalized treatment of men suffering from *shukra gata pitta* the herbal protocol is a mixture ashvagandhā 500 mg, vidārī 400 mg, gulvel sattva 300 mg, and moti bhasma 200 mg to be taken ½ tsp. TID with milk. For women with ārtava gata pitta, the herbal protocol is a mixture of shatāvarī 500 mg, gulvel sattva 400 mg, kāma dudhā 200 mg, and ashoka 300 mg taken ½ tsp. TID with kumārī. Use a topical application of tikta ghrita on the lips, nipples, belly button, and clitoris.

For tejas burning ojas as a complication of pitta ojo vyapat, women can take 1 tsp. BID of shatāvarī ghee, mahā tikta ghrita,[13] or shatāvarī *avaleha*[14] (syrup) orally. Men suffering from this condition can take 1 tsp. BID of ashvagandhā avaleha, 1 cup of almond milk, or have at least one ghee-soaked date per day.

## Vyakti Stage

Due to the light quality of pitta, in the vyakti stage, we will have the full-blown manifestation of pathologies and the treatment of those pathologies should follow the protocols of the sthāna samshraya stage.

## Bheda Stage

In the bheda stage, pitta will create a fleshy smell quality as at this stage there has already been inflammation, irritation, ulceration, and hemorrhage leading to abscess and gangrene. Therefore, in this stage it is crucial to have hospitalization as this stage is not to be treated at home.

---

12. Also known as ojo dushti, this is the qualitative disturbance of ojas by one or more doshas. It usually involves more than one dhatu. Ojo-vyapat affects the entire immune system of the body.
13. A classical formula described in *Sushruta Samhita, Chikitsā Sthana,* chapter 9.
14. A method of medicine preparation in which herbs and/or herbal extracts are mixed into a syrup.

# Chapter 4

# Shat Kriyā Kāla: Kapha
## Management of the Six Stages of Samprāpti for Kapha

Summer 2010, Volume 23, Number 3

THE THREE DOSHAS are the three organizations of the unique human physiology. Dhātus are the constructing, cementing material of the body and malas are the impurities. The doshas govern one's unique individual psychophysiology, which is called prakruti. At the time of fertilization, the prakruti of the father and mother create a unique genetic code that determines the individual's prakruti, or nature, their unique psychophysiology.

> *Dosha dhātu mala mūlam hi sharīram*
>
> *Sushruta Samhitā,* Sharīrasthānam

These three doshas are a qualified and quantified unit. The doshas have their own unique qualities, which all Āyurvedic students are familiar with. They also have a particular ratio, such as $vāta_1$, $pitta_2$, and $kapha_3$. This is quantification, but 10 individuals with a vāta-pitta constitution are 10 unique individuals because in these 10 people there will be a unique permutation and combination of the different gunas, or qualities. Therefore, whenever we discuss shat kriyā kāla, students should pay attention to both the qualities and quantities of the doshas that undergo change.

We have discussed in detail the shat kriyā kāla of vāta and pitta doshas in previous articles. In this chapter, we will switch our attention to shat kriyā kāla of *kapha dosha.*

We know that the main site of kapha is the stomach, but there are also other subordinate sites of kapha dosha. Kapha is present in the bronchial secretions in the chest, the lymphatic secretions of the lymph system, the saliva of the oral cavity and sinus secretions of the sinuses. Kapha is also present in the lubricating material of the joint, the synovia.

## Early Stages of Samprāpti

In shat kriyā kāla of kapha, we should pay attention to the main site of kapha dosha, which is the stomach. Sañchaya, or accumulation, is the first and most important stage of samprāpti. In *kapha samprāpti,* it occurs in the stomach. As we studied previously, sañchaya of vāta happens because of cold quality. Sañchaya of pitta is due to liquid and sour qualities, and sanchaya of kapha takes place due to the heavy and cold qualities. Students should pay attention to these two qualities: heavy, or *guru*, and cold, or *shīta*.

Due to the heavy quality, the person will have a subjective sense of heaviness. It may be generalized heaviness or localized heaviness. Whenever there is heaviness, there is kapha. In the sanchaya stage, excess *kledaka kapha* is secreted in the stomach. The heavy quality suppresses the agni and the cold quality cools down the agni. Because agni is suppressed by these two qualities that are the opposites of the light and hot qualities of agni, then naturally the person will feel no appetite. Due to low appetite and fullness of the stomach, there is also a lethargic feeling.

These expressions of kapha: no appetite, fullness of the stomach and lethargy are symptoms of the sanchaya stage of kapha samprāpti in the stomach.

For simple management, Āyurveda talks in terms of balancing the dosha. Kapha dosha accumulates in the stomach due to certain causes. The moment kapha accumulates in the stomach and agni is suppressed, then the person will get an aversion or repulsion toward the cause. Suppose every day a person eats foods with heavy, greasy, oily, and dull qualities. This will suppress agni and on the third day even a picture of these kinds of foods will make the person nauseated. Why?

Because the body has intelligence; it has wisdom. It happens in any condition—if someone who is not accustomed to smoking smokes a cigarette, he gets an aversion towards smoking. If someone drinks too much then the next day he doesn't even like to see the bottle of whisky or wine. Aversion towards the cause is the language of the body. That means listen to the body; don't continue with the same cause.

In the sanchaya stage of kapha, the treatment is simple: to strictly avoid the cause. If there is heaviness, fullness, low appetite, lethargy, and aversion toward the cause, then don't repeat that cause. That is also a treatment, called *nidānam parivarjanam,* avoiding the cause of the increased dosha.

*Vruddhih samānyaih sarveshām, viparītair viparyayah*

Vagbhata's *Ashtānga Hridayam Sūtrasthānam*

This sūtra says vruddhih samānyaih sarveshām—like increases like. On the other hand, opposite qualities heal the body and control the dosha. We use this same principle when dealing with the first stage of samprāpti. So, pay attention to the heavy, cool qualities. The first *kriyā kāla* of sanchaya is to use the opposite quality. The opposite of heavy is light, and light quality is present in fasting, so observing a fast is one treatment. Drink only warm water or drink nothing, and don't eat anything until normal appetite comes back.

Fasting can also be done by drinking warm or room temperature juice, like apple juice for kapha prakruti, pomegranate juice for kapha and pitta, and for vāta, orange juice or sweet lime juice. A juice fast is recommended so that a person doesn't get dehydrated. It will induce the light quality in the body. In that way the heavy quality can be controlled.

Not eating means not taking something inside. Our body also encounters these universal twenty qualities in the environment, in the atmosphere, in our relationships, and in our families and homes as well as in the diet. These qualities are constantly bombarding us.

Then there is cool quality. Cool quality can calm down the agni, so to kindle agni, one can take ginger tea. Take about 1 inch of fresh ginger root, chop it into pieces, and boil it in a cup of water for a few minutes. This is a simple home remedy. Sipping ginger tea will kindle agni and calm down the cool quality of kapha. Then the lethargy, heaviness, and low appetite will go.

For lethargy due to low agni, one can kindle agni by doing *dīpana* and *pāchana*. An example of dīpana is giving ginger tea. For pāchana, you can take a pinch of chitrak with a teaspoon of honey or trikatu, which is ginger, black pepper and piper longum (pippalī) in equal proportions. One-quarter teaspoon of this mixture can be taken orally with a teaspoon of honey, and it will definitely take care of agni and burn āma. It is the āma that creates lethargy.

Due to the accumulation of kapha dosha and suppression of agni, āma is produced. This āma clogs the channels. Lethargy happens because of lack of nutrition to rasa dhātu due to āma, which is clogging the *rasa vaha srotas*. To take care of that lethargy, trikatu chūrna is used. Take ¼ teaspoon with a tsp. of honey TID. In between one can drink hot water. This management will take care of the sañchaya stage of kapha, which is induced by the heavy and cool qualities.

During the sañchaya stage, you can conquer a dosha quickly. Sushruta says *'chayo jaye dosha,'* which means you should conquer the dosha in the first stage, sañchaya. However, most people are not aware of their own dosha. They eat emotionally and because of habit, without paying attention to their bodies, doshas, *nādi* (the pulse), breath, and tongue. That is how we create our own disease process. Sushruta is a great enlightened master. His explanation of shat kriyā kāla is a very practical guide for future generations.

T.I.D. = from the Latin means *ter in diem*, three times a day

B.I.D. = from the Latin means *bis in diem*, two times a day

Next is the prakopa stage. *Kapha prakopa,* or provocation, happens because of the liquid, slow, and dull qualities. Heavy and cool qualities create accumulation, sañchaya, but if the cause still continues because the person doesn't pay attention to the aversion, then it may induce other qualities of kapha such as liquid, slow, and dull.

Liquid, slow, and dull qualities will provoke kapha dosha. The liquid quality will create excess salivation, runny nose, cold, congestion, and mucus secretion. Excess salivation can suppress agni and create nausea. The person can also get mucoid vomiting. Prakopa also creates nausea, aversion towards food, anorexia, and loss of appetite.

These symptoms are obvious but, generally, when a person has a cold, he or she takes antibiotics or a decongestant and suppresses the symptoms. Antibiotics are okay if there is an infection, but in the prakopa stage of kapha there is non-specific cold congestion; and no bacteria are involved.

In the prakopa stage, the level of the dosha rises. In the sañchaya stage, kapha accumulates in the pyloric area. In the prakopa stage, kapha comes to the fundus of the stomach. Therefore, there is more fullness. Liquid quality creates excess salivation, cold, runny nose, congestion, and nausea. Slow quality creates stagnation, and dull quality dulls agni and the mind as well as the activity of the srotas, especially *anna vaha srotas*.

The herbal protocol for dealing with the prakopa stage of kapha is using certain drying herbs like sītopalādi, which is an expectorant, and tālīsādi, which is a decongestant. Use 500 mg of each, TID.

To deal with the slow, dull quality we can use herbs with a sharp quality—200 mg of either pippalī or trikatu. Take either of these with honey TID to take care of the liquid, slow and dull qualities and relieve the prakopa stage of kapha dosha.

If there is a runny nose during the second stage of kapha samprāpti, another treatment protocol is to inhale steam. Inhaling steam removes the liquid quality. The latent heat of the steam is much higher than boiling water, so when a person inhales steam, the liquid kapha will run out and that will help with decongestion.

In chronic runny nose or congestion, take hot water in a bowl, put a couple of drops of eucalyptus oil, cover the head with a towel, and inhale the steam. That eucalyptus steam inhalation is the opposite of liquid and dull quality, and it will relieve congestion.

When *sāma doshas*[15] are flowing out of the body, as in runny nose, let them go; don't stop them. If you use an antihistamine, decongestant, or anti-allergy medicine for a cold's congestion, it will suppress the movement of kapha and kapha will create more āma and more thick mucous. Prolonged usage of decongestants or antihistamine can create deviation of the nasal septum, nasal polyps, and thick mucus formation.

That is why Āyurveda says that to drain the nose in an acute cold, the best thing is to drink licorice tea. Boil one teaspoon of licorice in a cup of water for 3 minutes, and then add 5-10 drops of mahānārayana oil. Take one sip of this mixture every ten minutes. It will help to drain mucous without suppressing the flow of *sāma kapha* out of the body.

If we suppress the movement of sāma dosha, then this sāma dosha accumulates in the superficial and deep connective tissue as well as the subcutaneous tissue and can create other disorders like sinus congestion or even tumor formation.

Most of the time our approach is anti, anti, anti—we try to suppress. If there is pain, we use an analgesic painkiller; if there is a spasm, we use an antispasmodic. In an emergency, I'm not against suppression of symptoms but if we suddenly jump to an antihistamine for an acute cold, it will not only suppress the symptoms. Taking an antihistamine or decongestant every time can lead to complications such as nasal polyps, nasal adenoids, or snoring. By suppressing the sāma dosha, the accumulation can move into the deep tissues, creating other complications.

For example, if a person has boils, which is sāma dosha, and it is the first formation, then don't use an anti-inflammatory, just do an incision and the pus will come out. When

---

15. Sāma means a dosha with toxins; nirāma means a dosha without toxins.

the pus comes out, the symptoms of pain and fever will go away. There is no need to do suppression therapy.

In sāma kapha, the mucus is stringy, thick, and foul smelling. If that is coming out, let it go. During the sañchaya and prakopa stages in a healthy kapha person, you can do vamana under professional direction and supervision. That involves drinking licorice tea and vomiting it out.

Even a very mild vamana will bring the kapha out. Then the symptoms of sinus congestion, nasal polyps, and deviated nasal septum will disappear. After that, we can use Super Nasya Oil® or vacha oil nasya as a decongestant. These can remove both sāma and *nirāma kapha* and protect the nasal passage from complications.

In the first two stages of kapha samprāpti, dīpana and pāchana can be done. Dīpana will kindle agni and pāchana will burn āma. If sāma doshas are leaving the body, let them go. It may be beneficial to induce vomiting.

The next stage is the prasara stage. Prasara is when the dosha's site in the gastrointestinal (GI) tract is totally full with a particular dosha—vāta in the colon, pitta in the intestine, kapha in the stomach—and that dosha becomes further aggravated, then the dosha leaves the GI tract. It then enters bāhya mārga, the external pathway, or *shākhā mārga,* the blood vessels or lymphatic system. (see Vyādhi Mārga Illustration on page 16)

The prasara stage of kapha is created by the oily quality. If you put a drop of oil on the surface of some water, the oil spreads. In the same way, kapha spreads on the surface of rasa dhātu when kapha enters the shākhā mārga. The spreading stage of kapha is due to oily quality. Because of the oily quality, kapha spreads to the deep tissues.

In prasara stage, kapha enters the rasa dhātu and can affect the top most layer of the skin so there is water retention as well as lymphatic, capillary, and venous congestion. Prasara stage will also create cold, sinus congestion, slow heartbeat, excess salivation, and generalized heaviness. A ring on the finger becomes tight, the bra becomes tight, and there is pitting of the skin upon pressure. This is the book picture of the prasara stage of kapha.

The first two stages of kapha samprāpti are in our hands, because the doshas are still in the GI tract. Sañchaya is accumulation of kapha in the stomach; prakopa is aggravation of kapha in the stomach. But in prasara stage, kapha leaves the GI tract. We don't have as much control over this stage, but we can still do many things.

In prasara stage, kapha dosha travels and circulates in the body seeking a place to hide. As long as the dhātu agnis are healthy, kapha cannot enter into the dhātus and it will come back to the GI tract. However, one may be carrying a khavaigunya in some tissue, and we don't want to give kapha a chance to lodge in the khavaigunya and create a pathology.

To address this we can use 500 mg of punarnavā. Punarnavā is a dosha pratyanika as well as a diuretic. It will drain excess kapha out through the *mūtra vaha srotas.*

To kindle agni, use 200 mg of chitrak, and do pāchana using trikatu. Trikatu will kindle agni and chitrak will do *āma pāchana.* Dīpana and pāchana can be used mainly in the first three stages: sañchaya, prakopa, and prasara, because once we do dīpana and pāchana, the dosha loses its grip over the tissue and can come back to the GI tract.

One can use a formula of 500 mg punarnavā, 200 mg of chitrak, and 200 mg of trikatu, and take ½ teaspoon of this combination orally TID. It will help to liquefy kapha and take care of the prasara stage.

During the prasara stage, the oily quality is circulating in the rasa dhātu and there is not much oily quality in the GI tract, causing people to crave fatty fried food. Don't eat fatty, fried, greasy food when there is edema, swelling, lymphatic congestion, or capillary congestion. The body creates perverted desires because the bodily dosha wants to grow and enter into the dhātus.

The opposite of oily quality is dry. Dryness is created when kapha leaves the GI tract and goes into rasa dhātu. The dryness in the GI tract will attract the kapha back into the stomach. Trikatu performs dīpana and pāchana and creates more dryness in the stomach. That dryness will act like a sponge and help to pull the kapha back into the GI tract. That is why it is important during prasara stage of kapha to use punarnavā, chitrak, and trikatu. Take ½ tsp. of this combination TID with honey. The person should sip hot water in between so that āma is not produced.

These three stages—sañchaya, prakopa, prasara—belong to the first three stages of shat kriyā kāla, management of the six stages of samprāpti for kapha dosha.

## Deeper Stages of Samprāpti

Sthāna samshraya is the fourth stage. Sthāna samshraya takes place where there is a khavaigunya. If rasa dhātu agni is low, then āma and kapha have access to rasa dhātu and will get deposited there. If rasa dhātu agni is strong, then kapha cannot enter the rasa dhātu and it will attach to the next dhātu.

In sthāna samshraya stage, the dosha finds a weak spot. It may have been created by a previous trauma, a repressed emotion, a previous disease, or low dhātu agni. These factors, along with genetic predisposition, may be responsible for sthāna samshraya. Sthāna samshraya varies according to the site of the lesion, the site of the khavaigunya.

If sthāna samshraya happens in a vital organ, such as the heart, brain, lung, liver, or kidney then kapha will affect those areas. If sthāna samshraya happens in the bladder, the person will get polyuria, a bladder stone, or bladder atony, which is distention of the bladder. If sthāna samshraya happens in the genital organ then it will create blockage of the urethra. If sthāna samshraya happens in the testicles, it can create hydrocele. This is a bird's eye view of different types of sthāna samshraya.

Another possibility is that sthāna samshraya can happen within the GI tract itself. If sthāna samshraya of kapha happens in the stomach then it can create a tumor, or achlorhydria, which is suppression of gastric mucous secretion. If sthāna samshraya happens in the stomach itself, it will create chronic indigestion or chronic anorexia. Let us go step-by-step and look at the entry of kapha into the dhātus.

*Rasa Dhātu.* If kapha enters rasa dhātu due to low rasa dhātu agni, then in general it will create low grade fever, pallor, cough, common cold, catarrh, lymphatic congestion, edema, and hay fever. It will also create lack of nutrition and fatigue.

For low-grade fever and common cold, we can use 500 mg of sītopalādi, 300 mg mahāsudarshan, and 200 mg of abhrak bhasma. Sītopalādi is an expectorant and decongestant. Mahāsudarshan is anti-pyretic and good for low-grade fever. Abhrak bhasma is good for boosting the immune system and protecting ojas. Mahāsudarshan gana vati is good for catarrh. One can take ½ teaspoon of this herbal formula TID with a bit of honey or hot water to deal with lymphatic congestion, low grade fever, common cold, congestion, and cough.

Also in this stage, one can inhale steam and do nasya with Super Nasya Oil® or vacha oil to take care of common cold and catarrh. Punarnavā can be used if there is edema and sītopalādi is the best remedy for hay fever. This is a beneficial formula for entry of kapha into the rasa dhātu.

*Rakta Dhātu.* If rasa dhātu agni is strong and so there is no access to enter the rasa dhātu then kapha will try to enter rakta dhātu. If rakta dhātu agni is low, kapha can enter the rakta dhātu and create more swelling, plus megaloblastic anemia, high blood pressure, high cholesterol, and high triglycerides. The root of rakta vaha srotas is the liver and spleen. Excess kapha in the liver will create fatty changes in the liver and enlargement of the spleen. A person may also get hyperglycemia or any of the symptoms of diabetes.

For edema and swelling, a person can use 500 mg of punarnavā. For pallor, one can use abhrak bhasma, and for high blood pressure, one can use 200 mg each of passionflower, hawthorn berry, or rasagandha. For high cholesterol we can use 200 mg of triphalā guggulu, shuddha shilājit (purified shilājit), or trikatu.

For fatty changes in the liver, we normally use ārogya vardhini, but it may be difficult to find ārogya vardhini without mercury, so we can use 200 mg each of kutki, chitrak, and neem TID. That will take care of fatty changes of the liver as well as enlarged spleen. For diabetic patients one can use equal portions 200 mg each of turmeric and neem TID.

*Māmsa Dhātu.* These individual disorders can be treated as separate conditions created by the entry of kapha into rakta dhātu. If rakta dhātu agni is strong then kapha will leave rakta dhātu and go to the māmsa dhātu. If māmsa dhātu agni is low, kapha can enter the māmsa dhātu.

Entry of kapha into māmsa dhātu will cause māmsa dhātu agni to decrease even more. Then there will be increased *khamala* (earwax), tartar on the teeth, nasal crust, and smegma. Entry of kapha into māmsa dhātu can create myoma, or muscle tumor, muscle hypertrophy, fibroid tumor, or fibrotic changes in the breast or uterus.

We can take care of these conditions with the following herbal protocols. For earwax, clean the ear with medicated vacha oil diluted half-and-half in sesame oil and kindle māmsa dhātu agni with 300 mg of triphalā guggulu BID. For myoma, which is a muscle tumor, we should do *lekhana* (scraping) using kutki or chitrak. Vacha oil can be applied (see above) topically for myoma.

For muscle hypertrophy, one can use 200 mg each shilājit, triphalā guggulu, or chandra prabhā vati TID. For fibroid tumor, one can use 200 mg each of punarnavā, kutki, and chitrak TID. Kāñcanāra guggulu, 200 mg TID, is also quite effective for fibroid tumors, uterine fibroids, and muscle hypertrophy.

If a person develops tartar on the teeth, they should get their teeth cleaned by a dentist, no doubt, but tartar on the teeth is a sign of kapha entering māmsa dhātu. People who develop excess tartar on the teeth should also check their blood sugar, as they may be pre-diabetic. Using neem or triphalā toothpaste, or gargling with triphalā tea is quite effective for treating tartar. One can also hold a mouth full of sesame oil, swish it for one minute, and spit it out.

*Meda Dhātu.* If māmsa dhātu agni is strong, then kapha will not enter māmsa dhātu. It will leave māmsa dhātu and go to meda dhātu. If meda dhātu agni is low then kapha will enter the meda dhātu and create excess weight or obesity and cause cold sweating. If apāna vāyu is pulling kapha into the lower part of the body, then the person will get distended obesity. In this condition, they have a flat chest but enlarged thighs. If samāna vāyu is pushing kapha into the peritoneum and omentum then they will get truncated obesity and have a pot-bellied abdomen. If udāna vāyu is pushing kapha upward then there will be ascending obesity. In this condition, there is an enlarged face and pendular breasts, but the thighs are not enlarged. If vyāna vāyu is distributing kapha in the periphery, a person will have peripheral obesity. They will have enlarged thighs and arms but a flatter belly and chest.

One should pay attention to the different types of obesity. They each have a different protocol. In apāna vāyu obesity, or descending obesity, one can use triphalā guggulu and do dashamūla basti. In truncated obesity, which is *samāna vāyu dushti,* one can use chitrak guggulu. This will kindle agni and pacify samāna vāyu. In ascending obesity, where obesity affects the face and breasts, one can use trikatu, because it acts on the upper part of the body. If it is peripheral obesity, then treat vyāna vāyu with arjuna and vacha, or 200 mg each of arjuna and pushkarmūla. They can also use kaishore guggulu, which has an affinity for vyāna vāyu.

When kapha goes into meda dhātu a person can get gallstones. The treatment protocol for gallstones is 500 mg of punarnavā, 200 mg of chitrak, 200 mg of trikatu and 200 mg of shilājit, taken TID orally.

*Asthi Dhātu.* If meda dhātu agni is strong, kapha will go to asthi dhātu. If asthi dhātu agni is low, kapha can enter the asthi dhātu and create osteoma, tumors of the bones, swelling of the joints, effusion, bone spur, misalignment of the spine, and lordosis. These also go together with hypothyroidism. Hypothyroidism means kapha is at the junction between asthi and majjā. The endocrine system is majjā dhātu and glandular dysfunction can happen when kapha enters the junction between these two dhātus, which is the *dhātu dhāra kalā.* When kapha passes from the *asthi dhāra kalā* to the *majjā dhāra kalā* then hypothyroidism will happen.

In hypothyroidism, the patient has calcium in the blood so there may be micro-calcification. Kapha in the asthi dhātu reduces asthi dhātu agni further and then the bone starts losing calcium. Those calcium molecules can deposit in the breast because *poshaka kapha* and lactation are by-products of rasa dhātu. Even though kapha is in asthi dhātu, it still has an affinity to *stanya,* or breast tissue. Micro-calcification in the breast can create a pre-cancerous situation.

For osteoma, or bony tumor, we can use either 200 mg of yogarāja guggulu and 200 mg of kāñcanāra guggulu, or 200 mg of rāsnādi guggulu TID. For swelling of the joints, we can use punarnavā guggulu or the following lepanas topically to reduce the effusion— punarnavā lepana, gudūchī lepana, dashānga lepana. Lepanas are herbal pastes applied topically.

For bone spur, triphalā guggulu or yogarāja guggulu can be used TID. Traditionally, *agni karma* was done topically on the site of the spur. In agni karma, a red hot copper rod is used to do gentle branding. This has to be done with great skill. The counter-irritation of branding stimulates osteolytic enzyme,[16] and inhibits osteogenic enzyme.[17] This causes porosis in the spur. It also prevents spur formation by kindling asthi dhātu agni.

Misalignment of the spine may be due to kapha in asthi dhātu. Kapha is slow and sluggish, and people sitting around with bad posture develop misalignment. For that they have to correct their posture, do some yoga, and apply mahānārāyana tailam along the spine. Chiropractic manipulation or applying traction may also help.

When kapha is in the junction of asthi and majjā dhāra kalā and causes hypothyroidism, we can use 200 mg each of ārogya vardhini, chitrak, trikatu, and kaishore guggulu TID. Bhrāmarī and ujjāyi prānāyāma are also affective as well as specific *āsanas* that strengthen the spine.

***Majjā Dhātu.*** If asthi dhātu agni is strong, kapha will try to enter majjā dhātu. If majjā dhātu agni is low, kapha will enter majjā and create hypersomnia, or increased sleep, protruded eyes, hydrocephalus,[18] lethargy, and melancholy. These sound rather complicated, but they are simply kapha in the brain and nervous system.

Kapha in majjā dhātu can also create a pineal gland tumor, called pinealoma, or a pituitary gland tumor. It can also create petit mal epilepsy. These are serious conditions and they should be treated by experts.

For hypersomnia, increased sleep, we can use 200 mg each brahmī, jatamāmsī, vacha, shankha pushpī TID and vacha oil nasya. That will reduce kapha from the majjā dhātu. For a pineal or pituitary gland tumor, the dhātu treatment is the same because we are treating the dosha in majjā dhātu. For that, use 500 mg of punarnavā, 200 mg chitrak, 200 mg kutki, 300 mg brahmī, and 200 mg of shankha pushpī. One-half teaspoon of this formula TID will help. In both pineal and pituitary tumor, the following prānāyāmas are effective: bhrāmarī prānāyāma, *bhastrikā prānāyāma, anuloma viloma,* and *kapāla bhati.*

For lethargy, one should do pañchakarma with *shirobasti, shirodhāra,* and nasya. Internally we can use 200 mg each of punarnavā, brahmī, jatamāmsī, and shankha pushpī TID.

---

16. A bodily enzyme that breaks down bone cells.
17. A bodily enzyme that stimulates growth of the bone.
18. An accumulation of water in the subdural space or meninges.

***Shukra Dhātu.*** If majjā dhātu agni is strong then naturally kapha will go to *shukra dhātu.* *Shukra gata kapha* can create a tumor in the testicle or epididymis, benign prostatic hypertrophy, hydrocephalus, and semen leak. In all these disorders, there is a simple line of treatment: 500 mg of punarnavā, 200 mg chandraprabhā, 200 mg ashvagandhā, and 200 mg of ātma gupta; take ½ teaspoon of this formula TID.

A testicular tumor or benign prostatic hypertrophy could be cancer so in these conditions, one should consult with an expert to rule that out. Otherwise, benign prostatic hypertrophy has the same herbal protocol as above, and prostatic massage with medicated vacha oil or castor oil is also effective.

Shukra gata kapha can produce large amounts of semen, and the person may become sexually overactive. Even after prolonged sex, there is no satisfaction. These people may end up with depression. To strengthen shukra we can use 500 mg of ashvagandhā and 300 mg of vidārī TID. Shukra gata kapha can also produce raw, unhealthy semen that can get blocked in the prostate and produce prostatic calculi or prostatic stone. The herbal protocol for prostatic stone is 200 mg of punarnavā guggulu, 200 mg of gokshura guggulu, 200 mg of shilājit, and 200 mg of pāshana bheda TID. These herbs will help break down the prostatic calculi.

Kapha is dull and slow. In some individuals, kapha may produce low libido and premature ejaculation. The treatment protocol for low libido and premature ejaculation is 500 mg of ashvagandhā, 300 mg of balā, 200 mg of vidārī, and 200 mg of shilājit TID.

The pure essence of all bodily tissues is ojas. There are two types of ojas: *para* and *apara.* Para is superior ojas, which is present in the heart in a quantity of eight drops. There is half an *añjali* of apara ojas and it circulates throughout the body. If kapha enters shukra, it may slow down the process of dhātu metabolism and produce raw ojas. Increased raw ojas can create high cholesterol, high triglycerides, and hypertension with low libido. These people can also get albumin urea, protein in the urine.

The treatment protocol for ojovruddhi, increased raw ojas, is to treat kapha dosha with 500 mg of punarnavā, 200 mg shilājit, 200 mg of abhrak bhasma, and 200 mg of ātma gupta TID. This herbal protocol will create healthy ojas. These people should also take 1 teaspoon of tikta ghrita, which is bitter ghee, because the bitter taste can reduce kapha dosha.

Finally, to protect ojas, Ayurveda recommends madhu tailam basti, which is ½ cup of sesame oil and ½ cup of honey mixed together and given rectally. The subject is asked to retain this for as long as he can.

***Ārtava Dhātu.*** Lastly, if kapha dosha enters ārtava dhātu, it can slow down ārtava dhātu agni. The female egg becomes slow, sluggish, heavy, and enlarged, and can produce polycystic changes in the ovaries, known as polycystic ovarian syndrome or cystic ovary. This is accompanied by a hormonal imbalance with low estrogen and overproduction of testosterone. The patient develops male facial hair. This undue growth of the hair is due to male hormones, which are kapha in nature. The treatment protocol for polycystic ovarian syndrome is 500 mg of punarnavā, 200 mg of chitrak, 200 mg of kutki, and 300 mg of ashoka. Take ½ tsp. of this mixture TID. She should also do prānāyāma like kapāla bhāti, anuloma viloma, and bhrāmarī.

The entry of kapha in ārtava dhātu can also cause ectopic gestation, fibroid tumor, or cervical polyps. In all these disorders, the best remedy is 500 mg of punarnavā, 200 mg of chitrak, and 200 mg of shilājit TID. Don't use shatāvari or balā in these disorders, because these are anabolic and will induce kapha further. Instead of shatāvari and balā we can use ashoka with kumārī (aloe vera) as an anupāna.

Kapha dosha in *ārtava vaha srotas* may produce undue thickening of the endometrium, called endometriosis. Due to the increase of the heavy, thick, and stable qualities of kapha dosha, the endometrium grows through the fallopian tubes and ovaries. It can also spread into the pelvic cavity and create multiple adhesions. According to Āyurvedic principles, one should do *lekhana chikitsā* followed by 500 mg of punarvanā, 200 mg of kutki, and 300 mg of trikatu. Take ½ tsp. of this mixture TID. Also take 1 Tbs. of flax seed oil orally twice a day before breakfast and dinner.

The vyakti stage of kapha samprāpti is due to cloudy and soft qualities. Cloudy quality causes congestion and the soft quality causes discharge and oozing. During the vyakti stage, kapha can create various tumor formations related to the specific dhātu that has been affected in the sthāna samshraya stage.

In the bheda stage, we have a full-blown manifestation of pathogenesis, but the treatment of those pathogeneses should follow the protocol of the sthāna samshraya stage, because vyakti and bheda are related to the same site as sthāna samsraya. The vyakti stage may happen in any srotas or dhātu, so its signs and symptoms depend on the site of the lesion. For example, when sthāna samshraya happens in rasa dhātu, then the vyakti stage will create a growth such as lymphoma. If sthāna samshraya happens in rakta dhātu, then the vyakti stage will create will megaloblastic (pernicious) anemia or hemangioma, a tumor of the blood. Vyakti of meda dhātu will create lipoma. So, the manifestation of vyakti depends upon the dhātu. The protocol is the same as in the sthāna samshraya stage.

In the bheda stage, kapha creates structural changes in the tissue because of hard, dense, static, and gross qualities. Ultimately, the bheda stage of kapha will cause hardening, excess growth, and compactness of the tissue. There may be modified tumor, consolidation of the tissue, change of tissue structure and loss of tissue function. It can also create hard, calcified fibrotic nerves. That is why bheda stage is called *upadrava* stage, the stage of complications. The bheda stage should only be handled by a seasoned professional. Diet and lifestyle factors may help, but they will be limited, because the person has complications that may also require hospitalization, surgical intervention, chemotherapy, radiation, or other proper treatment from an oncologist.

The shat kriyā kāla opens a multi-factorial therapeutic approach. It moves students and practitioners to think about *vidhi samprāpti,* which involves the *dosha gati,* or movement of the doshas, and vyādhi mārga, the pathway of the disease. It also explains *vikalpa samprāpti,* the qualitative manifestation of the dosha. If a person follows shat kriyā kāla, they will hit the nail on the head. Their treatment will never go astray. Sometimes people think that Āyurveda takes a long time; I think that is not true. If a practitioner, student, or professional really puts these views of shat kriyā kāla into their practice, I am quite sure they will be great clinicians, healers, and practitioners. They will bring a positive result in their clinical practice.

This is my humble effort of expressing this shat kriyā kāla. It is briefly mentioned in Sushruta Samhitā but we have taken his wonderful idea and elaborated on it with our clinical data, making shat kriyā kāla a unique line of therapy.

# Chapter 5

# Pain

## Shūla

Winter 1997, Volume 10, Number 3 and Spring 1998, Volume 10, Number 4

In *Mādhava Nidānam,* one of the ancient Ayurvedic texts on clinical practice, *shūla* (pain) is treated as a separate *roga* (disease). However, many times we experience pain as a symptom of another disease. What is the difference between a disease and a symptom? A disease has its own samprāpti (pathological changes,) a definite etiology and specific signs and symptoms. It undergoes doshic changes, through the six stages of pathogenesis: accumulation, provocation, spread, deposition, manifestation and differentiation. Therefore, disease has a definite samprāpti.

On the other hand, a symptom isn't necessarily due to one particular disease process. A symptom may be caused when a dosha accumulates in its own site, without yet producing any disease. The dosha can then undergo changes and express different signs and symptoms in each stage of disease. When symptoms are incompletely manifested, they are called pūrva rūpa, which means warning bell symptoms. When signs and symptoms are completely manifested, they are called rūpa. When pain is constant, persistent and a major problem, it can itself be called a disease.

Vāta is the dosha primarily responsible for pain, because it is closely related to prāna, which governs the nervous system and all sensation. Vāta's main seat is in the colon and from there, vāta moves into different bodily *srotāmsi* (channels). *Prāna* also flows throughout the body, in every *srotas* (channel), organ, and *marma* point. If prāna becomes functionally disturbed, due to an imbalance in one or more of the qualities of *vāta dosha,* that results in pain in either the mind or body. Vāta is dry (*rūksha*), light (*laghu*), cold (*shīta*), rough (*khāra*), subtle (*sūkshma*), and mobile (*chala*). Extreme dryness or intense cold can create pain, as can excess roughness. The mobile quality of vāta can cause the pain to radiate, moving from one place to another.

Many times, vāta pain is seemingly causeless. The pain is mobile, radiating, fluctuating, and vague in nature. Vāta pain is aggravated at vāta times of day, which are dawn and dusk. It is also more intense during the vāta seasons, fall and winter, and is aggravated by exposure to cold, improper food combining and excessive movement. In addition, vāta pain is associated with flatulence, constipation, and bloating.

Next, look at the qualities of pitta—hot (*ushna*), sharp (tīkshna), spreading (sara), oily (*snigdha*), liquid (*drava*), and light (laghu). When these qualities are increased and pitta is blocking vāta, then these pitta attributes mix with vāta and create pitta type of pain. Increased hot quality causes burning and inflammation, sharp quality can create ulceration and perforation. Increased oily quality may increase congestion and produce nausea, and the spreading quality of pitta causes pain to flare, creating tenderness and pain on pressure. Pitta pain is associated with inflammation and increases during midday, midnight and during the summer season. It is often followed by nausea, vomiting and diarrhea. It is increased by exposure to heat and pacified by cooling treatments. Note that while heating treatments relieve vāta pain and increase pitta pain, both vāta and pitta pain are worsened by movement. Therefore fast walking or vigorous exercise can aggravate arthritic pain that is caused by vāta and/or pitta.

Kapha is heavy (*guru*), dull (*manda*), cool (shīta), oily (snigdha), sticky (*picchila*), static (*sthira*), and liquid (drava). When any of these qualities of kapha are disturbed and block vāta, the resultant pain will have kapha characteristics. Because of the heavy quality, kapha type of pain will be deep. Kapha is slow and dull, hence, kapha pain is a dull ache. It is also liquid and cool, so the skin in the affected areas will feel cold and clammy. Due to both the liquid and oily qualities, kapha pain is associated with congestion and swelling, and because kapha is static, the pain is localized, neither radiating like vāta, nor spreading like pitta. Pressure and deep massage can relieve kapha pain, as do movement and warming exercise. Kapha pain occurs more in early morning and early evening, which are kapha times of day, and during the winter and spring seasons.

Shūla is a complex subject, but we are presenting this information in a simplified way. Behind pitta or kapha pain there is always vāta, because a disturbance of vāta is always involved in any kind of pain. However, when vāta is blocked by pitta, the pain is colored by the qualities of pitta. The same is true for kapha. Pure vāta pain is pricking, gripping, spasmodic, colicky, and often excruciating. Psychologically, it creates nervousness, fever and insomnia. Pitta pain is hot, sharp and intense, and it creates irritability, anger and disturbed sleep. Finally, kapha pain is heavy, dull and static, and it creates attachment, depression and excessive sleep.

## The Qualities of Pain

Pain can be acute, subacute, chronic, radiating, and fluctuating. Whenever pain is present, we have to inquire into the qualitative changes that have occurred and determine whether the pain is mono, dual or triple-doshic.

*Mādhava Nidānam* speaks about sensory pain, motor pain and emotional pain. Sensory pain is related to prāna; motor pain to *apāna;* and emotional pain is psychosomatic. Pain is an interactive phenomenon that operates at the physical, mental, emotional and biochemical levels. It may be due to tissue damage, but remember that tissue damage is due to aggravation of the doshic qualities described above. A comfortable stimulus is called pleasure, whereas an uncomfortable stimulus is called pain.

Physiological, psychological, and social interactions can all create pain. For example, an argument with your spouse can precipitate pain. We have to see pain as a whole, having the qualities of vāta, pitta, and kapha. Understanding this basic concept helps us to deal with the pain directly.

Generally, there is a tendency for vāta pain to be acute, pitta pain to be acute or sub-acute, and kapha pain to be subacute or chronic. However this is not always true, as certain kapha pain is acute, such as a sinus headache. Kapha pain is always less intense; it doesn't create the agony caused by vāta and pitta pain. First, identify the doshic involvement: congestion is kapha; infection or inflammation indicates pitta; trauma, accident or neuralgia is vāta. Ask what time the pain occurs. Pain that worsens around midnight and midday indicates pitta. Morning and evening pain shows kapha, while pain that occurs at dawn and dusk is vāta. Also inquire about aggravating and relieving factors. Movement will aggravate vāta but relieve kapha. Application of heat, such as a warm castor oil pack, will soothe vāta but increase pitta. The usage of non- invasive measures, such as the application of heat, gentle manipulation, a splint or bandage, relaxation, yoga, prānāyāma, and meditation, will especially relieve vāta pain.

सर्वेष्वेतेषु शूलेषु प्रयेण पवन प्रभुः ।
मा. नि.

sarveṣveteṣu śūleṣu prayeṇa pavana prabhuḥ
*Mādhava Nidānam*

*Imbalanced vata affects the other doshas, creating pain. This sensory and emotional experience is associated with the psychosomatic response to actual or potential tissue damage. In all pains, vata is the main causative factor.*

Translation, Vasant Lad

### Associated Phenomena

Pain associated with symptoms such as fever, diarrhea, and vomiting is a sign of disturbed pitta dosha. Constipation and flatulence along with pain indicates a vāta disorder. Pain with heaviness and sleepiness is a sign of increased kapha. If there is extreme chronic anorexia (low agni) with epigastric pain, the cause may be cancer. Chronic low hydrochloric acid can also be indicative of cancer.

Vomiting is a common symptom that is associated with pain. Vomiting related to stomach or intestinal problems, such as gastritis enteritis, or peritonitis, is due to aggravated pitta. If there is also gas under the diaphragm, consider the possibility of a perforated ulcer. Vomiting may also be a sign of early appendicitis or cholecystitis, and meningitis can also cause vomiting. About ninety-five percent of vomiting is due to aggravated pitta, whereas only mucoid vomiting is a purely kapha disorder. In children, vomiting is often due to infection and projectile vomiting indicates pancreatitis. Sudden vomiting suggests an intracranial disease and if there is vomiting in the morning, during kapha time, think about pregnancy or alcoholic gastritis. Vomiting of large quantities of food in the later part of the day or night might be due to obstruction caused by a tumor, while involvement of the upper gut could be due to a pyloric obstruction.

Vomiting with heartburn could be caused by inflammation of the esophagus, another pitta disorder, and if there is regurgitation of food with pain, that might indicate an esophageal obstruction. Take the age of the person into consideration. If a man of 82 comes with a sense of obstruction while swallowing, think about cancer of the esophagus. However, if the person is in his or her twenties, the cause might be stress.

## Ayurvedic Pain Killers

*Shulāhara* or *shūlaghna* is the Sanskrit word for analgesic. Ayurveda speaks about many substances that can be used to alleviate pain.

*Opium (Papaver somniferum).* Ahiphenam or opium was used in ancient times as the most effective analgesic. Today it is a controlled substance and can only be prescribed by qualified physicians. It works as a painkiller and anti-spasmodic and it is effective for pain due to all three doshas. Even a small dose can relieve pain and insomnia, but there are many side effects. It is extremely addictive and causes severe constipation. Hence, it is vāta-aggravating. Perhaps the most serious side effect is that any form of opium is a respiratory depressant and an excessive dose can result in death.

*Dhattūra (Dhātura alba).* Although dhattūra is quite toxic to the liver and kidneys and may create extreme muscle spasm, in small doses it is a wonderful painkiller. The flower, which looks like a loudspeaker, is made into a tea. Dhattūra works best for vāta and kapha pain. Because it can create nausea and vomiting, it is not used for pitta.

*Yavānī (Trachyspermum ammi).* Yavānī is a special ajwan from Afghanistan. It is effective for vāta and kapha pain and also relieves stomach pain. Yavānī is not used for pitta, because it can create nausea and vomiting.

*Mustā (Nagar motha—Cyperus rotundus).* Mustā is effective for tridoshic pain. It is a muscle relaxant with an affinity for māmsa dhātu, so it is used for muscular-skeletal pain, but not for pain in the smooth muscles. Due to its diuretic action, it also relieves renal pain.

*Ashvagandhā (Withania somnifera).* Ashvagandhā pacifies vāta and kapha and it can stimulate pitta. This herb is effectively used for congestive and spasmodic pain, as well as neurologia and muscular pain. It soothes menstrual cramps caused by spasmodic dysmenorrhea, but if the cause is congestion, punarnavā is a better choice.

*Jatamāmsi (Nardostachys jatamāmsi).* This herb has an affinity for majjā dhātu and *mano vaha srotas*. Jatamāmsi is used for vāta and pitta disorders. Its actions are anti-inflammatory, analgesic and tranquilizing. It is particularly effective for pain caused by emotional or neurological or factors.

*Ajvain (Carum copticum—Wild Caraway).* Ajvain works on smooth muscles, including the muscles of the small intestine. It is heating and pungent and can be used for vāta and kapha, but it is too heating for pitta and may create bleeding. Ajvain is antispasmodic to the colon and stomach muscles and also relieves pain caused by congestion.

*Nutmeg (Myristica fragrans—jātīphalā).* Nutmeg is analgesic and a tranquilizer, similar to a mild version of opium. It may increase kapha. Therefore, excessive use can create depression. Nutmeg is used in diarrhea and it is effective for any generalized body ache, as it works on the nervous system. A pinch of nutmeg in milk, with a teaspoon of ghee added, acts on emotional pain. Nutmeg oil on the forehead will relieve a headache and it can be used in *marma chikitsā* for vāta and pitta.

*Ginger (Zingiber off.; adraka—fresh ginger; shunthi—dry ginger).* Ginger is tridoshic, but in excess may increase pitta. It has an affinity for māmsa, asthi and majjā dhātus. Note that dry ginger is more heating than fresh. Ginger paste is effective for sinus headaches and has many other uses as pain reliever. Ginger can be used if āma is lingering in rasa dhātu, as it has *āma pāchana* action. A ginger/baking soda bath will also help to remove this āma.

*Cinnamon (Cinnamomum zeylancium; tvak).* Cinnamon or tvak is used as a medicine for vāta and kapha, but not for pitta, because of its heating quality. It can be used internally and topically, and is good for relieving sinus headaches, stomachache and tooth pain.

*Guggulu (Commiphora mukal).* The various forms of guggulu are used for specific doshic pain. For vāta pain use yogarāja guggulu; for pitta, kaishore guggulu; for kapha, triphalā guggulu. Guggulu has a special affinity for the bones, so it is particularly good for arthritic pain.

*Jyotishmatī (Celastrus paniculatus).* This herb is used for vāta and kapha, but not for pitta dosha. Its actions are narcotic, tranquilizing and sedative. Jyotishmatī oil is used externally for arthritic pain.

*Clove (Syzigium aromaticum; lavanga).* Clove is used for vāta and kapha, but it can aggravate pitta. One drop of clove oil on an aching tooth will act as an analgesic and will also kill any bacteria. Clove is used for most types of dental pain and trigeminal neuralgia.

*Camphor (Cinnamonum camphora; karpura).* Camphor is the resin of a tree. It has an affinity to the nerve tissue and is a bronchodilator and analgesic. A pinch of edible camphor on an aching tooth will calm the pain. It is mainly used for vāta and kapha types of pain.

*Dashamūla.* This combination of ten herbal roots is widely used for vāta type of pain. Dashamūla has an affinity for asthi and majjā dhātus. Dashamūla oil can be used for massage and is effective for lower backache. Dashamūla tea basti is used to alleviate vāta pain in the abdominal area.

*Ajagandha (Cleome viscosa—Wild Mustard).* Ajagandha means male goat. This herb has a strong smell and is an aphrodisiac. It is used for vāta and kapha pain and for testicular pain in particular. Other uses include pain due to worms, parasites and indigestion.

***Kāma Dudhā.*** Kāma dudhā is a compound of anti-inflammatory and analgesic bhasmas and is effectively used for pitta pain.

***Vijayā (Cannabis sativa—Marijuana).*** Vijayā is marijuana. It is tridoshic when used in a small dose, but in excess it provokes all three doshas and overuse may particularly disturb vāta. Vijayā is a highly spiritual plant that is used by yogis and *tantric* people in India. It calms anxiety and gives a sense of well-being, as well as expansion of consciousness. However, it is addictive and toxic to the liver and lungs. Excessive consumption can lead to anxiety tachycardia, neurosis and schizophrenic changes. Because it slows metabolism, excessive use of this substance can also lead to weight gain. Vijayā guggulu is an effective treatment for rheumatoid arthritis and contains one-eighth vijayā.

***Bhangā.*** Bhang means 'to destroy worldly nature.' A mild preparation of marijuana made from young leaves and stems of the Indian hemp plant and drunk with milk or water as a fermented brew or smoked for its hallucinogenic effects. It is similar to marijuana and gives a beautiful perception of color vision. It pacifies vāta and kapha, but in excess it can increase all doshas. Although bhangā is a strong pain killer, it is highly addictive.

***Drākshā.*** Drākshā is an herbal wine and its alcohol base will increase pitta if used in excess. It acts as a diuretic and analgesic and it brings tranquility. It especially helps pain due to āma. Although drākshā can be used as a painkiller, alcohol is addictive and should be used with caution.

***Tobacco (Nicotiana tubacum; tamakhu).*** Tobacco is tridoshic when used in moderation as a painkiller, but it disturbs all three doshas in excess. Tobacco goes directly into the nervous system, and it is addictive and carcinogenic. A small dose brings a mild tranquilizing effect, causing stress-induced pain to subside. Those who smoke in moderation will hardly ever get Alzheimer's, because nicotine in a small dose is a vasodilator. However, if taken in excess, nicotine causes hardening of the blood vessels. Anything in its proper dose is medicine; anything in excess is poison.

***Arjuna (Terminalia arjuna).*** This herb is used for pain due to imbalanced vāta or kapha doshas. It relieves cardiac pain by increasing cardiac circulation.

***Pushkaramūla (Inula racemosis; Elecampane).*** Pushkaramūla is tridoshic. It is used for pleuritis and cardiac pain and combined with arjuna for cardio-pulmonary pain.

***Punarnavā (Boerhaavia diffusa).*** This herb is used for vāta and kapha disorders, and it is slightly heating, hence, not so good for pitta. Punarnavā is particularly effective for renal colic.

***Castor Oil (Ricinus communis; eranda).*** Castor oil is tridoshic when used appropriately and it is a strong laxative. A cup of ginger tea with one teaspoon of castor oil can help to relieve rheumatic pain.

Many of these substances are addictive. How and when should we use them? It depends on the skill of the physician as to the correct use of these addictive substances. The healer-patient relationship must be absolutely clear. With this clarity, the physician can use these strong herbs in small doses. The doctor-patient relationship is sacred and, unfortunately, in this modern age that relationship is rare.

For instance, ulcerative colitis responds well to a small dose of ahiphenam, but once the bleeding stops, one should gradually withdraw the drug before an addiction develops. In case of a psychic or stress headache, or even in anxiety, tobacco can be used along with nutmeg and rose. The patient can smoke three cigarettes a day with these special ingredients. Tobacco has an affinity to majjā dhātu, so in situations of stress, emotional crisis or phobias, appropriate use of tobacco induces a sense of well-being. These strong substances should be used with great caution but can be extremely helpful.

In this next section, we will discuss specific doshic treatments for various classifications of pain, as presented in *Mādhava Nidānam*.

## Part Two: Doshic Management

In the previous section, we explored the Ayurvedic concept of pain. We will now consider the management of pain according to the *doshic* involvement. The entire picture has to be considered before we can come to any conclusion about the appropriate form of treatment. The main question to ask is, "What is the nature of the pain—vāta, pitta, or kapha?"

Pain caused by vāta strikes intermittently, creating a period of time with pain followed by a period without. The symptoms may include breathlessness, tachycardia, and gas. The nature of the pain is excruciating, agonizing, colicky and intense. Vāta pain is relieved by the application of heat (svedana), oil massage (snehana), and dashamūla tea basti (medicated enema) as well as by pressure at the site of the pain.

Pitta pain is sharp, burning, and stabbing and it is increased by pressure. It is associated with nausea, vomiting, diarrhea, dizziness, and irritability. Cooling treatments, such as a cold compress or ice bag, relieves pitta type of pain. It is also relieved by virechana (purgation).

Kapha pain is dull, aching, and static. The pain is increased by bending over and lessened by standing up or otherwise moving against gravity. Movement of any kind generally relieves this type of pain, which is associated with stiffness and swelling. Kapha pain is relieved by dry and scraping treatments, such as dry brush massage or the application of dry heat, as well as vamana (therapeutic vomiting).

All types of pain can be relieved by snehana, using oils specific to the dosha involved. For vāta, use sesame oil or *ghee*. Pitta responds well to coconut, sunflower oil or ghee, all of which are cooling. For kapha, use a light and drying oil, such as corn or mustard oil. Vacha oil or dry vacha powder are also effective for kapha. In India, we use vacha oil as a nasya (nasal oil) for vāta or kapha types of sinus headache, and a vacha powder nasya is effective for kapha sinus congestion.

Essential oils can be used in svedana therapy. For pitta, use sandalwood or jatamāmsi oil added to a steam treatment. Kapha pain is helped by eucalyptus or cinnamon and vāta pain responds well to ginger, nirgundī, hina or amber in the steam.

Be sure to relieve or stop any severe pain before using the above treatments. Pain is an indication that something is wrong. One should always take it seriously and consider going to a doctor or even the hospital, especially if the pain is intense or prolonged.◆

## Classifications of Pain

*Mādhava Nidānam* speaks about various classifications of pain:

* *Udara shūla* – abdominal pain
* *Pārshva shūla* – pleuritic pain
* *Parināma shūla* – peptic pain during the process of digestion
* *Anna drava shūla* – pain during the process of liquefaction of food while it is still in the stomach
* *Hrid shūla* or *hricchūla* – pseudo-cardiac pain
* *Shira shūla* – headache[19]

### Udara Shūla

Udara shūla is abdominal pain. If it is present in the lower abdomen, the pain is usually due to vāta. Pain in the middle abdomen is generally from aggravated pitta and upper abdominal pain is often due to pitta and kapha. Whenever a patient reports abdominal pain, first determine the exact location of the pain. Pain in the right half of the epigastrium may be due to a duodenal ulcer, while pain in the left half possibly indicates a gastric ulcer. Generalized abdominal pain is commonly from āma; hence, it can be called āma shūla. In this case, there may be a history of indigestion or food poisoning and all associated symptoms need to be examined. If there is also abdominal distension and constipation, the cause may be an obstruction, which needs to be treated.

### Management

*Vāta udara shūla* occurs in the lower abdomen. First, apply a warm castor oil pack to that area. If this treatment relieves the pain, it is due to *vāta dosha*. Before proceeding with further treatment, one should be cautious and rule out the possibility of appendicitis. If the cause of pain is appendicitis, giving a basti could be dangerous. However, once appendicitis is ruled out, give a basti of dashamūla tea the moment the pain subsides.

If the person has had constipation for three or four days, give a basti or a glycerin suppository. If there is abdominal distension, find out if the cause is gas, constipation or an obstruction. A doctor can insert a flatus tube into the rectum and if the person passes countless bubbles, then there is no obstruction. If only a few bubbles or no bubbles pass through, send the person to hospital to determine the cause of the obstruction. Even worms in the colon can produce an obstruction, thereby creating an emergency. To treat shūla successfully may require a great deal of clinical experience.

Small stones may cause renal colic pain while passing them from the kidney into the urethra. If a stone becomes stuck somewhere, either in the beginning of the urethra near the kidney or at the end near the bladder, the entire urethra may spasm and create severe pain, causing attack after attack. It looks like vāta pain, but the pain moves from loin to groin, or vice versa. If you percuss the kidney area with your fist, it will increase the

T.I.D. = from the Latin means *ter in diem*, three times a day

B.I.D. = from the Latin means *bis in diem*, two times a day

---

19. Shira Shūla is covered in chapter 22, *Headache*, starting on page 165.

pain. Send the person to the hospital, as that patient needs a smooth muscle relaxant and intravenous flushing to assist in passing the kidney stone.

For management of vāta udara shūla, internally give:
Triphalā Guggulu       300 mg, 1 tablet TID
Hingvastak Chūrna      ½ teaspoon BID with warm water

Or make a tea using:
1 teaspoon Ginger
½ teaspoon Cinnamon
Pinch of Clove
Pinch of Rock Salt

Keep the colon clean by nightly giving:
½ teaspoon gandharva harītakī with warm water

**Pitta Udara Shūla.** If the pain is accompanied by nausea, vomiting, or peptic ulcer and the patient says food relieves the pain, the cause may be pitta.

Internally give the following mixture, ½ teaspoon TID after food:
Shatāvarī       500 mg
Shankha Bhasma  200 mg
Kāma Dudhā      200 mg

At night give:
Sat Isobgol     ½ teaspoon in 1 cup of water

Suggest a pitta soothing diet. Licorice tea with equal proportions of cumin, coriander and fennel is also soothing.
Many times pitta pain is accompanied by nausea and vomiting. For nausea, add jatamāmsi 300 mg to the above formula. Or quickly drink the following to relieve gas, improve digestion and soothe pitta pain:
1 cup warm water
¼ teaspoon baking soda
Pinch of salt
Juice of ¼ lime

**Kapha Udara Shūla.** Kapha pain is generally due to āma and the person feels dull with a sense of heaviness.

Internally give:
Lasunadi Vati   200 mg, 1 tablet twice a day after food
Or Shanka Vati  200 mg, 1 tablet once a day

If there is no āma, don't use shanka vati, because it is stronger than lasunadi vati.

At night give:
1 teaspoon bibhītakī with warm water

Once the kapha pain has subsided, induce vamana, but don't do vamana while there is pain.

In generalized abdominal pain, apply the appropriate paste around the belly button. For vāta, use ½ teaspoon dashamūla powder or ½ teaspoon garlic powder mixed with a little water. For kapha, use ½ teaspoon punarnavā powder and then sprinkle asafoetida powder on this paste.

## Parshva Shūla

Parshva shūla is pain in the sides of the chest, which is pleuritic pain. The patient has pain toward the end of each inspiration, along with shallow breathing and worsening of pain during the act of coughing, sneezing or yawning. Many times there is referred pain in the supraclavicle area around the C3 and C4 vertebrae, because of involvement of the phrenic nerve, which is connected to the pleura. If there is irritation of the pleura, there may initially be pain due to inflammation or vāta aggravation. Then if either pitta-type of inflammatory exudate or kapha-type of transudate accumulates in the pleural space, the pain is relieved. There may also be referred pain at the top of the shoulder, especially on the right side. Pain in this area suggests diaphragmatic pleuritis.

Pleuritic pain can be caused by vāta, pitta or kapha. The vāta type is called dry pleurisy and the pitta type is pleuritis, where the inflamed surfaces of the pleura rub against each other. Kapha creates pleurisy with effusion, with diminished movement on the involved side and a prominent sternal mastoid on the opposite side. With this kapha type of pleuritic pain, one must also consider the possibility of pneumonia.

## Management of Parshva Shūla

*Vāta Pārshva Shūla.* Internally give the following mixture, ½ teaspoon TID after food:

| | |
|---|---|
| Dashamūla | 500 mg |
| Mustā | 400 mg |
| Pushkaramūla | 300 mg |

If there is muscular pain, add yogarāja guggulu 200 mg to the above formula.

Apply a castor oil pack to the site of pain.

*Pitta Pārshva Shūla.* If there is inflammation, use the following mixture, ½ teaspoon TID after food:

| | |
|---|---|
| Gudūchī | 400 mg |
| Kāma Dudhā | 200 mg |
| Mustā | 300 mg |
| Pushkaramūla | 300 mg |

*Kapha Pārshva Shūla.* For the dull ache of kapha pleuritic pain use the following mixture, ½ teaspoon TID after food:

| | |
|---|---|
| Punarnavā | 500 mg |
| Tālīsādi | 300 mg |
| Tankana (Borax) | 200 mg |
| Mustā | 200 mg |
| Pushkaramūla | 300 mg |

## Parināma Shūla

Parināma shūla is pain created during the process of digestion. The entire gastrointestinal tract is divided into six areas relating to the six stages of digestion. The first stage is sweet and kledaka kapha is secreted in the upper part of the stomach. During the next hour, as the food passes into the middle part of the stomach, the sour taste is activated, created by pāchaka pitta. Then during the third hour, the food enters the duodenum and the salty taste is predominant. This is followed by the pungent and bitter stages in the small intestine and the astringent stage in the colon, which is governed by vāta dosha. The early stages of digestion are governed by kapha, while the middle stages are controlled by pitta.

It is important to know how long it is after taking food that the pain appears. Then the doshic cause can be identified. If there is an ulcer, its location can also be determined by how soon after eating the pain begins. To ascertain this, the stomach is divided into thirds.

If the ulcer is in the upper third, it is due to depleted kledaka kapha and will create pain within one hour, during the sweet phase of digestion. If the pain appears within two hours, the ulcer is in the middle curvature of the stomach and is due to pitta during the sour phase of digestion. An ulcer at this location may be caused by the over secretion of hydro-chloric acid. Pain within three hours, which occurs during the salty phase of digestion in the lower portion of the stomach and the duodenum, is due to pitta dosha. In the pyloric area, the enzymes are more alkaline and they try to regulate the acidity. If these alkaline enzymes are produced in excess, the ulcer will occur in the lower third of the stomach or the duodenum. We have to treat pitta in all three locations, but there is a secondary doshic involvement. The stomach is kapha, the small intestine is pitta and the colon is vāta. If the ulcer is in the upper portion, there is not enough kledaka kapha. If the location is in the middle section, there is too much pāchaka pitta. In the lower pyloric area, *prāna vāta* is involved in the disease process.

An ulcer may be a complication of parināma shūla, but parināma shūla doesn't just mean ulcer. Therefore, don't immediately jump to the conclusion that the pain is due to an ulcer. Acute pain in the stomach could be due to gastritis or food poisoning, which can aggravate pitta dosha. Or the person may have gone from doctor to doctor with no cause found for the pain. In that type of parināma shūla, the stomach pulse will generally reveal a kapha pulse and the pain will not respond to antacid treatments. This kapha pain is always present within the first hour of eating and the pain is dull, often with slight mucoid nausea. This condition can lead to cancer of the stomach, so always inquire about past history and present symptoms.

## Management of Parināma Shūla

*Āma Parināma Shūla and Kapha Parināma Shūla.* Pain will occur within an hour of taking food. The nature of the pain is heavy and dull and the quality of kledaka kapha is disturbed. Internally give:

Pāchaka Vati, 1 pill of 200 mg. This will burn āma and take care of the pain.

If Pāchaka Vati is not available use:
| | |
|---|---|
| Ajvain | 300 mg |
| Raw Sugar | 300 mg |

*Pitta Parināma Shūla.* Pain occurs about two hours after eating. Internally, give the following mixture, ½ teaspoon TID, in the middle of the meal:

Shatāvarī          500 mg

| Kāma Dudhā | 200 mg |
|---|---|
| Moti Bhasma | 200 mg |
| Yashthi Madhu | 300 mg |

At night give ½ teaspoon avipattikar churna, which contains nishottara. Do not give triphalā.

***Vāta Parināma Shūla.*** Pain occurs three hours after food. Internally give the following mixture, ½ teaspoon TID before food:

| Dashamūla | 500 mg |
|---|---|
| Hingvastak Chūrna | 200 mg |
| Shankha Bhasma | 200 mg |

At night give ½ teaspoon harītakī an hour before sleep, which is a specific remedy for high vāta in the abdomen.

## Anna Drava Shūla

Anna drava shūla means pain during the process of liquefaction of food, which is experienced while the food is still in the stomach. After chewing and swallowing the food, it enters into the stomach where kledaka kapha is secreted through the stomach wall and churning of the food breaks it up into smaller and smaller pieces. The food at this stage is called anna drava. In cases of low jāthara agni, there will be production of āma within the stomach. Āma and increased kledaka kapha suppress pāchaka pitta, which is hydrochloric acid, leaving insufficient agni to digest the food. The resultant undigested food further adds to the āma. When food is in the process of liquefaction (anna drava), this āma sticks to the stomach wall, which prevents absorption and creates pain in the stomach. As long as food is present in the stomach, there will be pain. The pain is due to hypochlorhydria, or diminished hydrochloric acid; hence, taking hydrochloric acid can help these people. This hypochlorhydric pain may indicate a pre-cancerous condition, so it should be taken seriously.

Internally give the following mixture, ½ teaspoon TID after food:

| Ajvain | 200 mg |
|---|---|
| Citric Acid | 5 mg |
| Chitrak | 300 mg |
| Punarnavā | 400 mg |

In addition, take one tablet of hydrochloric acid after food to maintain optimal acidity.

## Hrid Shūla or Hricchūla

Hrid shūla is pseudo-cardiac pain. Due to fermentation of food in the stomach, gases are created in the fundus of the stomach. Those gases back up and can create pain in the precordium. This pseudo-cardiac pain is not involved with the functioning of the heart, but rather with the digestive process. It has a specific cause and must be treated accordingly.

Internally give the following mixture, ½ teaspoon TID after food:

| Arjuna | 300 mg |
|---|---|
| Shringa Bhasma | 200 mg |
| Hingvastak Chūrna | 200 mg |
| Avipattikar | 400 mg |

# Chapter 6

# The Concept of Cancer in Ayurveda

Fall 2005, Volume 18, Number 2

## Tumors and Tissue Irregularities

IN AYURVEDIC LITERATURE, a detailed description is given of various types of tumors. Terms such as *gulma, granthi, utseda* and *arbuda* are used for specific tumor conditions.

A growth, enlargement or cluster is called gulma, which is specifically used to indicate a tumor. Gulma is a benign tumor that has defined borders. There are many types of gulma. For instance, *rakta gulma* means a fibroid tumor, or even a fatty tumor. *Māmsa gulma* is a tumor arising from the muscle tissue. *Vāta gulma* refers to diverticulosis or accumulated gases in the colon. It creates localized bunching, which moves from one part of the abdomen to another.

Granthi is the name given to a glandular tumor. *Rasa granthi* is a lymphoid tissue tumor arising from the lymphatic system (rasa dhātu). *Meda granthi* means lipoma, which takes place in meda dhātu, in the fatty tissue. *Jatru granthi* means a thyroid tumor, while *yakrut granthi* is a tumor arising from the liver or gall bladder and *kloma granthi* is a tumor of the pancreas.

The Sanskrit word utseda means bulging, referring to any kind of localized bulging underneath the tissue.

Finally, arbuda is a malignant tumor or cancerous growth. That means an uncontrolled growth of abnormal tissues, due to low dhātu agni, which is related to damaged nucleic acid within the healthy tissues—either locally or spread throughout the body. Arbuda can occur in the breast, prostate, lungs, colon or elsewhere in the body. The description of arbuda in Ayurvedic literature gives us a detailed picture of malignant tumors or cancer.

## Cellular Dynamics

According to Ayurveda, the cancer disease process happens at the subtle cellular level, called *ati anu srotas*. Agni is metabolic activity and there are thirteen main types of agni. Jāthara agni is the gastric fire, which governs gross digestion, absorption, assimilation and transformation of food into micro chyle. *Bhūta agni* is present in the liver and

49

governs subtle molecular digestion of food into the five elements: Ether, Air, Fire, Water and Earth. It is this molecular digestion that is affected by arbuda. Every tissue also has its own agni component, called dhātu agni, which refers to the enzymes and amino acids that govern tissue nutrition and cellular metabolic activity. The seven dhātus (tissues) are rasa (plasma), rakta (blood), māmsa (muscle), meda (fat or lipids), asthi (bones and cartilage), majjā (bone marrow and nerve tissue), and shukra (male reproductive) or ārtava (female reproductive tissue).

At the cellular level, each cell is a center of awareness, a conscious microscopic life. Every cell has cellular integrity and governs its own metabolic activity. There is a flow of communication from one cell to another, which is called prāna. *Tejas* is responsible for cellular metabolic activity and *ojas* governs immunity. These three (prāna, tejas, ojas) are the factors that control reproduction of arbuda at the cellular level.

Arbuda has its own tejas and it can produce new blood vessels (*sirā*) as part of the process of angiogenesis. Arbuda also has its own perverted prāna, which absorbs nutrients. It can produce agni (enzymes) and, with the help of prāna, it can invade the circulatory system and find a place to grow. Arbuda can also stimulate its own proteins to grow and multiply. It demands increased metabolic output; as a result, there is often severe weight loss in the patient.

### The Role of Ahamkāra

Why does a normal, healthy, life-maintaining cell become so crazy? That is a key point. According to Sankhya's philosophy of creation, *Purusha* is the conscious principle and *Prakruti* is primordial matter and creative potential. The first expression of Prakruti is *Mahat,* which is intelligence. Next comes *ahamkāra,* the 'I' former. Ahamkāra is a central energy field that is present in every substance, and it maintains that thing's form, shape, color, and consistency. For the past millions of years, mango seeds have never forgotten to produce mango trees, mango flowers, and mango fruits. The ahamkāra (or 'I' former) of the mango governs the specific forms of the tree, flower and fruit that are produced from the seed.

Ahamkāra is the energy that is responsible for the creation of all forms and the specific arrangement of their molecules. If we look at the human body, at the time of fertilization, a single sperm fertilizes a single ovum and mitotic division happens. Each cell is divided into two and continues multiplying to eventually create the beautiful form of a human mammal. What is true with the human being is also true in the rest of the animal and plant kingdoms. This philosophy of creation is applied at the cellular level. Every cell has definite form and functions, and the structure of the cell is maintained by cellular ahamkāra. Therefore white blood cells have a certain form, red blood cells have a typical form, the platelets and multiple nucleated muscle cells have specific forms, and so forth. These are all maintained by ahamkāra.

Ahamkāra can be called self-esteem. We all have this self, ego, 'I' or me. We all have consciousness, but it is the consciousness of millions and trillions of selves. Ahamkāra is the collective consciousness of trillions of cell bodies. There is some deep connection between ahamkāra at the gross physical level and at the cellular level. Disturbed ahamkāra can create a severe distortion of the physical body and individual identity. If someone doesn't have self-esteem and self-respect, that person may become depressed or have an inferiority complex, and he or she will become sad and miserable. That will slowly affect the immune system and the person's metabolism, distorting the whole psychosomatic identity.

---

## Arbuda Pūrva Rūpa: Warning Signs of Cancer

Cancer is a silent enemy in the beginning, with few signs and symptoms. The following is a list of the prodromal signs and symptoms of arbuda or cancer.

*Malāvashtambha* means repeated chronic constipation or absolute constipation. Changes in bowel habits are quite common after age 65, but if such a person does not have a bowel movement even after taking triphalā, one should think about cancer of the rectum as a possibility. It is helpful to do a colonoscopy just to rule out cancer.

*Mūtra krichra* means a change in bladder habits, repeated urethritis, or cystitis.

*Rakta gama* means bleeding. Say children are playing and a child who receives a pinch to the skin suddenly develops a balloon-like hematoma; that is an early sign of cancer. Rakta gama are bleeding disorders. One can rule out cancer when there are repeated attacks of bleeding from the nose, the ear, the vagina or the rectum.

*Srava* is a foul smelling discharge from a wound.

*Kāthinya* granthi means thickening of a tumor.

*Avipāka* is chronic indigestion, which is another preliminary symptom (pūrva rūpa) of cancer.

*Sakashta anna pravesha* means difficulty in swallowing. If a person feels like they have swallowed some food but it is stuck near the heart area, and especially if such a person is elderly, one can think about the possibility of cancer and encourage the person to have it checked out.

*Tīvra kāsa* is a nagging cough that doesn't respond to cough syrups. A nagging cough can be due to cancer of the lungs.

*Svāra bheda* means hoarseness of voice. A hoarse voice is due to dryness of the vocal cords and it is an important sign of cancer that is due to depletion of ojas. This may indicate a malignant tumor in the vocal cords, or a tumor elsewhere in the body. It is more common in the case of someone with a history of smoking. However it can also be a sign of pandu, which means anemia. In that case, the person looks fair and has low energy levels.

*Arbuda granthi* is a hard nodular mass. This is another pūrva rūpa that can occur in a person who has developed cancer.

*Deha laghutā means* extreme, severe weight loss. It is another warning sign of cancer.

---

The same thing is true at the cellular level. Each cell has its own self-esteem and self-importance and, if the cell membrane is clogged with āma, there is poor communication. Such a cell is an isolated cell that becomes lonely. A lonely cell starts to act independently, producing its own enzymes and its own agni. That cell goes on growing independently and, as a result, it becomes malignant. These arbuda cells have a distorted self and hyperactive metabolism, demanding more metabolic output and attacking their neighboring cells. They convert neighboring cells into cancerous cells.

Not every disease noticeably undergoes the standard process of samprāpti (pathogenesis) in its ordinary sequence. The cellular factors and pathological changes that occur in cancer may not appear to follow this process, yet they do. At the cellular level, there is defective tejas, which can be responsible for radical changes in cellular metabolic activity. This results in production of metabolic waste, creating cellular āma. This cellular āma covers the cell membrane, then it affects the defensive mechanism (ojas) and metabolic activity (tejas), and as a result there is a disturbance in the flow of intelligence (prāna) from one cell to another. Prāna, tejas, and ojas lose their functional integrity.

### Prognosis

A prognosis for cancer depends upon both the type of cancer and the stage of the disease. The type of tumor is important in this regard and understanding this can save a life. Cancers in rasa and meda dhātus are easier to treat, whereas the deeper tissues are harder to treat. Similarly, the prognosis will usually be better if there is early diagnosis, but most people ignore the warning signs and don't go to the doctor. As a result, the disease starts to spread, sometimes rapidly, and the prognosis is poor.

Warts and moles can become cancerous, if they start to be irritated. Hoarseness of voice (*svāra bheda*) and a nagging cough are warning symptoms for cancer and they may be specifically related to cancer of the trachea and lungs. Thickening of a lump in the breast can indicate breast cancer. Esophageal cancer can produce difficulty swallowing, while stomach cancer may manifest as low appetite, poor digestion and hypochlorhydria (extremely low stomach acidity). Colon cancer can lead to constipation, while cancer of the uterus may lead to profuse bleeding. Note that any sore wound that doesn't heal can be malignant. If cancer is detected in its late stages, it is bound to create a bad prognosis.

### Prevention of Cancer

Prevention is an important part of the Ayurvedic approach to arbuda. In the case of lung cancer in particular, it is most important to avoid the causative factors, such as smoking tobacco and exposure to asbestos and chemicals. It is also important for someone to regularly perform a self-examination of the body, with regard to early identification of possible cancer symptoms. This should include women examining their breasts and men checking their testicles. If there is a hard lump, immediately rush to the doctor. Don't wait for it to spread; just find out whether or not it is malignant.

## Arbuda Vyādhi Vinischaya: Diagnosis of Cancer

There are various ways by which Ayurveda can diagnose arbuda. First, prakruti-vikruti parīkshā is used, which means physical and pathological examination.

Second, the practitioner uses *ashtavidhā parīkshā,* which is the eight-fold examination process. This is comprised of assessing the nādī (pulse), *mutram* (urine), mala (wastes), *jihva* (tongue), *shabda* (voice), *sparsha* (palpation), *drig* (eyes) and *ākruti* (bodily form). All these ashtavidhā parīkshāna should be done in order to thoroughly diagnose the problem. An expert Ayurvedic physician should assess the prakruti by reading the pulse and also find out the vikruti and any weak organs.

Third is *srotas parīkshā,* the examination of the bodily channels. A srotas examination is a systemic examination of every channel. *Prāna vaha srotas* (the respiratory system), anna vaha srotas (digestive system) and *udaka vaha srotas* (the water metabolism system) are the first three important srotāmsi to be examined. The seven *dhātu srotas*—rasa, rakta, māmsa, meda, asthi, majjā and shukra or ārtava—and the three excretory channels of *mala, mūtra* and *sveda* (sweat) *vaha srotas* are also thoroughly assessed.

The fourth diagnostic tool used for arbuda is *granthi parīkshā,* which is examination of any abnormal growth. It may be a growth under the skin, the subcutaneous tissue, fatty tissue, muscle tissue, bone tissue, or nerve tissue, and this category also includes examination of the lymph glands. If one feels a tumor, one should feel whether it is palpable, movable, or fixed. Generally fixed tumors belong to māmsa and asthi dhātus, whereas a mobile tumor may be in the subcutaneous tissue or fatty tissue.

The fifth diagnostic technique is *vividha parīkshā,* which is a series of tests. In modern medicine, this includes X-ray, ultrasound, magnetic resonance imaging (MRI), cytological examination, and lab tests. In the past, they depended upon ashtavidhā parīkshā, the eightfold examination, and the diagnostic skills were totally based upon the ability of perception of the physician.

---

## Arbuda Rupani: Signs and Symptoms of Cancer

Once cancerous growth occurs, it produces various signs and symptoms that in Sanskrit are called *arbuda rupani.* The following are the most common signs and symptoms of arbuda.

*Rujā* (pain). A cancer patient has pain as a persistent symptom, because a cancerous tumor is irritating. There is no pain without the involvement of vāta dosha. In cancer, prāna vāta at the cellular level is constantly irritated and causes persistent pain.

*Daurbalya* (weakness). There is extreme fatigue and weakness, because ojas is depleted and the person's metabolism is affected. The healthy tissues start to suffer from lack of nutrition. Whatever nutrients the person takes in are absorbed by the cancerous cells. Even if the person takes a tonic, with rasāyana herbs such as shatāvarī, ashvagandhā and brahmī, it feeds the cancerous cells, because these have a greedy demand for nutrients. Cancerous cells suck the nutrients faster than healthy cells, leaving the healthy cells to starve. That is why a cancer patient has weakness.

*Alpa poshanam or Kuposhanam* (malnutrition). A cancer patient often shows a deficiency of iron, calcium, magnesium, vitamin B12 and folic acid. The reason is the same as above: most of the nutrients are absorbed by the malignant cells.

*Balakshaya* (extreme fatigue). This is due to defective agni, because healthy agni governs the biological strength of a human being. A malignant growth affects both cellular agni and dhātu agni, and it results in fatigue.

*Asthi Bhagnatā* (bone fractures). This symptom is due to malabsorption and malnutrition. This may lead to a spontaneous medical fracture or there may be a malignant tumor arising from within the bone. At the edge of the tumor, the bone tissue may become weak and that can lead to a fracture of the bone.

*Pakshavadha* (paralysis). Stroke-like paralysis is a complication of cancer and it commonly happens in cases of a cancerous tumor in the brain. A space-occupying tumor in the motor area of the brain can paralyze the opposite side of the body.

*Arbudam Prasaratvam.* Means cancer spreads and starts to metastasize. This metastasizing nature of cancer is due to pitta and rakta. *"Pittam tu sveda raktayo"* means pitta is present in sweat (sveda) and blood (rakta), so the cancerous cells spread throughout the plasma and blood stream, the lymphatic system and, in the case of skin cancer, they can even spread through the sweat.

## Arbuda Chikitsā: Management of Cancer in Ayurveda

The Ayurvedic approach to cancer is fundamental and radical. There is no standard treatment. The treatment varies from person to person. An Ayurvedic physician has to pay complete attention to the prakruti and vikruti of the patient, to determine which doshas are involved. It is also important to find out what dhātus and organs are affected. Based upon that understanding, one can then deal with arbuda by means of snehana, svedana and pañchakarma, using specific cleansing measures for each dosha. Typically, vamana (emesis) is used for kapha, virechana (purgation) for pitta, and basti (enema) for vāta.

Cancer care should be provided by a team of experts and your Ayurvedic physician should have great skill and experience in treating cancer, so that all aspects can be covered. Ayurveda has many treatment protocols that can be chosen according to the specific symptoms, including the following:

- *Shalya tantra* refers to surgically removing a tumor.
- *Sroto rodha* relates to clearing the obstruction of the vital pathways, which can be done either surgically or medically.
- *Shalya majjā* refers to cutting the nerves that carry the pain. This is actually a symptomatic form of treatment but when there is constant pain, a cancer patient may wish to commit suicide. This is sad and painful, so cutting the nerves results in that person being free from pain.
- Another type of protocol is *vyādhi pratyanika chikitsā,* which is specific treatment according to the specific disease. In modern medicine, chemotherapy, and radiation therapy have great value if done early enough. In Ayurveda, there is no chemotherapy or radiation therapy, but there is herbal therapy.
- Lastly, rasāyana or Ayurvedic immunotherapy is used to enable the patient's body to produce a substance that resists the growth of cancer. This is done through the use of naturally occurring substances that increase the activity of the immune system to increase ojas. The body's failure to detect and destroy the abnormal cancer cells is due to low ojas; in general management, we have to protect the patient's ojas.

### Ayurveda Management following Chemotherapy, Radiation, and Surgery

Ayurveda can also be used to alleviate the side effects of chemotherapy and radiation therapy. Radiation therapy creates anorexia, nausea and hair loss, while chemotherapy causes the same symptoms, plus bone marrow suppression, anemia and low grade fever. For example, in cases of low grade fever, Ayurveda uses laghu mālinī vasanta or mahā tikta ghrita, while for anemia; either mandhūra bhasma or abhrak bhasma is used. For bone marrow suppression, Ayurveda also suggests the use of brahmī oil or shatāvarī ghee, bringharaj oil for hair loss, and shankha bhasma and kāma dudhā for nausea.

The list below contains the main categories of therapies that are used in Ayurveda for the management of cancer patients who have undergone any of the therapies that are commonly used in modern medicine.

- Snehana (oleation therapy) is a useful treatment for this purpose. To choose the appropriate oil for snehana, look at the person's prakruti and vikruti. If vāta, one can use sesame oil or a medicated oil such as dashamūla oil or balā oil. For pitta, use sunflower or coconut oil, or any bitter oil. For kapha types, mustard, corn or sesame oil is a good choice. Neem oil is particularly good for snehana for pitta and kapha as it is both antipyretic and antiviral. Tumbī oil, also known as dāruharidrā, is also effective as an antipyretic and antipruritic. Guñjā is a detoxifier and it helps to grow the hair.

- Svedana (sudation therapy) is used for post-medical situations. For vāta types, it is best to use nirgundī essential oil in the steam treatment; for pitta people, sandalwood essential oil is good; and for kapha, lemon-scented eucalyptus essential oil can be added to the steam.
- Shodhana (detoxification program) is generally used following cancer treatment. If there is absolute constipation, one should administer basti (medicated enema). For pitta kinds of rashes, one can give mild virechana (purgation). If there is mucus formation and other kapha disorders, vamana (emesis) therapy may be given.
- Shamana (palliative therapy) is based upon pacifying the dosha in its site. Dosha pratyanika means a treatment that is pacifying to the dosha, *vyādhi pratayanika* is specific to the disease, and *dhātu pratayanika* means specific to the dhātu.
- Rasāyana (rejuvenation therapy) is important to use after *shodhana* or *shamana chikitsā,* so that the immune system is strengthened. Certain herbs and other powerful rejuvenative substances are given for this purpose.
- Lepana (application of paste) is generally used to take care of localized pain. Common examples for the kind of pain found in arbuda are kāñcanāra lepa, which is antiviral and reduces tumors; varuna lepa, which is anti-inflammatory; punarnavā lepa, which reduces swelling; and sandalwood and turmeric lepa.

## Herbal Adjuvants

Herbs that are frequently used in a shodhana detoxification program for arbuda are chitrak, katukā, and neem. Chitrak, with pungent and bitter tastes, heating *vīrya* (potency) and pungent *vipāka* (post-digestive effect), is a digestive herb that kindles agni and detoxifies āma. Katukā, which is known as kutki, has bitter and pungent rasa, cooling vīrya and pungent vipāka, is antipyretic, kindles gastric fire and aids in the scraping of abnormal tissue. Neem is bitter, cooling and pungent in vipāka. It is antiviral, antipyretic and also detoxifies āma.

Herbs used in shamana include gudūchī, guggulu, jatamāmsi, and tagara. Gudūchī is bitter and astringent in rasa, with a heating vīrya and pungent vipāka. It is anti-pyretic, an immune booster and a blood cleanser. Guggulu is bitter and pungent, heating and has a pungent vipāka. It scrapes āma and fat from the body, purifies the blood, and is a lymphatic cleanser and rejuvenative tonic.

Jatamāmsi and tagara are widely used as painkillers during arbuda. Jatamāmsi is bitter, astringent and sweet in taste, cooling in vīrya and with a sweet vipāka. It is antipruritic, antipyretic, analgesic and a tranquilizer. Tagara is astringent, heating and it has a pungent vipāka. It is a tranquilizer, analgesic and sedative.

For *rasāyana chikitsā,* which boosts the immune system, the herbal jam compound called chyavānaprāsh is widely used. Chyavānaprāsh contains various rejuvenative herbs, such as ashvagandhā, balā and vidārī. Ashvagandhā is bitter and astringent in rasa, has a heating vīrya and a sweet vipāka, and it is a rejuvenator for vāta and kapha, although it may overly stimulate pitta dosha. Balā is sweet, cooling and has a sweet vipāka, and it is tridoshic. Balā provides energy, vigor and vitality. Vidārī is sweet and bitter, cooling, and with a sweat vipāka, and it increases strength and stamina. Other common rasāyanas are pippalī rasāyana and punarnavā rasāyana. Pippalī is pungent in taste, heating in vīrya and sweet in vipāka. It is known for its antiviral and rejuvenating actions and it is generally good for pulmonary dysfunctions. Punarnavā is sweet and bitter, heating with a pungent vipāka. It is diuretic and it reduces tumors and is a rejuvenative tonic.

Herbs used in lepana chikitsā, which is the topical application of pastes, include kāñcanāra, varuna and haridrā. Kāñcanāra is astringent, cooling, and has a pungent vipāka. It is antiviral and reduces tumors. Varuna is sweet, bitter and astringent in taste, heating in vīrya and has a pungent vipāka. It reduces swelling and is anti-inflammatory. Haridrā is bitter, astringent and pungent in taste, heating in vīrya with a pungent vipāka. It is beautiful in reducing tumor.

## Conclusion

Students of Ayurveda should know the dynamics of arbuda and pay attention to the three doshas, seven dhātus and three malas, and their involvement in the pathogenesis of this disease. Based upon the individual samprāpti (pathogenesis), the treatment plan will change. That is why there is no standard treatment for cancer in Ayurveda. What is statistically common in a thousand people is the standard according to modern society, whereas Ayurveda gives emphasis to the individual and says that one cannot judge that person based upon statistical data. By virtue of this unique approach, some cases of arbuda, along with the complications of both the cancer and the related treatments, can be effectively treated with Ayurveda.

## Arbuda Nidāna: The Etiology of Cancer

References in the ancient text, *Mādhava Nidānam,* give us the etiological factors that are still, today, the true causes of arbuda. This gives us a complete picture of the etiological factors that can lead to cancer.

*Ātapa seva* means overexposure to solar radiation, and in this case refers to ultraviolet light in particular. Overexposure to ultraviolet radiation may disturb tejas at the cellular level.

*Vidāhāni annapānāni* is another cause of arbuda. *Vidāhi* means burning and irritating, *anna* is food and *pana* is drinks. This refers to a cause of cancer being food, drinks, and other substances that have irritating or burning properties. This includes alcohol, marijuana, tobacco, and many other carcinogenic chemicals and substances.

Another cause is *tīkshnāni aushadhāni,* which means sharp or penetrating cytotoxic drugs.

A fourth factor is cellular āma, which is toxic metabolic waste at the cellular level.

*Viruddha āhāra* means incompatible food, such as a pitta person eating too much hot, spicy food, or a vāta person eating too many beans or raw vegetables, or a kapha person consuming excessive amounts of dairy products and hydrophilic substances. These foods may be incompatible to someone's prakruti and also to the person's vikruti.

*Viruddha vihāra* means wrong lifestyle and this is another important etiological factor in the production of cancer.

Next, the *Mādhava Nidānam* says *bīja dosha* is a cause of arbuda. Bīja means seed and it refers to genetic predisposition. If someone's father died of cancer of the colon and his grandfather also died of the same type of cancer, it indicates an increased likelihood that the person himself may develop colon cancer. In a certain family, there may be racial or genetic factors that predispose them to a particular type of arbuda and this is called bīja dosha.

*Sūkshma krumi* means invisible parasites or micro-organisms in the blood that provoke arbuda. Perhaps there may even be a cancer virus.

*Vyavasāya* means occupational hazards and exposure to toxic substances. There are certain carcinogens or 'arbudogens,' if I may call them that, that are important substances in the etiology of cancer. Tobacco, asbestos, radioactive substances and any irritant substances that aggravate are examples of this category. People working in chemical factories, mines or asbestos factories may develop arbuda. Exposure to contactants also falls into this category.

*Mano vedana* means psychological and emotional factors, such as unresolved grief, sadness and other emotions, which can be called stress. If a person has intense grief, sadness, sorrow, stress and so forth, it may lead to arbuda. It is true that if a woman loses her loved one during middle age, she is more likely to get breast cancer or uterine cancer.

*Vārdhakya* refers to old people (over age 65), who are more prone to cancer of the prostate and colon.

*Paryāvartanam* means pollution. A polluted environment, maybe due to cars emitting carbon monoxide, can poison the air or water. Polluted water, air and food are all factors that can lead to arbuda. Pollution is a factor that is difficult for the individual to difficult to control, especially in third world countries.

# Chapter 7

# The Ayurvedic Perspective on Diabetes
## Prameha

Winter 2001, Volume 14, Number 3 and Spring 2002, Volume 14, Number 4

*PRAMEHA* (WHICH MEANS PROFUSE URINATION), *prakrushta meha,* and *prakarshena meha* are names indicating a dysfunction in mūtra vaha srotas (the urinary system) and *ambu vaha srotas* (the water carrying channels). In this chapter, we will discuss prameha as diabetes syndrome and its associated disorders.

In prameha, there is a disturbance in ambu vaha srotas, mūtra vaha srotas, rasa vaha srotas, rakta vaha srotas and medo vaha srotas. The *kloma* (pancreas), *tālu* (palate) and choroid plexuses are all connected to ambu vaha srotas and are all affected by prameha. *Medo vaha srotas* (the channel of fatty tissue) and *rasa-rakta vaha srotas* (lymph and blood carrying channels) are affected by prameha due to their affinity for the water element. In fact, any system or tissue in the body that is associated with water will be affected.

It is very important to understand that Ayurveda sees prameha not as one disease, but as a multifaceted syndrome with various, complex metabolic disorders. Prameha describes a syndrome of varied symptoms and complications related to or causing diabetes. It includes the prodromal symptoms and disease conditions of diabetes mellitus types one and two and diabetes insipidus. However, it is important that we understand the doshas and systems involved, not just the modern medical definition of this disease.

The Ayurvedic picture is based on the concept that all dhātus (tissues) have a normal level of *kleda* (moisture or liquid). One function of kleda is to maintain the body's water-electrolyte balance. It also nourishes and lubricates all tissues. It is associated with kledaka kapha in the stomach and, in the prasara (spreading) stage of prameha, kledaka kapha overflows from the gastrointestinal (GI) tract and enters the rasa dhātu (blood plasma). This kledaka kapha disturbs the kleda present in all dhātus. The function of urine is to remove excess liquids, so when kleda is increased, urination is also increased, called polyuria. Hence, prameha, or prakrushta meha, indicates this profuse urination.

Polyuria may be present in other conditions, such as hysteria, renal disorders, hyperparathyroidism (which may lead to hypercalcemia and then polyuria), or potassium deple-

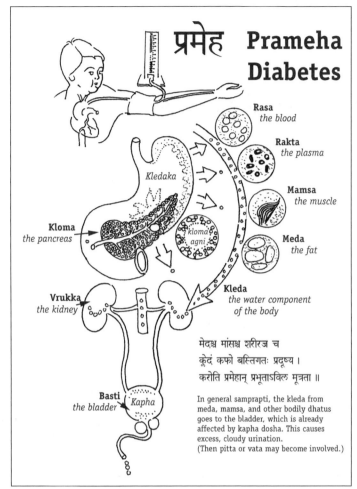

प्रमेह **Prameha Diabetes**

**Rasa**
*the blood*

**Rakta**
*the plasma*

*Kledaka*

**Mamsa**
*the muscle*

**Kloma**
*the pancreas*

*kloma agni*

**Meda**
*the fat*

**Vrukka**
*the kidney*

**Kleda**
*the water component
of the body*

**Basti**
*the bladder*

*Kapha*

मेदश्च मांसश्च शरीरज च
क्लेदं कफो बस्तिगतः प्रदूष्य ।
करोति प्रमेहान् प्रभूताऽविल मूत्रता ॥

In general samprapti, the kleda from
meda, mamsa, and other bodily dhatus
goes to the bladder, which is already
affected by kapha dosha. This causes
excess, cloudy urination.
(Then pitta or vata may become involved.)

tion, which is a kidney disorder. Due to these etiological factors, one or more of the doshas increases, leading to progression of the diabetic disease process.

The first three stages of any disease are called sanchaya (accumulation), prakopa (provocation) and prasara (spreading). High blood sugar is described in Ayurveda as increased kapha in the prasara stage of disease, affecting the *rasa-rakta dhātus* (circulatory and lymphatic systems). The increased kledaka from the dhātus starts leaking via the digestive system, through the kidneys and into the bladder, causing the prodromal signs and symptoms of diabetes. These are called pūrva rūpa and occur after the dosha enters the third stage of the disease process.

During this period, the person commonly accumulates tartar on the teeth and notices that they have to go to the dentist more frequently to clean the teeth. Generally there is sticky sweat, even after a bath, and an increase in kha mala (nasal crust, ear wax, sebaceous secretions and smegma). There is excess urination, nocturnal urination and when one is passing the last drops of urine, the urinary sphincter muscles constrict and create goose bumps. It is common for the person to have a sweet taste in the mouth and for the breath to smell like vinegar. Charaka says that these are all early or prodromal signs and symptoms of prameha.

The general samprāpti (pathogenesis) of prameha almost always begins with increased kapha, as seen in most of the signs and symptoms. Later, vāta and pitta can enter the picture, because prameha is a complex syndrome that can involve all three doshas.

## Causes of Prameha
Prameha is most often due to hyperglycemia (increased blood sugar) caused by diminished insulin production by the kloma (pancreas). It is a chronic endocrine disorder that affects the metabolism of carbohydrates, proteins and fats as well as the water-electrolyte balance. It can cause functional and structural changes in the bodily cells, creating complications of the eyes, kidneys, nervous system and other organs.

Some other causes of prameha are:

- It may be a secondary condition to pancreatitis, which is a pitta disorder. Viral infections such as mumps or staphylococcal infections can create pancreatitis.
- Heredity plays an important role in the predisposition to destruction of beta cells in the pancreas. This can cause pancreatitis or neoplasm or tumor of the pancreas, leading to diabetes.
- A tumor of the pancreas, which is a pitta-kapha condition.
- Autoimmune dysfunctions, whereby tejas burns ojas and antibodies affect the pancreas.
- Obesity, which is almost always associated with non-insulin-dependent diabetes. This is a metabolic disorder of kapha dosha.
- Diet, emotional overeating, and excess consumption of sugar.
- Pregnancy. During pregnancy there is an excessive demand for insulin and if the pancreas cannot provide that insulin, it becomes stressed. This can lead to gestational diabetes, a type of diabetes mellitus. Also, there is a natural physiological increase in kapha dosha because kapha is responsible for the creation of the new baby and placenta. This increased kapha can inhibit the pancreatic function, which can also lead to gestational diabetes.
- Liver diseases, including hepatitis and cirrhotic changes, can lead to portal hypertension and affect the pancreatic function, resulting in diabetes.
- Corticosteroid therapy is an iatrogenic (drug- induced) cause of diabetes. Steroidal hormones are kapha provoking and steroid toxicity often creates underactive thyroid, water retention, hypertension (high blood pressure) and obesity. It also compromises kidney functions and causes 'moon face,' which results in a swollen and fatty appearance of the face.

The famous Ayurvedic author, *Mādhava*, says that worry, anxiety, fear, and anger are all connected to cerebral kloma and these can affect glandular functions, leading to prameha.

## Types of Diabetes

The modern definition of diabetes differentiates two main types, mellitus and insipidus. Diabetes insipidus, at least in the beginning, is an imbalance of the diuretic hormone vasopressin. It is rare and occurs most often in young people.

Diabetes mellitus is a metabolic disorder characterized by increased blood sugar and passing of sugar in the urine, due to a dysfunction of *kloma* (pancreas) *agni*. It is classified as either insulin-dependent diabetes (IDD) or non-insulin-dependent diabetes (NIDD). Insulin-dependent diabetes is type I diabetes mellitus and is also known as juvenile-onset diabetes, because it generally

**PURVA RUPA OF PRAMEHA**
**(Prodromal Signs and Symptoms)**

- Excess tartar on teeth
- Burning hands and feet
- Excess thirst
- Frequent, excess urination
- Nocturnal urination
- Goosebumps during and after passing the last drops of urine
- Sweet, sticky saliva
- Acetone-like smell to the breath
- Sticky sweat and increased kha mala (nasal crust, earwax, etc.)
- Pulse becomes slow and sluggish; the stomach pulse shows a kapha spike

begins prior to 30 years of age. The cells of the islets of Langerhans in the pancreas are unable to produce enough insulin and the person usually requires external sources of insulin for the rest of his or her life.

Non-insulin-dependent diabetes is type II diabetes mellitus. It is the most common form of diabetes and is found throughout the world, but especially amongst affluent people and therefore in Western countries. Type II mellitus is also known as late-onset or adult-onset diabetes, because it usually begins from age 40 to 50 or above. It can also occur in pregnancy. Women are more prone to this condition, especially obese women and those who have had many pregnancies.

Many of the signs and symptoms of type II diabetes relate closely to the various kapha types of prameha mentioned in Ayurveda. In this condition the functions of the pancreas are affected by fat clogging the cell membranes. These pancreatic cells then become resistant to insulin, resulting in the body not being able to process sugar. Unlike type I diabetes mellitus, type II does not require insulin injections. Promoting the pancreatic functions and controlling blood

> **RUPA OF PRAMEHA**
> **(Cardinal Signs and Symptoms)**
>
> - Polyuria (excessive urination) - the person may pass 10 to 20 liters of urine per day
> - Low specific gravity of the urine
> - Polydipsia (excessive thirst)
> - Fatigue
> - Disturbed water-electrolyte balance
> - Potassium depletion, which leads to kidney
> - malfunction
> - Hyper-parathyroidism
> - Excess water consumption, which inhibits anti-diuretic hormone and leads to water toxicity and low agni. Note: A vāta or pitta person typically needs 5 to 10 glasses of water per day, whereas a kapha person may require less than this.

sugar, primarily through diet and lifestyle, can treat it.

In diabetes mellitus, the Earth and Water elements are not properly digested, leading to excess sugar in the urine and blood. These are known as hyperglycemia (high blood sugar) and glycosuria (excess glucose or sugar in urine). Sushruta calls the condition *rakta sharkarā,* which means high blood sugar.

## Ayurvedic Classification of Prameha

There are twenty types of prameha identified by Ayurveda, which correspond to the various signs and symptoms found in diabetes syndrome. Diabetes is included in prameha, but prameha is more than diabetes. We can say that all 20 types of prameha may end up within one of the Western classifications of diabetes. Alternatively, we can state that the 20 types of prameha can be seen as different stages or conditions that may lead to one of these types of diabetes.

Prameha is a metabolic disorder of agni, the energy of transformation. The stomach is the seat of jāthara agni, which is the central bodily fire; the liver the seat of bhūta agni; the pancreas has kloma agni; and each dhātu (tissue) has its own agni. When there is a dysfunction of these agnis, especially kloma agni, the carbohydrate metabolism is disturbed.

Ayurveda classifies prameha according to the primary dosha involved. There are ten kapha, six pitta, and four vāta types related to this complex syndrome.

- ◆ Kapha Prameha — 10 types; relatively easy to cure; non-insulin-dependent
- ◆ Pitta Prameha — 6 types; difficult to cure; may be insulin-dependent
- ◆ Vāta Prameha — 4 types; incurable or very difficult to treat; insulin-dependent

In kapha type of prameha, kledaka kapha slows down agni so that the kleda goes partly unprocessed into rasa dhātu. Rasa, rakta, meda and shukra dhātus are all involved in kapha prameha. In pitta type, rakta is the major dhātu affected. In vāta prameha, all dhātus can be involved, but complications involve mainly majjā, as in diabetic neuropathy.

We will now examine these twenty types according to the signs and symptoms and appropriate treatments for each.

## Ten Kapha Types of Prameha

These kapha types of prameha fall into the category of type II (non-insulin-dependent) diabetes mellitus, or may be a precursor to that disease. These conditions commonly begin with low meda dhātu agni, which can cause obesity and other kapha disorders.

*1.* **Ikshu meha:** digestive or alimentary glycosuria. Ikshu means sugarcane juice and the urine looks cloudy like sugarcane juice. This condition is due to weak jāthara agni and kloma agni. The person eats too many sweet substances and the GI tract gets overloaded with sugar. Kleda is then unprocessed, which creates the glycosuria.

The function of urine is to carry kleda and there is functional integrity between urine and kleda. Kleda from the stomach and pancreas add to the quantity of urine, producing excessive urination, which makes the person feel tired and also leads to constipation. It is necessary to increase agni and eliminate toxins, so a good formula is:

| | |
|---|---|
| Gudūchī | 300 mg |
| Neem | 300 mg |
| Tumeric | 200 mg |
| Chitrak | 200 mg |
| Trikatu | 200 mg |

Take ½ tsp TID with warm water.

> T.I.D. = from the Latin means *ter in diem*, three times a day

*2.* **Sitā meha:** sita means rock candy. This type of prameha can be compared to renal glycosuria, which means the presence of sugar in the urine. It is a kidney dysfunction due to depleted agni of the glomeruli. Apāna vāyu governs glomeruli filtration, which maintains the concentration of urine. Because of disturbed apāna the glomeruli permeability increases, which is responsible for leaking kleda and causing renal glycosuria. This causes the urine to become more diluted, so the person passes cool, clear, water-like urine that feels like frozen water and looks like rock candy dissolved in water. Diagnostically, you will find the kidney pulse is weak. Sitameha can be helped by taking the following formula:

| | |
|---|---|
| Punarnavā | 500 mg |
| Gokshura | 400 mg |
| Gudūchī | 300 mg |

Shilājit            300 mg
Take ½ tsp TID with warm water.
Also useful is Chandraprabhā, one tablet daily.

*3.*   **Udaka meha:** diabetes insipidus. This is due to a dysfunction in the posterior pituitary gland that produces the anti-diuretic hormones arginine and vasopressin, which constrict the blood vessels of the glomeruli in order to prevent the elimination of excess water. There is polyuria (excessive urination) and polydipsia (excess thirst). The urine looks like water and excess water retention can cause water toxicity. This slows agni and lowers kidney energy.

This condition occurs mostly in young people. It begins with disturbed kledaka kapha, leading to over-secretion of kleda into the rasa dhātu, which is the prasara stage of this disease. This can affect *tarpaka kapha* in the posterior pituitary, causing inadequate secretions of vasopressin and anti- diuretic hormone. This in turn results in excess kapha and kleda going into the kidneys, which creates polyuria (excess urination) and other symptoms. Remember that prameha means profuse urination.

Diabetes insipidus may be due to a growth hormone disorder such as acromegaly (gigantism), pituitary tumor, excess ACTH hormone, excess thyroid hormones that affect carbohydrate metabolism, diminished glomeruli threshold in the kidneys, or diminished production of anti-diuretic hormone. It might also be due to vāta pushing pitta in the majjā dhātu, which can manifest as encephalitis, basal meningitis, syphilis, or a trauma (cerebral concussion, compression, or contusion). These disturb the functioning of tarpaka kapha and become kapha prameha.

This posterior pituitary dysfunction, which causes the inadequate secretion of vasopressin, happens in young people at a kapha age. Anti-diuretic hormones can be compared to tarpaka kapha, because of their cold and stable qualities. For this condition, we can use the following formula to promote secretions of anti-diuretic hormone:

Parijata            300 mg
Mustā               300 mg
Vanga Bhasma        50 mg
Arka Patra (calatropis)  1 drop
Take ½ tsp TID with cumin, coriander, and fennel (CCF) tea.

Yashthi madhu (licorice), the herbal compound tikta, and cumin, coriander and fennel tea also promote the secretion of vasopressin and maintain the glomeruli function.

*4.*   **Pistha meha:** phosphate urea. Pishta means refined white flour and the urine looks cloudy and pale, like a mixture of water and flour. The urine is alkaline and the phosphate molecules start to leak through the glomeruli filtration system in the kidneys, which can lead to renal calculi. This condition may be associated with diabetes.

Chandraprabhā       300 mg
Dāruharidrā         300 mg (a special kind of turmeric)
Shilājit            200 mg
Take ½ tsp TID with warm water.

**5.   Shukra meha:** shukra is the male reproductive tissue (semen). Kleda from shukra dhātu passes through a weak prostate gland and sperm starts leaking into the urine, which is called spermatorrhea. This predisposes one to diabetes and is part of the prodromal symptoms that develop about six months before diabetes. There is a biochemical dysfunction of *ashthīlā agni,* the enzymes that maintain the functions of the prostate. Spermatorrhea may be due to gonorrhea, syphilis, trauma, excess sexual activity, anxiety, fear of sex and excessive or forceful masturbation, which can all deplete shukra agni and weaken the prostatic sphincters. The person can also get constipation, pass mucus in the stools and strain to pass urine or feces. The condition may also be associated with amoebiasis.

We can use certain herbs to improve the prostate tone and control the spermaturia:

| | |
|---|---|
| Ātma Guptā | 300 mg (kapikacchū) |
| Shilājit | 300 mg |
| Cardamom | 200 mg |
| Asafoetida | 100 mg |

Take ½ tsp TID with warm water or guñjā tea.

Guñjā (abrus precatorius) is a plant with small, tamarind-like leaves. It enhances the tone of the prostate and helps to prevent semen from leaking. The leaves can be made into a tea by boiling with water or milk. Use as an anupāna (a carrier or vehicle).

Note that ātma guptā works on the male reproductive and nervous systems and is indicated for Parkinson's Disease.

**6.   Lālā meha:** *lālā* means drool, and lālā meha means that the person's urine becomes thick like saliva. This is also called prostate urea, because it occurs when a man passes stringy, prostatic secretions in the urine and gets spasms and goose bumps. There is also leakage of prostatic secretions during the day, which indicates that he could become diabetic. It is common in males from about age 55 on. The same type of thing can also occur in women, but instead of prostatic secretions they have profuse secretions from the Bartholin's glands that can mix with the urine. Additionally, the vagina becomes overly lubricated.

| | |
|---|---|
| Tulsi | 300 mg |
| Turmeric | 300 mg |
| Pātthā | 300 mg |
| Agaru | 200 mg |
| Shilājit | 200 mg |

Take ½ tsp TID with warm water.

Men can also do a daily massage over the prostate region.

**7.   Sikata meha:** *sikata* means sand, so sikata meha means lithuria or crystalluria. The urine has a crystalline dust or coarse sand made up of phosphates, calcium, uric acid, or oxalate crystals. A person with lithuria may become diabetic. The glomeruli allow these crystals to pass through the urine, so the condition is associated with kidney stones. When the person passes kidney stones he feels great pain from the loin to the groin. If a baby boy cries incessantly and pulls the penis while peeing, consider the possibility of urinary stones. A female gets a radiating pain from the loin to the labia (renal colic), indicating it may be kidney stones.

If the stone is just silently sitting in the kidney, it will create a typical tenderness in the renal angle. At the time of passing the stone, when it is coming through the urethra, or even coming through the ureter into the bladder, it is extremely painful. In sikata meha, the person passes broken down stones that look like gravel. When a baby with this condition passes urine, you can see the stain of minerals (yellow for oxalate, white for phosphate).

For this condition we can use:
Punarnavā          500 mg
Gokshura          400 mg
Chitrak          200 mg
Take ½ tsp TID with warm water.

Also give kidney bean flowers, steeped in warm water, which are a good astringent. Alternatively take cumin, coriander and fennel tea.

**8.    Shanaih meha:** this means increased frequency of urination. The person has frequent urination during both day and night, because they cannot completely evacuate the bladder due to an obstruction. This may be due to enlarged prostate, stricture of the urethra, or kidney stones. It is also necessary to rule out benign prostatic hypertrophy. The bladder loses its tone, so when the person goes to bed it stretches and creates the desire for urination, but the blockage doesn't allow urine to easily pass.

For frequent, profuse urination we use catechu (khadira), which is astringent and helps to control urination. If there is a blockage of the urethra, which is generally a secondary complication to syphilitic urethritis, surgical intervention is needed. If it is a prostate problem, one must treat the prostate. A good formula is:

Arka Pushpa          200 mg
Vanga bhasma (tin ash) 200 mg
Take ½ tsp TID with warm water.

**9.    Sāndra meha:** turbid urine. The urine looks turbid and dense because of protein. When the nephron lining is compromised, there is a tendency to get urinary tract infections. Sugar is the best medium for bacteria to grow, so the excess sugar in the system combined with the disturbed nephron lining will cause the patient to lose his or her natural resistance. That is why diabetic people are prone to infection. The person also passes minerals into the urine.

For this condition we use the juice of fresh saptaparnī, a bitter, seven-leaf plant that is one of the ingredients of mahāsudarshan.

Saptaparnī          300 mg
Shilājit          300 mg
Gokshura          300 mg
Take ½ tsp TID with warm water.

*10.* **Surā meha:** *surā* means alcohol and surā meha is acetone urea. This condition exists when a person passes acetone without consumption of alcohol. The urine smells like alcohol and ferments.

| | |
|---|---|
| Kutki | 300 mg |
| Tikta | 300 mg |
| Chitrak | 200 mg |
| Take ½ tsp TID with aloe vera. | |

These are the ten types of kapha prameha. The following can also be associated with kapha prameha:

***Lāsikā meha or phena meha.*** Albumin urea. When passing urine there is lots of foam, which indicates a change in the specific gravity. The urine looks like carbonated water or beer. This is due to albumin and the person passes protein in the urine, due to kidney infection, pre-diabetes, a high protein diet, or toxemia in pregnancy. It can lead to nephrotic syndrome. A good formula is:

| | |
|---|---|
| Punarnavā | 500 mg |
| Gokshura | 300 mg |
| Triphalā | 200 mg |
| Shilājit | 200 mg |
| Take ½ tsp TID with warm water. | |

For all types of kapha prameha, a kapha pacifying diet and small sized meals is recommended. Take 1 teaspoon of triphalā each night at bedtime. Do regular exercise and also yoga, including spinal twist, bow, boat, bridge, and peacock poses.

**Table 2: Etiological Factors of Prameha**

| Primary | Secondary |
|---|---|
| Kapha provoking diet — especially excess sugar consumption | Viral infection |
| Obesity | Pregnancy — excess demand for insulin |
| Sedentary lifestyle | Thyroid gland disorder — excess production of thyroid hormones |
| High cholesterol and high triglycerides | Pituitary gland disorder relating to ACTH or growth hormone |
| Emotional overeating | Pituitary tumor |
| Stress | Liver diseases — hepatitis, cirrhosis, etc. |
| Genetic predisposition | Encephalitis |
| Pancreatic disorder: pancreatitis is pitta, tumor is kapha | Basal meningitis |
| Auto-immune disorder | Syphilis |
| | Corticosteroid therapy |
| | Diminished glomerular threshold |
| | Physical or psychological trauma |

This covers the principle kapha-related prameha conditions, which are non-insulin-dependent and relatively easy to treat. Next, we will discuss the pitta and vāta-dominant disturbances, both of which are more difficult to treat. This is according to the Ayurvedic concept of prameha as it relates to the western syndrome of diabetes.

## Six Pitta Types of Prameha

In these six pitta types of prameha, the pancreas may or may not be directly involved, depending on whether the person has a khavaigunya (weak space). Management of the doshas can control the metabolic imbalance if there is not pancreatic involvement, so for these six types of prameha, pitta must be pacified. The moment the pancreas is severely affected, the person can develop type I diabetes mellitus, which is primarily a vāta type of prameha. Once this happens, the person needs to severely limit the intake of sweet foods and support the pancreas, as well as manage the doshas.

In pitta prameha, it is common to have complications such as diabetic neuropathy, diabetic retinopathy and diabetic nephropathy. Patients are prone to repeated infections, boils, abscesses and other inflammatory disorders. The six pitta prameha follow.

*1.* **Kshara meha:** alkalinuria. *Kshara* means salt, which is alkaline, and here the urine becomes alkaline. Acids can burn, but a substance that is alkaline may also cause inflammation, because it fosters infection. There are two types of pitta: *sāma pitta,* which is pitta with āma (toxins) and is acidic; and *nirāma pitta,* which is pitta without āma and is alkaline. Hence, alkalinuria is related to nirāma pitta and is common when there is a liver dysfunction. Bile is alkaline, so if a patient has excess bile passing through the urine, it too becomes alkaline. This condition is also known as non-specific urethritis and is treated with āmalakī. Āmalakī is acidic, so it neutralizes the alkali. Take ½ teaspoon TID with hot water.

*2.* **Amla meha:** aciduria. *Amla* meha means aciduria, where the urine becomes acidic, and it is the opposite of kshara meha. For this, use bibhītakī or harītakī. Or if you're not sure which, just use triphalā and it will bring balance. This condition can also be helped by:

| | |
|---|---|
| Shatāvarī | 500 mg |
| Gulvel sattva | 300 mg |
| Kāma dudhā | 200 mg |
| Take ½ tsp TID with warm water. | |

*3.* **Nila meha:** *nila* means indigo, and here the urine looks purple-blue, which is known as urocyanosis or indicanuria. It is a sign of congestive heart failure and happens because of central cyanosis. In chronic congestive heart failure, the heart fails to fully pump blood out of the chamber and there is stagnation of venous blood, so the visceral organs look cyanotic. If you look at the tongue it is purple-blue and in this case even the urine looks purple or indigo. The person passes unoxidated blood cells in the urine. To test the color, put the urine in a glass jar or vial and hold it up to the light. This is a serious condition that is due to a chronic pitta disorder. However, another cause of indigo urine is iron toxicity. If the liver doesn't process iron efficiently, it can be stored in the liver. Liver disease is a serious complication of diabetes, as are vascular and heart problems.

The best herb for both causes of nilameha is kutki (also called katukā), because it enhances iron metabolism and scrapes excess cholesterol from the arteries. For iron chelation, katukā is the herb of choice. For both these you can give 200 mg TID. A good formula is:

| | |
|---|---|
| Kutki (Katukā) | 200 mg |
| Neem | 200 mg |
| Raktachandana | 200 mg (red sandalwood) |
| Turmeric | 200 mg |
| Take ½ tsp TID with warm water. | |

*4.*  **Rakta meha:** hematuria, which occurs when the person passes blood in the urine. It may be due to oxalic acid crystals, or a hemorrhage into the kidneys. First, rule out all other causes for hematuria, such as stricture of the urethra, kidney stones, or polyps. If these causes are eliminated and the person still passes some red blood cells in the urine, it means that he or she is likely to develop pitta type of diabetes. For this condition we use hemostatic herbs.

| | |
|---|---|
| Gudūchī | 300 mg (or gulvel sattva) |
| Manjishthā | 300 mg |
| Arjuna | 300 mg |
| Karanja | 300 mg |
| Take ½ tsp TID with warm water. | |

*5.*  **Manjishthā meha:** *manjishthā* means red, so this is red urine or hemoglobinuria. The person passes microscopic oxygenated red blood cells in the urine. This means that disintegration of red blood cells has already happened.

| | |
|---|---|
| Manjishthā | 300 mg |
| Chandana | 300 mg (white sandalwood) |
| Ushīra | 300 mg |
| Take ½ tsp TID with warm water. | |

*6.*  **Haridrā meha:** haridrā means turmeric, and in this type of prameha the urine looks dark yellow, the color of turmeric. It can be caused by bilirubinuria, chronic hepatitis, or cancer of the liver. One of the causes of diabetes is a liver dysfunction. The liver doesn't process carbohydrates and there is an overproduction of bilirubin that passes through the urine, so the person has dark colored urine, called haridrā meha. The best medicine for this condition is:

| | |
|---|---|
| Shankha pushpī | 400 mg |
| Tulsi | 300 mg |
| Kutki | 200 mg |
| Bilva | 200 mg |
| Take ½ tsp TID with aloe vera gel. | |

For all these pitta types of prameha, a pitta pacifying diet and regular meals is recommended. Regular exercise and yoga is good, along with a teaspoon of triphalā at bedtime. Triphalā is particularly helpful for pitta prameha because it balances the acid-alkaline balance (pH) of the urine and removes toxicity from the bladder. If it causes excessive urination at night, it may be an indication of low glomerular threshold in the kidneys, which can predispose the person to diabetes or reflect a family history of diabetes.

## Four Vāta Types of Prameha

These four vāta types of prameha can fall into the category of type I (insulin-dependent) diabetes mellitus, or may be a precursor to that disease. They are the most difficult to treat and some texts even list them as incurable. However there is much we can do to help these conditions.

*1.* **Vasa meha:** *vasa* means subcutaneous fat, so this is lipiduria. The person passes lipids in the urine, which show as oily droplets. It is a severe disorder of the fat metabolism that is often seen in the later stages of type I diabetes mellitus. The individual loses fat so rapidly that there can be severe emaciation and extremely dry skin. There is often high cholesterol, fatty diarrhea and fatty degenerative changes in the liver.

It is caused by disturbed apāna vāta, which allows lipid molecules to leak through the glomeruli and Bowman's capsule, resulting in either lipiduria or heavy proteinuria.

The treatment needs to strongly pacify vāta dosha:

| | |
|---|---|
| Dashamūla | 500 mg |
| Ashvagandhā | 500 mg |
| Katukā | 300 mg |
| Agni mantha | 200 mg |

Take ½ tsp TID with warm water.

*2.* **Sarpi meha:** *sarpi* means ghee. This condition is known as chyluria and it is a disorder of rasa dhātu. Chyle is the end product of digested food and the precursor of all bodily tissues. It is a milk-like alkaline substance containing lymphatic secretions that normally flow through the blood stream. In this condition, the astringent phase of digestion that happens in the colon is disturbed, creating vāta aggravation due to the dry, light and rough qualities of astringent taste. Disturbance of apāna vāta affects the pelvic organs and rasa and rakta dhātus. The glomerular threshold is also so disturbed that, instead of filtering kleda, it also filters chyle. This results in the person passing chyle into the urine, which can lead to emaciation.

In this disorder, vyāna vāta is disturbed and the chyle is pushed through the glomeruli of the kidneys, which makes the urine look like liquefied ghee. Note that in vasa meha, the urine appears to contain oil droplets, but here the whole urine looks like ghee.

A good formula is:

| | |
|---|---|
| Balā | 500 mg |
| Pātthā | 300 mg |
| Katukā | 300 mg |
| Hing | 200 mg |
| Kutaja | 200 mg |
| Kushtha | 200 mg |

Take ½ tsp TID with warm water.

*3.* **Madhu meha:** the person gets a sweet taste in the mouth, which later becomes sour, then salty, pungent, bitter and ultimately astringent. That indicates a very serious condition. Initially, the sweet taste from āhāra rasa (the food precursor of the tissues) cannot be converted into *sthāyi rasa dhātu* (fully processed plasma), so that dhātu becomes depleted. Sweet is the most nourishing taste and also the heaviest to digest, so it is the first to be unprocessed. Eventually even astringent, the final taste in the sequence, cannot be digested. At this point, agni has weakened to the extent that it cannot digest any of the tastes. Hence, the rasa dhātu becomes very depleted causing severe emaciation and all seven dhātus can also be affected in this way. This condition can then turn into type I diabetes mellitus.

Madhu meha means sweet urine, which is called glycosuria. There is also hyperglycemia (high blood sugar levels), due to diminished effectiveness of insulin. It is an endocrine disorder that affects carbohydrate, fat and protein metabolism, plus the water-electrolyte balance in the body. However the glomerular threshold is not directly affected. Madhu meha is a chronic condition that generally involves all three doshas, but ends up being a predominantly vāta imbalance. Insufficient insulin can be confirmed by a vāta spike on the pancreas pulse, which is found at the site of the spleen pulse.

It is a difficult condition to treat, but certain herbs do help. Shardunikā regulates carbohydrate and sugar metabolism and thereby helps to control blood sugar levels. Karela is bitter gourd (or bitter melon) and it is most effective for madhu meha. Vasant kusumakar contains purified gold, silver, pearl and mercury ash, so it is not allowed in the United States. However in India, most patients with type I diabetes mellitus take one pill daily to regulate blood sugar, so they do not require insulin.

| | |
|---|---|
| Shardunikā | 200 mg (or Gurmar or Madhuharini) |
| Bitter Gourd | 200 mg |
| Neem | 200 mg |
| Turmeric | 200 mg |

Take ½ tsp TID with warm water.

Also: Vasant Kusumakar 200 mg once daily

4. **Hasta meha:** *hasta* means elephant. The patient passes astringent urine and has incontinence. There is extreme polyuria, with gushing of urine like an elephant. The best formula is:

| | |
|---|---|
| Palash | 300 mg |
| Kapittha | 200 mg |
| Arjuna | 300 mg |
| Vangeshvara | 200 mg (contains vanga bhasma, along with other ingredients)[20] |

Take ½ tsp TID with warm water.

For all four vāta types of prameha, a vāta pacifying diet with regular, small meals is recommended. Gentle exercise, such as yoga, and basti (medicated enema) can also be helpful, as can taking a teaspoon of triphalā at bedtime each night. If it causes excess urination during the night, the triphalā can be soaked overnight and drunk the following morning. Overall, treatments for vāta prameha can generally only alleviate the symptoms, because vāta prameha is extremely difficult to cure.

---

20. A tin-lead oxide compound. This is of the types known as a rasa shastra product, alchemical combinations that usually include metals, some of which are considered toxic in their raw forms.

## Summary of Treatments for Prameha

These are the twenty major categories of prameha and we have to treat each one according to the doshas involved. Herbs, or insulin if necessary, can regulate blood sugar, but there needs to be a holistic treatment program to treat this syndrome. That usually includes proper diet, daily exercise, yoga, hygienic measures, an appropriate lifestyle and pañcha-karma cleansing, all according to the individual's constitution and the particular type of prameha.

It is also necessary to rebalance agni (metabolic fire) to regulate carbohydrate, fat and protein metabolism, and restore the water-electrolyte balance. Kapha types need to focus on controlling their weight and treat any edema. Pitta types must be vigilant about preventing infection and acidosis and should be particularly careful about cuts and abrasions. Vāta types should have a nourishing diet and not overdo things. Finally, anyone with prameha should keep a close watch on associated conditions such as glucose levels in the urine, hyperglycemia, high blood pressure, bacterial infections, blurring vision, glaucoma, cataracts, insulin shock, and diabetic nephropathy.

Prameha is a metabolic disorder, but if you manage the doshas you can control the pathogenesis. Find out the person's prakruti, vikruti, and the organs involved. When making an herbal formula, keep in mind that it has to be dosha pratyanika (specific to the doshas involved), vyādhi pratyanika (specific to the disease), and *dhātu poshaka* (supportive to the tissues).

Physical exercise is very important for improving circulation, glucose utilization, and agni. Diabetes patients can take part in athletics and high-level activities, although insulin-dependent diabetics should not do intense exercise.

Yoga postures can also help, particularly the camel, cobra, boat, bow and peacock poses. Ujjāyi prānāyāma, *udara bandha* (abdominal lock), *nauli* (an abdominal intestinal movement that massages the pancreas), and alternate nostril breathing with retention of the in-breath are all effective for most types of diabetes. These should all be learned from an experienced yoga instructor and done gently.

Doing pañchakarma for five or seven days a week can help prameha conditions immensely. In pañchakarma, the client receives snehana (oleation) and svedana (sweating therapy), which help to bring the doshas stuck in the tissues back to the gastrointestinal tract. If it is vāta type of prameha, do basti (medicated enema); for pitta type, virechana (purgation); and for kapha type, do vamana (vomiting therapy). Vamana can be very helpful in certain kinds of kapha prameha, especially diabetes insipidus. The uvula is connected to the pineal gland, so if you drink a cup of licorice tea and then rub the tongue to create a gag reflex, this induces vomiting, thereby releasing vasopressin and antidiuretic hormones from the posterior pituitary.

One of the therapies used in pañchakarma is shirodhāra. It consists of pouring a constant flow of warm oil onto the forehead area, on the third eye. Use a mix of base oil and jatamāmsi oil for vāta, brahmī oil for pitta or vacha oil for kapha. Pouring these medicated oils onto the forehead creates a situation where the head is surrounded by warm oil, which is similar to a baby being surrounded by the amniotic fluid inside the mother's womb. This calms the nervous system and helps to rebalance the doshas. Shirodhāra directly helps patients of diabetes insipidus by acting on the cerebral kloma to rebalance the hormones.

When the body receives oil during abhyanga massage and shirodhāra, the oil penetrates through the skin and into the fascia and affects the nerve endings, stimulating the secretion of hormones, neurotransmitters and neurological peptides, including acetylcholine and serotonin. Neurotransmitters are the functional integration of tarpaka kapha, *sādhaka pitta* and prāna vāta. These subtypes of the doshas are responsible for maintaining optimal neurological and cerebral functions and play an important role in hormonal balance. Oil massage can improve communication in the nervous and glandular systems, thereby helping to address the cause of prameha. Shirodhāra also regulates the hormonal balance in the body.

After pañchakarma, Ayurveda recommends rasāyana, or rejuvenation therapy. There are a number of good rejuvenative tonics for the pancreas, including shilājit, kutki, neem, gokshura, and karela (bitter gourd). In India, they make a cup out of wood from the jambul tree, put water in it overnight and then drink that water to regulate blood sugar. Licorice and manjishthā are two herbs that have a diuretic action, which is useful for kapha type of prameha. Note that although licorice is very sweet, it does not increase blood sugar.

Ayurveda believes that our bodily cells carry the memory of our parents' and grandparents' illnesses. This includes our glandular and nervous systems, which are part of majjā dhātu and therefore heavily involved in prameha. By treating majjā dhātu in the ways we have described, we can address these underlying genetic factors and manage diabetes.

Prameha or diabetes often has associated emotional factors, such as psychological trauma, abuse, depression, or deep-seated grief and sadness. Diabetes and depression often go together. If we manage the doshic imbalance that is responsible for these factors, there will be a radical improvement in the condition, both physically and mentally. Diabetes is often a chronic disorder, yet the patient can live a long, happy life.

# Chapter 8

# Celiac Disease with Reference to Grahani Roga

Spring 2009, Volume 21, Number 4

CELIAC DISEASE (ALSO CALLED CELIAC SPRUE) is a chronic intestinal malabsorption disorder. It is caused by intolerance to foods that are rich in gluten, or more specifically to gliadin and gliadin-like protein fractions in wheat, rye, barley and possibly oats. Most people call these gliadin and gliadin-like proteins gluten.

The word sprue comes from the Dutch word 'spruw,' which means mouth blisters. These were highlighted by the Dutch physician Vincent Ketelaer as a noticeable symptom of celiac disorders in 1669, almost three centuries before a reaction to gluten was found to be the cause of celiac disease. Note that tropical sprue is an infectious disease, due to bacterial infection. It is different from celiac disease and gluten sensitivity.

Ayurveda categorizes this disorder as being due to an imbalance of agni. Celiac disease falls under *grahani roga,* because *grahani* is the name for the small intestine. Grahani is the container, while agni is the content. If one is affected, the other is also bound to be disturbed.

The functional unit of the small intestine is the villus. The intestinal villi hold food molecules during the digestive process. If agni is strong, the villi are strong and healthy. They maintain their tone, coordination, and rhythmic movement, and correctly perform their actions in the process of digestion, absorption, and assimilation.

When there is agni imbalance, the functioning of the villi are affected and the person can get either gluten enteropathy or non-tropical celiac sprue. Any food substances that are heavy, fatty, and gross can suppress agni. Gluten is gross, heavy, sticky, dull, and oily in nature, so it can cause low agni and result in the production of āma.

According to Ayurveda, cellular agni maintains cellular intelligence and selectivity. In cases of a chronic agni disorder, the bodily cells lose their intelligence, which affects their selectivity. These cells react to gliadin molecules as if they are a bacteria or virus.

Gliadin acts as an antigen. To fight with this antigen, the cells of the intestinal mucous membrane produce antibodies, creating an immune reaction. The aggregation of killer T lymphocytes attacks the neighboring mucous membrane, causing mucosal damage and loss of some of the villi. This leads to poor assimilation and malabsorption of foodstuff. The affected person typically has low iron levels, malabsorption of fat-soluble vitamins A, D, E and K, and possibly dehydration. If gluten is removed from the diet, the patient's health can show noticeable improvement.

After someone with celiac disease eats wheat or another gluten-containing grain, the food enters the small intestine and, once it reaches the jejunum, antibodies in the intestinal wall are stimulated. These antibodies destroy the villi. This is one theory behind celiac disease.

The other theory is that due to a chronic agni imbalance, the undigested gluten acts like a toxin (āma). This āma clogs the channels of the villi and creates a thick coating of toxic matter over the intestinal mucosa, resulting in malabsorption.

Irritable bowel syndrome (IBS) is another form of grahani roga, producing abdominal pain when passing stools as well as bloating, gas, abdominal distension, mucous in stools, and episodes of alternating diarrhea and constipation. More women are affected by this condition than men and there is no weight loss. In IBS, the symptoms disappear when the patient is asleep. This is partly because IBS is sometimes related to a history of sexual or physical abuse. In sprue syndrome or celiac disease, there is usually weight loss and the symptoms are always present.

## Diagnosis

Various tests can be performed to determine if someone has celiac disease. A biopsy has historically been the main diagnostic tool. Blood tests taken after eating wheat or other gluten foods can reveal if there is a reaction to gluten as well as whether there are low levels of minerals, vitamins and other nutrients. However, not everyone with gluten intolerance has celiac disease.

The only way to tell if you have celiac sprue is through biopsy and laboratory tests. It is important to rule out other causes of nutritional deficiencies, so consult with a gastroenterologist if you want an accurate analysis.

Ayurveda uses examination of the intestinal pulse to discern whether someone has celiac disease or gluten sensitivity. If the intestinal pulse is extremely feeble, it may mean celiac disease; whereas if it is strong, it can indicate food sensitivity.

Celiac disease has hereditary factors. In certain families, the family members carry a low agni disorder from one generation to another. The affected children may be born with a khavaigunya (defective space) in the small intestine. In such cases, these individuals can often develop gluten sensitivity and may have a genetic predisposition to celiac disease.

People with northwestern European ancestry are most often affected by celiac disease. It equally affects men and women. Ayurveda says that pitta and kapha types mainly get this disorder: either pitta predominant and kapha secondary, or kapha predominant and pitta secondary.

In terms of vikruti, celiac disease can involve all three doshas. Either increased vāta suppresses agni by its cold quality, aggravated pitta disturbs agni due to its liquid quality, or increased kapha suppresses agni by its heavy and dull qualities.

In vāta celiac disease, there is more atrophy of the villi, causing pain, bloating, gas, and hyper-peristalsis. The person commonly feels fear and anxiety, and suffers from insomnia. Pitta type of celiac disease causes significant inflammation, leading to burning, pulling, and sucking sensations in the intestines. It often produces rashes, urticaria, and irritability. Kapha celiac disease features clogged and hypertrophied villi, smooth intestinal walls and bulky, pale, fatty stools (steatorrhea). The person may have feelings of heaviness, dullness, sleepiness, and depression. This Ayurvedic symptomatology gives us a clear picture of the various types of celiac disorder.

*Children.* The general signs and symptoms of celiac disease can begin in children during infancy, when the child starts to eat cereals or other foods with gluten. The affected baby or child does not thrive and may cry after eating because of painful gas and bloating. The baby may pass pale, foul-smelling, bulky stools and he or she might have abdominal distension.

Malabsorption of iron and other minerals can cause to the child to look pale. Poor protein absorption can result in edema (swelling). The child will be underweight, with stunted growth and little fat on the body, and there may be bony deformity. These babies don't sleep soundly and awaken at night crying, due to abdominal gas.

Children tend to develop celiac symptoms during the fourth to sixth month after eating cereals. If there is a family history of celiac disease, one has to take great care with the children's diet. Be very careful about feeding gluten-containing foods to these children. A gluten-free, anti-doshic diet should be given at the first sign of symptoms. Basmati rice and mung dal kitchari are great alternatives to the gluten-containing grains.

*Adults.* In adults, the signs and symptoms are similar to those in children. Common symptoms include:

- Bulky, fatty, foul-smelling stools that sink
- Weight loss
- Diarrhea
- Malnutrition (vitamin and mineral deficiency)
- Paleness
- Anemia
- Fatigue
- Headaches
- Aches and pains in the bones
- Epigastric fullness or abdominal distension
- Mouth blisters

- Burping
- Pricking pain
- Tingling sensations or numbness in the hands or feet
- Untimely cessation of menstruation
- Mood changes
- Atrophy of the intestinal villi
- A biopsy will show no villi or damaged villi, and a disorganized network of blood vessels.

## Management by Following a Gluten Free Diet

The treatments for celiac disease can also be used to manage other gluten intolerance disorders. The main line of management is a gluten-free diet.

This means no wheat, rye, or barley, and possibly also no oats. Refer to a dietician for a full list of foods to avoid. It includes no hamburgers, hot dogs, or sausages, which often contain gluten fillers. The person should also avoid candy bars, baked goods, ice cream, and canned foods, because these contain ingredients that slow down agni.

Eat a healthy diet that is relatively high in calories and protein and low in fat. Most celiac patients do not digest fat very well. Ghee is an exception because it kindles agni, promotes ojas, and calms down immune reactions.

The best foods are basmati rice, mung dal, quinoa, blue corn, millet, and buckwheat as well as vegetables such as broccoli, asparagus, zucchini, lettuce, sprouts, leafy greens, Jerusalem artichoke, bitter melon, gourd, and banana flower. The best fruits are berries and pomegranate. Avoid dairy products other than ghee and *takra* (buttermilk). End each meal with a glass of takra with a pinch of cumin powder.

The Ayurvedic approach to management of celiac disease is basic, fundamental, and radical. Determine the client's prakruti and vikruti, i.e., which dosha is out of balance. Then give *dīpana* and *pāchana chikitsā* to kindle agni and eliminate āma. For dīpana, give trikatu (ginger, black pepper, long pepper). Then as pāchana, give the person chitrak, fennel, cumin, and takra (buttermilk).

### For vāta-type sprue syndrome

| | |
|---|---|
| Dashamūla | 500 mg |
| Ashvagandhā | 400 mg |
| Trikatu | 200 mg |
| Sanjīvanī | 200 mg[21] (to digest āma and fat in the stools) |

Give ½ teaspoon of this mixture TID with warm water.

Additionally, one teaspoon of ashvagandhā ghee should be taken during each meal.

Finally, the person can take ½ teaspoon of sat isabgol with a cup of warm water at night.

### For pitta-type sprue syndrome

| | |
|---|---|
| Shatāvarī | 500 mg |
| Gulvel Sattva | 400 mg |

---

21. Can substitute kutaja (*Holarrhena antidysenterica*).

Kāma dudhā      200 mg
Kutaja          200 mg, when there is diarrhea
Give ½ teaspoon of this mixture TID with 1/3 cup of cranberry juice.

Take one teaspoon of shatāvarī ghee or bitter ghee (tikta grihta) during each meal.

### For kapha-type sprue syndrome
Punarnavā                     500 mg
Yashthi madhu (licorice) 300 mg
Trikatu                       200 mg
Chitrak                       200 mg
Give ½ teaspoon of this mixture TID with honey and/or hot water.

> T.I.D. = from the Latin
> means *ter in diem*,
> three times a day

The person should also take one teaspoon of licorice ghee or bitter ghee (tikta grihta) during each meal.

## General Management

For all celiac or sprue patients, an herbal tea made of equal parts of coriander, cumin, fennel, khus, ginger, and bilva is effective as dīpana and pāchana. This is called *dhanyaka-dhi kashayam* and it is useful for kindling agni.

Once the sprue symptoms are under control, the person should undertake pañcha-karma treatment. Vamana is good for kapha type of sprue syndrome, virechana for pitta type of celiac disorder, and basti for vāta type.

Get plenty of rest by going to bed early. Avoid heavy exercise, such as weightlifting and jogging, as this will further aggravate vāta. Yoga is very beneficial, including camel, cow, cobra, boat, bow and bridge poses as well as leg lifts. Anuloma-viloma, kapāla bhāti, and ujjāyi prānāyāma are also helpful when done under the guidance of an expert.

In old people particularly, grahani can be very difficult to cure, and it can lead to complications. Common complications that result from celiac disease or severe gluten intolerance include:

- Vāta type: malabsorption, weight loss, irritable bowel syndrome, degenerative arthritis
- Pitta type: rashes and skin disorders, gout
- Kapha type: diabetes, edema, steatorrhea and multiple lipoma

In severe cases, corticosteroid drugs are recommended to reduce inflammation and manage the symptoms. However, these medicines can produce many adverse side effects. Ayurveda traditionally recommended the use of licorice or licorice ghee as an alternative to synthetic steroid therapy.

### Prognosis
Celiac disease can be helped by dietary therapy that is further supported by herbal programs, pañchakarma, and rasāyana. The best rasāyana for grahani is parpati, a medical preparation of mercury and sulphur as well as various herbs. However, these compounds are not allowed in the West.

This ailment is usually completely treatable through an Ayurvedic protocol. The prognosis is good for most patients, especially if young, with only a few exceptions. Recovery can be dramatic in children, whereas in severe, chronic cases, a complete return to normal intestinal functions can take months or years. Then again, it may never fully resolve in some cases. Success in treatment depends upon restoring the strength of the person's agni.

Chapter 9

# The Ayurvedic Perspective on Allergies
## Asātmya

Summer 2002, Volume 15, Number 1

ALLERGY AND INTOLERANCE are explained in the Ayurvedic literature as the concept of *asātmya*. *"Aushadha anna viharanam upayogam sukhavaham sahi satmyam"* is an ancient Ayurvedic phrase saying that *sātmya* is when a person's doshas accept and adjust to medicines, dietary, and environmental changes. Sātmya means tolerance. Asātmya, or intolerance, is when one or more doshas do not accept these things and they react, often as an allergy. Intolerance and allergy are conditions of hypersensitivity, a reaction of one or more doshas to a causative factor. The root cause is imbalanced agni.

Sātmya is natural tissue tolerance, or specific immune response. The two most significant factors determining one's resistance to infection and allergy are agni (metabolic fire) and the specific qualities of a person's prakruti. Agni maintains our natural resistance and immunity by producing balanced ojas, tejas, and prāna, which destroy or neutralize any invaders. Certain specific immune responses may produce unpleasant and sometimes very severe hypersensitivity (allergic reactions). The substance (either food or medicine) may be eaten, inhaled, or brought into contact with the skin and cause the individual to develop a reaction or allergy.

Each dhātu agni in the human body regulates the physiological functions of its particular tissue. The elemental components of cells—ether, air, fire, water, earth—govern the structural aspects of the cells, while their derivative doshas—vāta, pitta, kapha—organize and govern the functional activities of the cells and intercellular communication.

When bacteria or toxic substances invade the tissues, prāna promotes the secretion of ojas and tejas in the cells. These three subtle energies move to the affected region and either destroy the bacteria or neutralize the toxins with the help of the respective dhātu agni. Ojas is the essence of all tissues and it plays a primary role in maintaining immunity. It is derived from kapha molecules, but it functions along with tejas and prāna. If the dhātu agni is inadequate, the invading substance may damage the cells and produce toxic material, called āma. This āma affects the doshas according to the characteristics of the invading substance and the individual's constitution.

Each of the three doshas interacts with āma to produce local or general reactions of a vāta, pitta, or kapha nature. The substances that produce these reactions are called allergens. The form an allergy takes depends upon the specific type of allergen and the aggravated dosha (vāta, pitta, or kapha).

Circulating throughout the body in the bloodstream are molecules of vāta, pitta and kapha, proportionate to the ratio of the doshas in a person's prakruti and vikruti. An allergen may be absorbed into the bloodstream and come into contact with these doshic molecules. If *rasa* or *rakta agni* is low, the doshas will react to the allergen, depending upon the strength and qualities of the allergen. This is called *dosha rūpa,* which is the doshic reaction of the allergy.

The factors that determine whether or not there is an allergic reaction and its severity are:

- *Prakruti dosha* (the amount of any dosha at conception)
- *Vikruti dosha* (current state of a dosha)
- Dhātu agni
- Quantity of allergen that enters the body

An important point is that the dosha rūpa of a prakruti dosha will create a mild allergic reaction, while the dosha rūpa of vikruti doshas creates severe allergic reactions. For instance, suppose two people have weak rasa dhātu agni and they get exposed to a moderate amount of kapha-type pollen. If person A has balanced kapha, he or she will have no reaction or only a mild reaction to the allergen. If person B has high kapha, he or she will have a much more severe reaction, possibly even going into anaphylactic shock if exposed to a large quantity of the substance.

It is the production of toxins (āma) due to poor agni that causes an allergy. There are four types of āma that can be produced:

1. *Rasa āma* – from unprocessed āhāra rasa
2. *Mala āma* – from improper elimination
3. *Āma dosha* – from imbalanced doshas in the 3rd stage of pathogenesis onwards
4. *Mano āma* – mental toxins from unprocessed, unresolved, and suppressed emotions. It is due to low sādhaka agni and it reduces clarity.

All occur only if there is low agni in that particular process. Hence, if there is *dosha dushti* (qualitative disturbance of a dosha) but strong agni, there will be no āma, just nirāma (no āma) doshic disturbance.

Note that a person with strong and robust dhātu agni will generally not have an allergic reaction at all, even if there is vikruti dosha. The only exception is if the person is exposed to a huge amount of the particular allergen and it overwhelms the dhātu agni.

## The Role of the Thymus and Spleen in Asātmya

Agni is the first protective barrier against allergens. When foreign organisms or allergens invade the tissues, the bodily cells often respond by releasing substances that cause local blood vessels to dilate and become more permeable. The cell membrane actually secretes an irritant chemical substance that is toxic to the body, a type of āma. This is due to low agni in those particular cells.

These substances that are released are a manifestation of tejas. As they are produced, the tissues become reddened, leaking excess fluids into the interstitial space due to the local reaction of pitta. The swelling produced by pitta is an allergic, inflammatory reaction that is a protective barrier to delay the spread of the invading allergen or microorganism into other tissues.

At the same time, ojas liberates more kapha molecules at the site of the lesion. Thus, ojas and tejas act together to detoxify the foreign substances that enter the tissues through the lungs or intestinal tract. In this defense mechanism, the thymus and spleen play an important role.

The thymus is a soft, bi-lobed gland located in the chest in front of the heart, behind the upper part of the sternum and just above the pericardium. In Ayurvedic texts, this gland is called jatru granthi. It is a predominately kapha gland, located in the kapha site of the chest and is relatively large in children during kapha age. After puberty, it tends to decrease in size and in adult years it may be quite small. The agni of this gland helps to produce ojas, which includes T-lymphocytes that either destroy a bacteria or virus or neutralize toxins. Weakness of this gland may be one of the causes of allergies and can be detected as low energy at the pericardial pulse level.

---

**THE ROLE OF OJAS IN ASATMYA**

| | |
|---|---|
| Ojovisramsa | Mild allergies |
| Ojovyapata | Moderate allergies |
| Ojokshaya | Severe allergies |

Allergy is the great effort of ojas to reach the heart. In ojo visramsa, a normal amount of allergen only causes a mild reaction, whereas in ojo kshaya the same amount of the allergenic substance can cause a more severe reaction. However even in ojo visramsa, a very strong allergen may not allow the processed ojas to stabilize in the heart. This causes very severe allergies and even anaphylactic shock. Hence the emphasis in Ayurveda to protect ojas at all costs. This is accomplished through proper lifestyle and appropriate use of rasāyana.

---

The spleen, an organ made up largely of lymphoid tissue and located in the upper left portion of the abdominal cavity, is called *plīhā* in Sanskrit. Its role is to remove bacteria from the blood. The spleen lies beneath the diaphragm and a little behind the stomach. It is the root of rakta vaha srotas (the hematopoietic system) and is filled with rakta (blood) and *rañjaka pitta*. It acts as a blood reservoir and stores and filters blood.

Embryologically, the spleen produces red blood cells, but in an adult that function is transferred to the bone marrow. The subtle molecules of rañjaka pitta present in the spleen destroy foreign particles and microorganisms. A defective spleen can cause depleted immunity and such individuals may be prone to allergies.

### Assessment of Asātmya (Allergies and Intolerances)

Atopic allergy is defined as a tendency for hypersensitivity to a specific allergen that is inherited as part of the person's genetic predisposition. This khavaigunya (weak or defective space) can also be due to childhood trauma and suppressed or unresolved emotional issues accumulated into the organs.

Repressed emotions—such as anxiety, fear, or anger—produce stress. This stimulates the secretion of toxins in the body. Repressed fear, anxiety, and insecurity aggravate vāta dosha. Repressed anger, hate, and envy aggravate pitta dosha. Repressed greed, possessiveness, and attachment aggravate kapha dosha. Meditation, breathing exercises (prānāyāma), and stress management are particularly effective in minimizing allergies due to repressed emotions.

Ayurveda places emphasis upon clinical observation of the signs and symptoms of allergy. The pulse, tongue, nails, skin, heart and lung sounds and other bodily systems are examined thoroughly. The prior health of the individual as well as the family history must be taken into account along with the present problem. The person is carefully observed in order to assess prakruti (constitution) and vikruti (the doshic imbalance, which in this case is the type of allergy).

Vāta type of allergy is due to *vishama agni* (irregular digestion), causing gas, bloating, distention, discomfort, and breathlessness. It may create headaches, arthritic changes, sciatica, or hemorrhoids. Pitta type is due to *tīkshna agni* (sharp digestion), which causes sudden symptoms such as stomach ache, diarrhea, nausea, vomiting, hives, rashes, urticaria, eczema, or psoriasis. Kapha type of allergy is due to *manda agni* (slow digestion) and results in hay fever, cold, congestion, cough, wheezing, or asthma.

## Chikitsā (Treatment)

*Nidāna parivarjanam* means to avoid the cause. If we know the most common allergens, we should teach the client how to identify them and thereby eliminate the causative factors. These can include household sprays and cleaners, fabrics, animals, and foods. However, depending upon the specific nature of the allergic reaction, this may not always be possible. Hence, a comprehensive approach to treatment along doshic lines is needed.

Modern medicine treats allergies with antihistamines and steroids, but this is best used to handle acute emergencies. Certain Ayurvedic herbs contain natural antihistamines and steroids. These include ashvagandhā, shatāvarī, and licorice (yashthi madhu), which are good for vāta, pitta, and kapha respectively as well as aloe vera, cilantro, hibiscus, and tikta ghee.

The Ayurvedic approach falls under two categories of *chikitsā:*
- Shamana – palliative therapy for acute phase of allergies
- Shodana – detoxification program (including pañchakarma) to remove doshic causes of allergies. Pañchakarma is only done once the acute symptoms are under control.

## Pañchakarma and Allergies

Vāta from the colon, pitta from the small intestines and kapha from the stomach, can all undergo accumulation, provocation, and then spread (prasara). During the prasara stage, the dosha moves into the rasa and rakta dhātus. Longstanding, lingering doshas in rasa-rakta cause sensitivity to allergens.

By doing snehana (oleation), svedana (sudation), and massage according to the doshic type, the dosha moves back from rasa and rakta dhātus to its site. One can see this clinically and feel it in the pulse. Once the dosha has returned home, it can be eliminated by pañchakarma (the five actions):

* Basti (medicated enema) for vāta
* Virechana (purgation) for pitta
* Vamana (therapeutic vomiting therapy) for kapha
* Rakta moksha (blood-letting) for blood cleansing
* Nasya (nasal administration) to remove the residual doshas

During this process, the person eats a cleansing mono-diet such as kitchari and drinks herbal teas in accordance with his or her constitution. Pañchakarma should be carried out under the supervision of an experienced Ayurvedic physician or technician. It helps to detoxify the body and build the resistance of the tissues by gradually rebalancing agni. Pañchakarma is also very helpful in stress management and accelerates the natural healing processes.

Pañchakarma helps to eradicate the internal causes of allergies, so that there will not be any future recurrence. A proper rasāyana according to the person's prakruti and vikruti is also important following pañchakarma.

### Rejuvenation Program (Rasāyana)

Ayurveda teaches the art of rebuilding and revitalizing tissues through proper lifestyle, diet, herbs, yoga, and meditation. When a subject is suffering from allergies, it is said to be the weeping cry of the tissues to change one's lifestyle, diet, and habits and thereby bring clarity and compassion to relationships. Allergy is nature's demand for physical, mental, and emotional cleansing through radical change.

Harītakī is a specific rasāyana for vāta type allergies, āmalakī for pitta allergies, and bibhītakī for kapha allergies. The combination of all three is called triphalā, which is balancing for all three doshas. Triphalā is a natural antioxidant that removes free radicals and helps to maintain doshic balance by detoxifying cells, thereby increasing longevity. It is a good cellular food and actually rejuvenates the cell.

## Management of Kapha Type of Allergies

Kapha allergy results in rhinitis, colds, cough, nasal congestion, wheezing, sneezing, asthma, or edema. The person is often sensitive to milk and dairy products, wheat, red meat, and other kapha aggravating foods. It is better to avoid these things and follow a kapha pacifying diet. Certain herbal teas, like ginger, cinnamon and coriander, are very effective to pacify kapha dosha. Regular kapha-reducing yoga postures and prānāyāma are also advisable.

Finally, an effective herbal formula to minimize kapha type of asātmya is:

| | |
|---|---|
| Sitopalādi | 500 mg |
| Mahāsudarshan | 300 mg |
| Licorice | 300 mg |
| Pippalī | 200 mg |

Abhrak bhasma       200 mg
Take ½ teaspoon with warm water after meals.

Note: Kapha type of allergy can also cause increased white blood cell count, which may be associated with worms. If there is krumi (worms) add Vidanga 200 mg and Shardunikā 200 mg.

## Management of Pitta Type of Allergies

Pitta allergies result in hives, rashes, urticaria, dermatitis, eczema, psoriasis, diarrhea, nausea, vomiting, headache, inflammatory responses, or even severe anaphylactic shock. When a person eats pitta-aggravating foods such as peanuts, strawberries, bananas, citrus fruit, cranberries, eggs, garlic, onion, hot spicy foods, pork, yogurt, and hard cheeses, pitta allergies can occur. Insect bites, strong sunlight and exposure to heat may also be causes of pitta allergies. Environmental chemical sensitivity also falls under pitta-type of allergy. Susceptible individuals should avoid these influences and follow a pitta pacifying diet.

In the case of recurrent allergic dermatitis, eczema, or psoriasis, Ayurveda suggests rakta moksha (bloodletting). It can be performed by either the application of leeches at the site of the lesion, or by aspirating approximately 100 cc of blood from the vein. This kind of bloodletting can improve the detoxifying function of the spleen, as more phagocytes (kapha cells) are attracted to the site of the lesion. At the same time, fresh ojas and tejas molecules are released by the cells to help neutralize the toxins. Rakta moksha is very effective in pitta individuals, but it should be done under the supervision of a medical doctor.

Pitta type of allergy symptoms may be associated with anger, hate, and irritability. To reduce these stressful factors, it is beneficial to practice *shītalī prānāyāma **or** chandra bhedana* (inhaling through the left nostril and exhaling through the right). Deep, quiet meditation can also accelerate the healing process. A useful herbal formula for pitta type of asātmya is:

Shatāvarī                    500 mg
Gudūchī or Gulvel Satva     300 mg
Kāma dudhā                   200 mg
Take ½ teaspoon with warm water or cilantro juice after meals.

Note: Severe allergies and even anaphylactic shock are more common in pitta individuals with pitta type of asātmya. If a severe allergic reaction occurs and the subject needs antihistamines or steroids, a medical doctor should be consulted immediately.

## Management of Vāta Type of Allergies

People having vāta type allergies may be sensitive to vāta aggravating foods such as night-shades (potato, tomato, eggplant), beans, and certain dry or bitter foods and herbs. After eating these substances, they have symptoms such as gas, bloating, headache, muscle spasms, palpitations, insomnia, and nightmares. Emotionally, people with *vāta asātmya* experience anxiety, fear and insecurity and they may become hyperactive. It is best to avoid all these causes and to eat vāta reducing foods and follow a vāta-pacifying lifestyle.

An effective herbal formula for vāta asātmya is:
Dashamūla              500 mg

Yogarāja Guggulu   300 mg
Triphalā Guggulu   300 mg
Trikatu            200 mg
Take ½ teaspoon with warm water after meals.

# Remedies for Specific Types of Allergies

## Skin Allergies (Hives, Rashes, and Urticaria)

These are all pitta disorders. One simple remedy is cilantro juice. Take a bunch of fresh cilantro (coriander leaf), chop it into pieces, put into a blender, add a couple of teaspoons of water, blend it, strain it through cheesecloth, and collect the fresh juice. One to two teaspoons of cilantro juice TID, will take care of hives and rashes. You can also apply the pulp onto the skin.

A second remedy is to drink coconut water, which is cooling to pitta. Alternatively, burn a dried coconut (not in the shell) so that it turns black. This tarry black carbon accumulated on the surface of the burnt coconut is the best medicine for rashes and urticaria. Apply topically.

Take bitter ghee (tikta ghrita) or just plain ghee. Add a pinch of black pepper and apply the mixture topically on the rash or urticaria.

You can mix equal parts of sandalwood and turmeric with just enough water to make a paste. Apply that paste to affected areas of the skin.

A cooling yoga exercise called the Moon Salutation is very helpful.

Watermelon has two uses for skin allergies: eat the red part of the melon, then rub the white part onto the skin.

Finally, a cool shower or bath can help to reduce aggravated pitta in the skin.

## Respiratory Allergies

In respiratory allergies, the agni of the respiratory tract (prāna vaha srotas) is depleted. The chest and sinuses are main seats of kapha, so kapha-type of respiratory allergies are more common. Examples are cold, congestion, cough, sneezing and wheezing.

For these types of allergies, use vacha (calamus root) oil nasya to remove the mucus. Once the mucus or kapha dosha from the lungs, throat and sinuses is clear, you can definitely control much of the respiratory allergy. For elimination of kapha, one should drink flax seed tea. At night boil one teaspoon of flax seeds in a cup of water and drink it, the tea along with the seeds. That will eliminate mucus and help the respiratory allergy.

In vāta-type of asthma or wheezing, udāna vāyu and *prāna vāyu* are affected and there is narrowing of the bronchial trees causing wheezing.

Another good remedy is to drink a cup of licorice tea with ten drops of mahānārāyana oil mixed in thoroughly. To make licorice tea, boil one teaspoon of licorice powder in a cup of water. Take one sip of this tea every ten minutes as needed. Also rub mahānārāyana oil on the chest and apply heat (such as a hot water bottle) to the chest.

Hay fever is a kapha or pitta disorder, where individuals are hypersensitive to pollen, dust, and debris. There are two types of hay fever.

| Spring Type Hay Fever (Kapha) | | Summer Type Hay Fever (Pitta) | |
| --- | --- | --- | --- |
| Allergy to airborne pollens such as oak, juniper, elm, hickory. Produces sinus congestion, watering of eyes, catarrh, and coryza. | | Allergy to airborne pollens such as grasses, sorrel, hay, ragweed, house dust, combined with excess heat. Produces sinus congestion, inflammation of upper respiratory lining, headache, bronchitis. | |
| Punarnavā | 400 mg | Kāma Dudhā | 200 mg |
| Ginger | 200 mg | Gulvel Sattva | 200 mg |
| Turmeric | 200 mg | Sudarshan | 200 mg |
| Pippalī | 200 mg | Moti Bhasma | 200 mg |
| Take ½ teaspoon of this mixture TID, plus vacha oil nasya (nasal drops) | | Take ½ teaspoon of this mixture TID with aloe gel, plus ghee nasya. | |

## Food Allergies and Intolerance

Generally food intolerance directly results from disturbed digestive fire (agni). In vāta people, agni commonly becomes irregular and creates intolerance to vāta-provoking foods such as beans, chickpeas, raw vegetables, and nightshades (potato, tomato, eggplant). These all aggravate vāta, causing gas, bloating, stomachache, abdominal discomfort, burping, breathlessness, and pains. You may use triphalā guggulu and trikatu 200 mg of each. Take ½ teaspoon of this mixture TID with warm water.

When pitta affects agni, there is strong appetite but poor digestion, causing intolerance to pitta foods such as sour fruit, citrus fruit, cheese, yogurt, fermented food, and hot spicy food. These things aggravate pitta and result in acid indigestion, heartburn, nausea, vomiting, diarrhea, hives, rashes, and urticaria. A good formula is:

| | |
| --- | --- |
| Shatāvarī | 500 mg |
| Gulvel Sattva | 300 mg |
| Mahāsudarshan | 200 mg |
| Kāma Dudhā | 200 mg |

Also see the remedies for hives, rashes, and urticaria.

> T.I.D. = from the Latin means *ter in diem*, three times a day

If kapha slows down agni, immediately after eating the stomach becomes heavy and the person feels dull, sluggish, and sleepy. There is excessive mucus and it can cause kapha disorders such as cold, congestion, cough, asthma, obesity, hypertension and diabetes.

## General Management of Allergies

Once the acute phase of allergy is over, one should treat agni to prevent future recurrence. For vishama and manda agni, use agni tundi 200 mg, chitrak 200 mg, and trikatu 100 mg. Take ½ teaspoon of this mixture TID with honey. If agni tundi is unavailable, use agni tea or ginger tea. For contactant allergies, apply tikta ghrita, sandalwood paste, neem oil, and cilantro pulp. For injectant allergies, treat according to the doshas.

*Important:* If one has serious complications, such as asthma, laryngeal edema causing breathlessness or choking, anaphylactic shock, severe rash, or urticaria, then prompt medical attention should be sought.

Chapter 10

# Bronchial Asthma

## Shvāsa

Fall 1993, Volume 6, Number 2

IN THE ANCIENT Ayurvedic literature, *shvāsa* (asthma) is considered a kapha disorder; hence, it may start in the kapha time of life: childhood. Early onset asthma is more common in males having a kapha prakruti or vikruti and those with kapha-type allergies from external sources. The male reproductive tissue, shukra has many kapha characteristics. These individuals prone to early asthma may have allergic rhinitis (acute stuffy nose), kapha-type eczema, or a family history of such conditions.

Late onset asthma is more common in females. The female reproductive tissue, ārtava, has mostly pitta characteristics. This kind of asthma is not necessarily caused by external allergens, but is triggered by the intrinsic cause of high pitta. The cause of the high pitta may be a pitta-provoking diet, which can cause bronchial constriction and inflammatory reaction within the respiratory passage.

Allergic asthma is triggered by allergens such as pollen, house dust, feathers, animal hair, and fungal spores. Food allergies may also become aggravating factors in some individuals. Kapha increasing food, such as wheat and dairy, may stimulate bronchial congestion leading to asthma. Much less frequently, similar effects may be produced by ingested allergens derived from foods such as fish, eggs, nuts, and yeast.

A third category of asthma involves vāta aggravating substances such as dust, tobacco smoke, dry weather, and emotional stress like grief, sadness, and fear. This type of asthma can also be triggered by strenuous exertion, sexual activities, or exposure to cold air. Incompatible food combinations such as milk with banana, meat with dairy, or melons with grain can also provoke an attack. These causative factors inhibit agni (the gastric fire) by producing āma (toxins), which eventually enter the respiratory track and cause a constriction of the respiratory passages.

The general pathogenesis of asthma starts in the stomach. Owing to the etiological factors, kledaka kapha undergoes accumulation and provocation, and during the spreading stage it moves into the lungs. Kapha is heavy, cold, slimy, and unctuous in nature while prāna vāta has dry, cold, rough, and active attributes. Within the lungs, kledaka kapha and prāna vāta intermix and alter each other's qualities in the respiratory passage. Due to the dry, rough qualities of vāta, the kledaka kapha becomes sticky and thick and adheres to the walls of the bronchi, causing narrowing of the bronchial tubes. This leads to breathlessness or an asthmatic attack. The prāna becomes stagnated within the alveoli, causing diminished air entry. Because the kapha is heavy, it accumulates at the bottom of the lungs. The person with this kind of asthma feels better in a sitting position where she/he can breathe through the less congested upper parts of the lung. When the person lies down, kledaka kapha moves to the middle and upper parts of the lungs, and causes congestion in the entire lung, leading to more obstruction and difficulty breathing. This is why a person with asthma sits propped up with pillows and often craves hot drinks during attacks. The cold attributes of kapha and vāta create this craving for heat. Though pañchakarma is the main line of treatment for asthma, one has to understand the strength and the stage of asthmatic attack. Pañchakarma should be done when the strength of the person is good and kapha is well-provoked in the stomach. Massage warm oil gently into the chest and give a pint or two of licorice tea (made from chopped licorice root, one teaspoon per cup of water) or a salt-water solution (one teaspoon to a pint of water) and induce vomiting to eliminate the kapha. This often provides instantaneous relief.

Individuals with low energy are not healthy enough for pañchakarma during an attack, and they need a gentler approach. But if a person is strong and kapha is provoked in the stomach during an attack (if this is the case, one will feel heaviness in the stomach and have excess salivation and nausea), drinking sip-by-sip a cup of hot licorice tea with 5 to 10 drops of mahānārāyana oil is advisable. This mixture liquefies the kledaka kapha. And, although not the goal of this treatment, the tea may also induce vomiting and eliminate some of the kapha, relieving the spasm of the bronchial tree and calming down the prāna vāta. The person usually feels better immediately.

Taking a mixture of sitopalādi 500 mg, trikatu 200 mg, punarnavā 400 mg, and abhrak bhasma 200 mg with one teaspoon of honey TID can be beneficial. This formula eliminates the pathogenesis of asthma from the stomach. Drinking a cup of flax seed tea at bedtime also eliminates the residual kapha from the stomach.

There is a specific management for each specific type of asthma in the Ayurvedic literature. To regulate the normal physiological func-

> **Shvāsa (bronchial asthma)** is characterized by sudden attacks of short, gasping breath accompanied by wheezing. This is due to narrowing of the bronchial tree caused by muscle spasms, mucosal swelling or thick, sticky secretions. The normal free movement of air is obstructed within the lungs. Gaseous exchange is hampered and the lungs get stagnated with carbon dioxide which causes undue stimulation of the respiratory center, profuse mucous secretion and an acute awareness of respiratory distress. During shallow expiration, air gets trapped in the lungs and can not be expelled, causing the breathlessness to be more marked. The narrowed bronchi can no longer allow the mucous to be cleared or thrown out by the act of coughing. In a severe, acute asthma attack the bronchi become obstructed by the accumulated tenacious secretion of mucous. This eventually leads to the sensation of tightness in the chest. Progressive alveolar hypo-ventilation (shallow breathing) results in a lack of sufficient oxygen in the blood, possibly culminating in cardiac arrest.

tions of each srotas (channel), the human body utilizes a type of agni called sroto agni. In asthmatic conditions, the agni of prāna vaha srotas becomes low, which is why a person with asthma gets repeated attacks of wheezing and chest colds. In order to kindle this sroto agni, Ayurvedic literature suggests pippalī rasāyana (rejuvenative). Daily take 2 pinches of pippalī (long pepper) with a teaspoon of honey in the morning on an empty stomach. This will help to prevent future asthma attacks.

When the attack is over, the subject should follow the doshic regime properly, do *yoga āsanas,* prānāyāma, and get accurate advice from an experienced Ayurvedic physician.

# Chapter 11

# Urah Shūla

## Chest Pain

Spring 2005, Volume 17, Number 4

HERE WE PRESENT an understanding of the Ayurvedic approach to chest pain, called *urah shūla* in Sanskrit. However, before we study chest pain, we should understand the Ayurvedic concept of pain. *Shūla* means pain in the general sense, but there are synonyms that refer to specific types of pain. For instance, *rujā* means a dull aching pain, *vedana* is radiating pain, and *dukkha* is deep aching or excruciating pain. Pain may be a sign of infection, but there is also non-inflammatory pain, such as congestive pain, stagnation pain, and pain due to physical trauma or psychological factors.

A famous sūtra says: *'Nahi vāta drute shulam,'* which means there is no pain without disturbance of vāta dosha. Vāta is the active, dynamic force that is behind all psycho-physiological and pathological changes. One aspect of vāta dosha is prāna vāyu, which is the life force that governs inhalation and many subtle, mental functions. Udāna is the upward moving form of vāta that brings energy, vitality and memory, and regulates exhalation. Samāna is the subtype of vāta that creates appetite and directs the movements of the gastro-intestinal tract and the processes of digestion, absorption and assimilation of food-stuff. Apāna is located in the pelvic cavity and helps in the elimination of urine, feces and flatus. Finally, vyāna is the type of vāta that governs bodily circulation and movements of the joints. These five subtypes are different vectors of vāta dosha that bring changes in structure and function as related to the physiological activities of vāta. When vāta is *anuloma,* which means it has normal movement, it supports the bodily functions. However, if vāta gets blocked, it becomes *pratiloma* and this creates pain.

Both quantitative and qualitative changes of vāta dosha cause pain. Dry, light, cold, rough, subtle, mobile, clear, and astringent are the qualities of vāta. Any attribute that goes out of balance can create pain. For example, too much exposure to the dry quality can create pain. The opposite of dry is oily, so pain caused by excessive dryness can be decreased by an oil massage. Likewise, if vāta is exposed to extreme cold, that can also create pain. In such a case, the application of local heat will relieve that pain.

Pain is nothing but disturbed vāta dosha, but vāta can be disturbed by a blockage created by pitta, kapha, or āma (metabolic toxins). In all cases, the pain is due to vāta, but if pitta, kapha, or āma is involved, it can be categorized as pitta pain, kapha pain, or āma pain.

Vāta pain means no other dosha is primarily involved. It includes shifting, fluctuating, spasmodic, excruciating, or colicky pain. Vāta pain occurs more during dawn and dusk and it causes fear, anxiety, and insecurity. It is increased by movement and often relieved by the application of heat and oil as well as by rest.

Pitta pain is usually sharp and it can be burning, sucking, or pulling pain with tenderness, which is pain upon pressure. Pitta pain is present in cases of inflammation, ulceration, and even tissue perforation and it is more common during midday and midnight. For instance, a silent peptic ulcer may become violent at midnight. Pitta pain can create irritability, anger, and frustration, and it can be relieved by the application of a cold compress or cooling paste, such as sandalwood or khus.

Deep, dull aching indicates kapha-type of pain. A person can sleep with kapha pain, which manifests due to kapha disorders such as congestion, stagnation and swelling of the tissues. Dry massage, exercise, and other forms of movement can relieve kapha pain. Also helpful is the application of a dry paste, such as vacha powder or ginger powder.

When āma blocks vāta, it creates pain due to indigestion, constipation, and other forms of toxic build-up. Āma pain is aggravated during dawn and dusk, on cloudy days and when it snows. It is also increased by indigestion, constipation, and gas, whereas it can be relieved by fasting and by drinking hot herbal teas such as ginger, cinnamon, and cardamom with a pinch of rock salt. Dīpana and pāchana herbs, such as chitrak and trikatu, are helpful when there is pain due to āma.

## Pain and the Organs and Channels

Ayurveda talks a great deal about doshic pain, but pain is also related to the organs and bodily channels. One common area of pain is chest pain, which may be caused by any dosha and be related to any chest structure such as the heart, lungs, pleura, and intercostal muscles. I will discuss simple treatments for some of the disorders that cause chest pain. All herbal formulas listed below are recommended for use three times daily unless otherwise stated.

The first category of chest pain is pain related to disorders of the lungs and respiratory tract. Some chest pain worsens during inhalation, exhalation, coughing, sneezing, or yawning. This is related to the pleura. Pleuritic pain can be relieved by topical application of an herbal paste that will pacify the disturbed dosha.

Dry pleurisy (vāta) is best treated by the following formula:

| | |
|---|---|
| Dashamūla | 500 mg |
| Pushkaramūla | 400 mg |
| Tagara | 200 mg |

Local application of a turmeric poultice is also useful for dry pleurisy or even a poultice made of fine oatmeal cooked together with turmeric and mustard seeds. This gruel or porridge can be put on a clean cloth or handkerchief and applied topically.

Pitta type of pleuretic pain is pleuritis. It can be treated with:

| | |
|---|---|
| Shatāvarī | 500 mg |
| Gulvel Sattva | 400 mg |
| Pushkaramūla | 300 mg |
| Tagara | 200 mg |

If pleuritis is not treated effectively, it can become pleurisy with effusion, which is a kapha disorder. Mild pleuritic pain is usually accompanied by fever, breathlessness, and diminished air entry, and it can be confirmed by an x-ray. For treatment, give a mixture of:

| | |
|---|---|
| Sitopalādi | 500 mg |
| Punarnavā | 400 mg |
| Pushkaramūla | 200 mg |
| Abhrak Bhasma | 200 mg |

If the pain is severe and there is breathlessness, it is necessary to refer the patient for aspiration. However, the above formulation is suitable for general management of mild kapha-type pleuritic pain.

If there is pleural pain with high fever and tachycardia and the patient looks toxic, it indicates acute pneumonia. Don't treat that person at home. Refer them to a hospital because he or she will need antibiotics. When there is intercostal pain, diminished air entry, mouth breathing, and prominent sternocleiomastoid muscles, think about the possibility it is emphysema and advise the patient to seek expert advice. Finally, any time there is severe breathlessness, immediately send the person to a hospital for a full investigation.

The second category of chest pain is related to the chest wall, due to an injury, trauma, or physical hurt. If this is muscular pain, the intercostal muscles can become extremely painful. Intercostal muscular chest pain can be relieved by topical application of heat and the use of a lepa (paste), such as garlic paste or dashamūla paste. Alternatively, one can rub mahānārāyana oil onto the painful area. Additionally, the person can take shūlah vati (analgesic compound) or shanka vati.

One relatively common injury that causes chest pain is a rib fracture, which gives rise to tenderness in that area and serial pain on breathing. With a fractured rib there will be a history of trauma and there is always a local tender spot. It may be either a recent fracture or an old fracture. If you press the sternum and the backbone together with two hands, the pain worsens with the pressure because the ruptured ends of the ribs actually rub together to create the pain. This is a simple but important clinical test for a fractured rib. Of course, you can also confirm the fracture with an x-ray. Strapping to immobilize the chest may be required for this condition.

During winter or in cold weather, costochondritis is a common cause of anterior pain in the second, third and fourth ribs, giving parasternal or retrosternal tenderness along the border of the sternum. This is a condition of *asthi gata vāta* and giving the following mixture can treat the pain:

| Kaishu Guggulu | 300 mg |
|---|---|
| Tagara | 200 mg |
| Pravāl Pañchāmrit | 200 mg |

Topically, one can apply dashanga lepa, darushatak lepa,[22] or mahānārāyana oil to the chest and place a hot water bottle on the area. This is a simple way to deal with costochondritis with parasternal tenderness.

When the chest is barrel-shaped with intercostal tenderness (along the intercostal muscles) and possibly retrosternal tenderness (behind the sternum) as well as diminished air entry, this is a book picture of emphysema, which is common in chronic smokers. One can give:

| Sitopalādi | 500 mg (for expectoration) |
|---|---|
| Tālīsādi | 400 mg (for decongestion) |
| Mahāsudarshan | 300 mg |
| Abhrak Bhasma | 200 mg |
| Pippalī | 200 mg |

Latākaranja lepa can also relieve the emphysema.

The next category of chest pain is pain in the lower right chest. This indicates an amoebic hepatic abscess, which is related to a liver abscess. Here, an ultrasound can rule out a liver disorder, such as hepatic abscess or cholecystitis. If an amoebic hepatic abscess is the cause, use a combination of Liv 52®, ārogya vardhini, and sūkshma triphalā. Sometimes the person has to be referred to a surgeon to open and drain the abscess.

If there is scarring from healed herpes, there may be post-herpetic pain. Even though the symptoms of herpes zoster have healed, it can leave reddish-brownish spots along the line of the intercostal nerve and cause chest pain. In that case, one has to use the following formula:

| Shatāvarī | 500 mg |
|---|---|
| Gudūchī or Gulvel Sattva | 300 mg |
| Tagara | 300 mg |
| Mahāsudarshan | 300 mg |
| Kāma Dudhā | 200 mg |

Additionally, one can apply a topical paste of sandalwood and turmeric, which are both pitta-soothing herbs.

Chest pain after a meal usually indicates indigestion and gas. However, it could be due to angina. (see cardiac conditions below)

Retrosternal pain that increases when swallowing food may be due to esophagitis or hiatus hernia. Esophagitis is a pitta disorder, so treat the condition with:

| Shatāvarī | 500 mg |
|---|---|
| Gulvel Sattva | 200 mg |
| Shankha Bhasma | 200 mg |
| Kāma Dudhā | 200 mg |

22. Contains, dāruharidrā, mustā, shunthi, red sandalwood, sandalwood, haridrā and other ingredients.

The same treatment can be used for hiatal hernia but you should also teach the client beneficial yoga exercises such as camel pose, cobra pose, and breathing with pressure on the epigastrium, so that the hernia pain is relieved during exhalation.

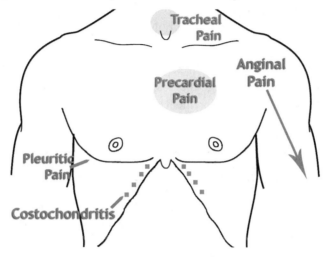

## Hrid Shūla (Cardiac Pain)

A number of disorders can be included in the final broad category of cardiac pain. A common form of cardiac pain is precardial pain (pain in front of heart area) that is usually centered a little to the left side of the chest. Pain may radiate down the left arm or up to the jaw.

If someone presents with cardiac pain, give first aid treatment as appropriate. If the cardiac pain is associated with sweating, restlessness, and falling blood pressure, one should suspect myocardial infarction. If it appears to be aggravated by exertion and relieved with rest, it is angina pain. If any cardiac pain does not subside, send the person to a doctor or hospital. One must take immediate action because a cardiac condition can damage the brain and the person may become unconscious.

Once any severe pain subsides or someone has taken care of an emergency, one can use this formula for cardiac chest pain:

| | |
|---|---|
| Dashamūla | 500 mg |
| Arjuna | 300 mg |
| Abhrak Bhasma | 200 mg |
| Shringa Bhasma | 200 mg |

The best paste is shringa shunthi lepa, which contains deer horn and dry ginger.

For anginal pain, Ayurvedic literature says to rub hema garbha and lakshmī vilas paste onto the tongue. Rub one hema garbha tablet on a sandstone in a circular motion for seven circles of about one-inch diameter, and then do the same for a lakshmī vilas tablet. Mix with just enough water to make a paste and rub it onto the person's tongue. That can immediately relieve angina pain.

Please note, chest pain that appears after a meal could be angina pain, it could be pain due to indigestion and gas, or it could even be cervical spondylosis. Pain in the neck area and jaw down to the chest, along with dizziness when the person looks up, indicates cervical spondylosis. When there is chest pain, a student of Ayurveda must bear in mind all these conditions. Do not take any chest pain lightly, as it may be an acute emergency.

In this chapter, we briefly examined the Ayurvedic understanding of pain and some common causes of chest pain. We also discussed some simple treatments that can be used to effectively ease the pain and manage the doshas, thereby treating the cause of the pain. This is beauty of Ayurvedic pain management.

## Table 3: Understanding Chest Pain

| Nature of Pain | Specific Symptoms | Condition |
|---|---|---|
| Retrosternal pain on left side (precardial pain) | Sweating, restlessness, falling blood pressure | Myocardial infarction |
| Retrosternal pain on left side, radiates down left arm or up to the jaw | Appears on exertion and reduces with rest | Angina |
| Severe unilateral chest pain while breathing, coughing, sneezing or yawning | Causes patient to support chest with palm; shallow breathing | Pleuritis |
| Pain when breathing, coughing, sneezing or yawning | Mild fever and breathlessness | Pleuritis with effusion |
| Pain when breathing, coughing, sneezing or yawning | High fever, tachycardia, toxins | Pneumonia |
| Intercostal pain | Diminished air entry, mouth breathing, and prominent sternocleiomastoids | Emphysema |
| Right side chest pain | Pain mainly in the lower right chest, tender liver | Amoebic hepatic abscess |
| Pain along margin of ribs | History of trauma | Rib fracture |
| Mid-sternal pain | Occurs when swallowing | Esophagitis or Hiatus hernia |
| Neck and jaw pain | Dizziness when looking upwards | Cervical spondylosis |

# Chapter 12

# The Heart

Fall 1996, Volume 9, Number 2

THE HEART IS a maternal muscular organ that contracts and relaxes regularly in order to receive and pump blood through the body. It is closely connected with thoughts, feelings and emotions and is the substratum of individual consciousness. The mental functions of love, devotion and intelligence are related to the heart. It is a vital organ, the abode of ojas and life. The Sanskrit word *hridayam* means the individual heart. Its three root syllables convey the meaning of the word quite significantly. *Hri* means to carry, to convey, to receive; *da* means to give, to donate and *yam* (pronounced yum) means to circulate or to distribute. The heart receives, donates and circulates blood and nutrients throughout the body.

The heart in the Ayurvedic literature is not only an anatomical organ but it includes the concepts of the heart *chakra,* represented by the cardiac plexus, and the heart as the seat of awareness, the substratum of consciousness and consequently the abode of mind. It is a maternal organ, as it is the site of ojas and prāna. It governs the functions of prāna vaha srotas—the system in the body for respiration and the flow of intelligence—and rasa vaha srotas—the system in the body for nutrition and nourishment including blood plasma, the right chamber of the heart and the ten great vessels. The heart is the main reservoir of blood in the cardiovascular system and is essential in the distribution of rasa and rakta dhātus. In the heart, vyāna vāyu, sādhaka pitta, and *avalambaka kapha* express the feeling of self.

अर्थे दश महामूलाः समासक्ता महाफलाः
महद्यार्थश्च हृदयं पर्यायैरुच्यते बुधैः
षडङ्गमङ्गं विज्ञानमिन्द्रियाण्यर्थपञ्चकम्
आत्मा च सगुणश्चेतश्चिन्त्यं च हृदि संश्रितम्

*Ca. Su. 30, 3-4*

The sūtra above, from Charaka Samhita, is quite significant. In it Charak describes the six main parts of the body: the trunk, the four extremities, and the head. The center of these six divisions is the heart. The functional aspects of *buddhi* (intellect), *vijñānam* (specialized knowledge), and the senses are closely connected to the heart. In Sankhya's philosophy mahat is the principle of universal intelligence while, in Ayurveda, it is the individual's reasoning capacity or intellect, whose abode is the heart. Therefore, the heart is also called mahat.

Around the heart is a special membrane called the pericardium, which contains a fluid known as avalambaka kapha. Within the heart, a thin basement membrane, called the endocardium, secretes kapha to aid in the easy passage of blood nutrients throughout the body in order to protect and support all systemic kapha. Avalambaka kapha indirectly nourishes the doors of perceptions through the heart.

In the Charaka Samhita, the commentator goes on describing the heart as:

- a maternal organ
- the site of ojas
- the location of prāna
- the dwelling of vyāna
- the seat of sādhaka pitta
- the source of avalambaka kapha
- the root of rasa vaha srotas
- the beginning of prāna vaha srotas
- the reservoir of blood
- the center of consciousness
- the place of mind
- the seat of feelings and emotions
- the home of self

The ancient Vedic concept of heart is as a mystic lotus with twelve petals, each having its own seed sound, as shown in the picture on the cover. It is a seat of the god Shiva or Rudra. The heart is connected to the ten nadis, which are the five pairs of sensory pathways. These manifest psycho-physiologically as the five cognitive organs existing in pairs—two ears; two eyes; two nostrils; even the tongue is divided in half, the right and the left sides; and the tactile sense of the skin is also located on the right and left sides of the body. Anatomically, there are ten important blood vessels related to heart. The ten great vessels which carry the vital fluid ojas throughout the body are:

- the superior vena cava vein
- the inferior vena cava vein
- the aorta
- the right and left subclavian
- the right and left carotid artery
- the right and left brachial artery
- the coronary vessels

## Ojas and the Heart

These vessels carry ojas (the vital fluid) to individual dhātus (tissues) and to their respective cells to maintain the activities of life. On the subtle cellular level ojas acts as a fuel, where tejas transforms ojas into immunity in order to protect the life energy of cells, called prāna. The heat maintained by the heart acts as the radiant energy of tejas. The flow of life energy is prāna. Without this functional harmony between ojas, tejas, and prāna, the life of a creature is not possible.

The biological essence of all tissues is ojas, which is essential to male and female reproductive tissues. In each sperm and ovum, ojas, tejas, and prāna are present as the cell's basic essential material. These cellular principles are needed for fertilization and later they protect and help the growth of the fetus in the womb. Ojas coordinates the formation of the fetal heart during the third month of pregnancy. That is why the heart is considered the seat of ojas and ojas is the mother of the heart. As the pregnancy progresses, ojas continues to move back and forth from the mother's heart to the heart of fetus. Gradually, the baby begins to communicate to the mother through this flow of ojas. The child in the womb slowly expresses his or her likes and dislikes and this is reflected in the mother's cravings. Ayurveda says that it is quite important to satisfy the pregnant mother's desires at this time, because it will promote the baby's ojas, tejas, and prāna and help the child to develop a healthy heart. On the other hand, if the mother suppresses her cravings and doesn't satisfy her natural biological longings, it may affect the fetal heart and can cause congenital heart conditions.

There are two aspects of ojas. One is apara (raw and unprocessed) and other is para (processed and superfine). The processed and refined ojas is the sustainer of the life of a cell. If a living cell is removed from the body and put under a microscope, it will die in a minute or two because it does not receive ojas to maintain it's life functions. The life sustainer, para ojas, needs raw apara ojas to nourish it. That is why cells perish so quickly when removed from the body.

Superfine, processed ojas is the pure essence of all the tissues. It is formed in the body during the metabolic process. The ingested food undergoes the process of grosser digestion in the gastrointestinal tract due to gastric fire. Later, bhūta agni from the liver begins a more subtle process of digestion culminating in āhāra rasa, the food precursor for the tissues. This food precursor is the *maha phala,* referred to as the juicy fruit in the first line of the sūtra at the beginning of this article. The ten great vessels of the heart carry this maha phala, the fruit of food nutrients, into the six parts of the body—the head, trunk and four extremities. The fire component of individual tissues, called dhātu agni, creates the superfine ojas from the systemic raw ojas. This transformation is governed by the tejas of the individual cell and occurs during the further stages of cellular metabolism, called *pīlu pāka* and *pithara pāka*. The ultimate product of food nutrients after digestion, the pure essence, is ojas, which is a vital factor established in the heart.

## The Etiology of Heart Disorders

The Sanskrit word dhamanī is described in the sūtra as a pulsating, red-colored blood vessel—known today as an artery—that carries blood away from the heart. The word sirā is described as a non-pulsating, bluish-colored vein that carries blood toward the heart. The systemic ojas flows through arteries and veins with the help of vyāna vāyu and maintains the essential movement of life. Excessive worries, anxiety, and stress affect the normal flow of ojas. The ojas may be consumed too fast and weaken the heart. Ayurveda says that the causes of heart disease are overwork, excessive eating, overindulgence in sexual activities, intense grief, sadness, and biochemical stress. When the heart is stressed, ojas becomes depleted and gradually, or suddenly, an individual begins to have signs and symptoms of heart disease, depending upon the severity of the causative factors. Other pathological conditions such as obesity, diabetes, hypertension, and rheumatic conditions may affect the heart. Ayurveda talks about bacterial infections under *krumi hridroga* as one of the etiological factors of heart disease. Functional defects of rasa and rakta vaha srotas can be a major root cause. In spite of these elements, the constitutional doshic imbalance of vāta, pitta and/or kapha is the leading initial causative factor in heart conditions. Diet, lifestyle, genetic factors, and emotional reactions in daily relationships play an important role in many conditions of heart disease mentioned in Ayurvedic literature.

All symptoms can be classified according to vāta, pitta, and kapha. When vāta is predominant, there will be twisting pain, palpitation, breathlessness, and mental confusion. The individual experiences sleeplessness and doesn't tolerate loud noise. Anxiety, fear, and insecurity are the cardinal signs of imbalance in vāta subjects; while nausea, vomiting, fever, and syncope are due to pitta. The pitta individual may feel smoke-like heat in the heart and have profuse sweating and fever with dizzy spells. Increased kapha may be responsible for cough, swelling, dull pain and excess salivation. A sense of heaviness in the heart, anorexia, excessive sleep, and a cold and/or cough may manifest in kapha-type individuals. A sudden heart attack that comes and goes is vāta type. In connection with heart disease inflammation, fever and profuse sweating indicate a pitta type of heart condition. While slow, progressive congestive cardiac failure with edema belongs to kapha-type heart problems. Owing to the nature of causes, dual or triple symptoms may manifest. If the cause is worms, then the individual may get a throbbing, cutting pain in the heart with fever, anorexia, and cyanosis. Congenital mitral valve prolapse is a vāta-type heart disease as well as rheumatic valvular heart diseases.

### Samprāpti (pathogenesis)

If there are causes that provoke vāta, then vāta from the colon undergoes sanchaya (accumulation), prakopa (aggravation) and prasara (spread), thereby entering into general circulation. If the heart has been weakened by the factors mentioned above, the circulating dosha finally lodges in the heart and produces vāta-type heart conditions indicated by one or more of the following symptoms: churning, pricking, or stabbing pain in the heart area, breathlessness, fear and cold sweat. On the other hand, if the causes are pitta-provoking, then pitta from the intestines undergoes the same changes of sanchaya, prakopa and prasara and lodges in the heart, producing typical pitta symptoms such as sharp, burning pains in the heart, nausea, vomiting ,and syncope. Kapha dosha, owing to its causative factors, also moves away from the stomach and enters the heart producing a sense of heaviness, tightness in the heart, anorexia, edema, or congestive heart failure. On entering the heart, these doshas affect ojas, tejas, and prāna within the heart. Initially the presence of the aggravated doshas in the heart creates functional changes and subsequently more serious structural changes.

The cardinal signs of heart disease are:
* *vaivarnya* – discoloration, cyanosis, due to poor circulation
* *mūrchā* – syncope, transient loss of consciousness, owing to sādhaka pitta disorder
* jvara – fever, due to the entry of pitta into the rasa dhātu

- *kāsa* – cough, congestion of prāna vaha srotas
- *hikkā* – hiccough, owing to ischemia of diaphragm
- *shvāsa* – breathlessness, prāna vatadysfunction
- *āsya vairasya* – perverted taste in the mouth, due to bodhaka kapha dysfunction
- *trushnā* – excess thirst owing to congestion of palate
- *pramoha* – mental confusion due to lack of pranato the brain
- *chhardi* – vomiting, pāchaka pitta disorder
- rujā – cardiac pain, congestion of heart muscles

## General Management

Even though heart disease is a serious condition, with the help of your cardiologist you can monitor your heart condition while using the Ayurvedic remedies that follow in a preventative manner.

Arjuna powder enhances the tone of the heart muscle.

Katukā powder improves coronary circulation.

Ashvagandhā helps to protects the ojas in the māmsa dhātu.

Punarnavā a mild diuretic that helps to regulate blood pressure.

Gudūchī is anti-inflammatory and anti-pyritic.

Shatāvarī is a general rejuvenative tonic for the heart muscle.

Triphalā is a colon cleanser and detoxifier.

Pippalī is a broncho dilator and relieves pulmonary congestion.

Shringa Bhasma is a specific cardiac tonic that improves the tone of the heart muscle, increases oxygenation of the heart and relieves cardiac ischemia.

Dashamūla is a general tonic for all bodily dhātus, but is specifically effective for calming vāta and reduces palpitations.

Lasuna (garlic) is used as a seasoning in the food, reduces cholesterol and has pain-killing properties.

Onion (cooked) is also used as a seasoning in the food and reduces heart rate, acting in a manner similar to digitalis.

Gold Water improves coronary vaso-dilation, coronary circulation, and protects the heart muscle from dying. It is made by boiling 24 carat gold (coin or your own jewelry) in 2 cups of water. Boil this down to one cup of liquid. Take 1 teaspoon every 15 minutes.

Yashthi Madhu is a decongestant, expectorant and helps ease breathing.

Yoga Postures: Sun Salutations (10 postures done in a specific order) is an ancient Vedic cardio-vascular exercise. One should gradually work up to repeating the cycle 12 times per day. Yoga postures increase the movement of prāna and help the processing of ojas by tejas into the protection of prāna. Every yoga posture has therapeutic value as it enhances tone, coordination and power of the muscles. Some that are helpful in cardiac conditions are: camel, cobra, cow, boat, bow, bridge, tree, triangle, and corpse poses.

Mantra meditation: Sound is energy and every cell has an affinity toward certain sounds. When one repeats a particular sound, the cell recognizes it and becomes harmonious. Cellular function becomes rhythmic, bringing a balance in the rhythm of the cell. To balance vāta, the mantra is *hrim*, pronounced "hreem." For pitta, *aim*—"I'm." For kapha, *klim*— "kleem." And for the heart chakra, *yam*—"yum."

Walking for ½ an hour is good cardio-vascular exercise. It helps to improve circulation, kindles fire and reduces cholesterol. It is an exercise that is mild enough for anyone to perform.

Rudrāksha beads have a spiritual energy to protect the heart chakra. They improve coronary circulation and give spiritual support to the patient of heart disease.

Rose Quartz bead necklaces improve warmth in the heart and are recommended for vāta- and kapha-type conditions.

Limited sexual activity decreases the wasting of vital fluid which is eliminated during the secretion of orgasmic fluid. This will indirectly protect one's ojas and prāna.

Herbal wines, like *drākshā,* kindle agni, performs vaso-dilation, improves circulation and is good for the heart. Take 4 teaspoons with an equal amount of warm water before meals.

Regular checkups with your doctor.

# Chapter 13

# An Ayurvedic Perspective on Fevers

## Jvara Roga

Fall 1997, Volume 10, Number 2

The concept of fever in Ayurvedic literature is interesting. The Sanskrit quote, *"Jvara deha indriya manasa santapa"* means that fever is heat in the mind and senses as well as the physical rise of body temperature. *Deha* is the physical body; *indriya,* the senses; *manas,* the mind; and *santapa* means heat.

There is a wonderful Vedic story about fever. Lord Shiva was in deep meditation on Mount Kailas. There was a demon known as Tripurasura. *Tri* means three and *pura* means city, so his name refers to the 'three cities' of body, mind, and consciousness. This demon was destroying these cities and only Shiva could stop Tripurasura. But Shiva was in deep *samādhi,* a transcendental state of meditation. Who would disturb his samādhi? All the gods were worried. When Shiva is in samādhi, no one should disturb him. So the God of Love, Madana, said, "I will disturb the samādhi of Lord Shiva." By his magnetic power, Madana created a wonderful garden with birds, swans, a lake, lotus, peacocks, and beautiful fragrant flowers.

Then Madana started throwing arrows of flowers toward Lord Shiva. Symbolically, an arrow is an object of perception. Arrows of flowers are symbolically arrows of senses— sight, smell, sound, taste and touch. In other words, the God of Love was stimulating Shiva's senses while he was in a deep state of meditation. Shiva opened his third eye, the eye of wisdom, and fire came through it and burned Madana. Madana's wife, Rati, whose name means romance, came to Shiva and prayed, "Lord Shiva, you have killed my husband and I am now a widow." Lord Shiva, being full of mercy and compassion, looked at the ashes with intense love and Madana came back to life. The Fire God, who had been burning Madana, came out of his body and said to Shiva, "Where can I go now? You have created me through your third eye and my job is to burn. Where can I go?" Lord Shiva said, "Go to the earth and afflict those people who do not follow the laws of nature, the laws of health." Those laws of nature refer to following a daily and seasonal routine, eating a proper diet, and avoiding abuse of the senses. Those who do not follow these rules become ill.

Since then, fever has been on this planet. This is a mystic story, but it tells us the truth that fever happens to those who eat the wrong food, indulge in excessive physical activity, and otherwise burn their ojas. Fever also happens to those who are consumed by excessive sensual temptation, which burns the body's intelligence and immunity.

## The Stages of Fever

Anger, hate, envy, jealousy, and criticism provoke a kind of fire in the consciousness. This is a type of feverishness that affects the mind. According to Ayurveda, fever begins with judgment and criticism. For example, when you feel that your husband or wife is support-ive of you, fever is absent. However, the moment you feel that your partner is confused or critical or that the relationship is not working in your favor, you become furious. That furiousness may become a physical fever. There is even a fever of love. When you fall in love and sing, "I'm crazy for you, I'm dying for you," it is a sort of fever. A newly married couple can get honeymoon urethritis or cervicitis and may even develop a fever called *kāma jvara*.

Before the rise of body temperature, the senses become agitated and then the mind gets confused. This confusion leads to improper food choices. For example, in the summer you may work all day in the hot sun and your body may become hot. Then if you come home and drink chilled water, it is a shock to the system. Ayurveda says to drink warm or room temperature water, even in summer. When you are hot from working outside, wait a bit before rushing to the refrigerator. Give your body time to cool down and then take a sip of room temperature water. People tend to drink cold fluids when the body is hot. This shock to the system affects agni and displaces ojas.

Consuming fluids in this way is similar in its effects to incompatible food combining, such as eating bananas with milk, yogurt with fruit, melon with grains, fruits with cheese or milk, and eating dairy products with meat. Such combinations affect agni and create āma (toxins). Then samāna vāyu pushes āma and pāchaka pitta (the gastric fire) out of the stomach into rasa dhātu and produces fever.

### Explanations of Fever: Modern and Ancient

Fever is a disease in itself, but it can also be the symptom of another disease. Accord-ing to ancient Vedic science, the entry of dosha and āma into rasa dhātu creates fever. Whichever dosha goes into the rasa tissue will create a specific type of doshic fever.

According to Ayurveda, there are many kinds of fever, including continuous and interrupted fevers, such as when a person runs a fever every second or third day. Fever is classified as mono, dual or triple doshic—vāta, pitta or kapha type, or vāta-pitta, pitta-kapha, or kapha-vāta, or even vāta-pitta-kapha type of fever. Triple doshic fever can be compared with septicemia in modern medicine.

When fever is itself the disease, modern science calls it a fever of non-specific origin. In such cases, there is no septic infection in the body, urine and blood cultures are normal, and there is no strep throat. This fever of non-specific origin is called *jvara roga* in Ayur-veda. It is caused simply by the entry of āma into rasa dhātu, the plasma-protein pathway. There is an origin, but it is different from that understood by the modern definition, which has a septic focus. According to modern medicine, fever is a sign of infection such as

Samāna vāyu pushes āma and pāchaka pitta (the gastric fire) out of stomach and into rasa dhātu, producing fever.

acute conditions of tonsillitis, pharyngitis, bronchitis, pneumonitis, hepatitis, cystitis, or meningitis.

Some people feel feverish but the thermometer doesn't show a rise of temperature. They are running an internal fever. This is called internal jvara. Such a person has the cardinal signs of fever—headache, bodyache, and malaise, but the skin is cool to the touch. According to the thermometer, there is no fever, but Ayurveda says the person has an internal fever.

How can there be internal fever without a rise of temperature? This condition causes a subjective feeling of feverishness, whereby the person may feel heat going out of the eyes or ears and even the breath becomes hot. The person *feels* on fire, but the external temperature is cool. In these cases, āma and pitta are moving in the sthāyi rasa dhātu, the fully processed rasa tissue. Some people have a burning sensation while passing urine without a clinical diagnosis of urethritis. That is also a symptom of internal fever. Internal fever creates canker sores, fever blisters, or aches and pain in the lymphatic system. When the samprāpti of fever affects mano vaha srotas, the mind becomes irritable, judgmental, critical, and even furious. This is a fever in the mind. There are people who have an internal fever but they do not know it. They continue to take fever suppressants, such as acetaminophen and aspirin, and the cause is never treated.

## Signs and Symptoms of Fever

Ayurveda says that kapha fever begins in the stomach, pitta fever starts in the small intestine, and vāta type in the colon. In a fever, the dosha undergoes sanchaya (accumulation), prakopa (provocation) and prasara (spread).[23] When the dosha goes into the second stage, prakopa, it will disturb agni, creating toxins. In the third stage, prasara, the dosha will push that āma into rasa dhātu and create fever.

During a fever there is no appetite, because jāthara agni is pushed into rasa dhātu and is no longer present in the stomach. This lack of fire in the stomach creates āma. However there is too much fire in rasa dhātu, which enters into mano vaha srotas, the mental channels, and causes fever in the mind. Mental fever can be due to incompatible food combining, wrong lifestyle and diet, and the application of extremes of hot and cold, such as a hot shower followed by cold shower. If it is vāta fever, the person experiences fear and anger together. Anger has the qualities of fire, while fear is vāta. If a person has a kapha fever, he or she experiences greed or attachment along with anger. Pure pitta fever is mainly anger and irritation.

In fever there is no sweating—except in pitta type of fever—because āma clogs *sveda vaha srotas,* the channels of perspiration. This āma also creates generalized bodyache. A function of rasa dhātu is nutrition. Because rasa dhātu is not functioning properly during a fever, there is poor cellular nutrition and the tissues suffer from lack of nourishment. When nutrition of the dhātus is affected, the body and the internal organs start aching. Even the hair aches, because āma in rasa affects the skin at the roots of the hair. These three signs must happen together: internal heat, lack of perspiration, and generalized bodyache. Then you can say that it is jvara. These cardinal signs of fever indicate that the dosha and āma are moving in rasa and looking for a place to stay.

### Prodromal Symptoms

Two of the symptoms of fever are low appetite and feverishness. What are the prodromal symptoms before a fever begins? The person feels exhausted and fatigued. He or she doesn't feel OK with his or her life or with anything. There is no charm in life. A smoker doesn't feel like smoking. A drinker doesn't feel like drinking. There is an aversion toward external sensory stimuli. If it is a vāta type of fever that is coming, the person's skin looks dark. If it is pitta type, the skin appears flushed. If kapha type, the skin is pale. This discoloration is because of āma moving in rasa dhātu. There is no sense of taste in the mouth, because taste comes from agni. The taste of food lies not only in the food but also in the quality of agni.

Frequent yawning and goosebumps also presage a vāta fever. Hot flashes, burning, and dizziness as well as a burning sensation in the eyes indicate a potential pitta fever. Chills, runny nose, and loss of appetite are present before kapha fever manifests. Apathy can lead to fever, as can too much sympathy. Intense crying and grief can also create a fever.

Another indication of fever is constant lacrimation or tears in the eyes. Those tears are hot at one moment and cold the next. At one moment the person wants food, while the next moment all desire to eat has gone. Or the person feels like watching TV and then loses that desire. At one moment the person feels chilled and sits by the fire, then the next moment he becomes hot and throws off the blankets. Or craves cold things, but the

---

23. See Table 1, "Gunas (Qualities) Relating to Each Stage of Samprāpti," on page 7.

moment he touches cold, he craves heat. In the prasara stage of āma, when toxins are circulating, these opposite symptoms occur. Some people can experience these prodromal symptoms of pūrva rūpa for a considerable period of time.

*Vāta Fever.* In vāta fever there is constipation, shivering, and a craving to be bundled in many blankets. There is also generalized bodyache, headache, ringing in the ears and muscle stiffness. The symptoms are similar to malaria. Vāta fever creates insomnia, anxiety, headache, muscle pain, and joint ache. Many times vāta fever is diagnosed as rheumatic fever. The pulse is fast and temperature is not that high, just 99.5 to 99.7 degrees Fahrenheit.

*Pitta Fever.* In a pitta type of fever, there is a high temperature of 102 to 103 degrees, bloodshot eyes, and temporal headache. The person is irritable and throws off the blankets. There is nausea, vomiting, nosebleed, and dark yellow urine. The body is hot. Some pitta prakruti children get convulsions when they have fever. There is photophobia and sometimes diarrhea or dysentery. In pitta fever there is sweating, but that sweat doesn't bring down the temperature.

*Kapha Fever.* Kapha fever is accompanied by a cold, congestion, and cough. The temperature is not that high and sleep is not a problem, because a person can sleep with a low-grade kapha fever. There is a runny nose, excess salivation and no appetite.

*Other Fevers.* Continuous fever is present in acute rheumatic fever, typhoid, septicemia, and tuberculosis. In typhoid, fluctuations of temperature are also present. In the morning there is a rise of temperature and in the evening the temperature comes down. Sometimes the high temperature appears twice, in the morning and evening, and the temperature comes down only during midday. This is typical of a vāta type of fever. The interruption is due to fluctuations of the dosha. Some people will have a fever on every second or third day.

# Fever in the Dhātus

Fever can go into each of the biological tissues, or dhātus: rasa (plasma), rakta (blood), māmsa (muscle), meda (fat and adipose), asthi (bone), majjā (bone marrow and nerve), and shukra/ārtava (male/ female reproductive). By studying the fifth level radial pulse you can find exactly where the fever is lodged.

*Rasa Dhātu.* When fever is in rasa dhātu, the person has kapha symptoms—heaviness in the heart, congestion in the lungs, generalized bodyache, and excess salivation. The by-product of rasa dhātu is stanya (lactation) and *raja* (menstruation) and the waste product of rasa is kapha—hence, the kapha symptoms. When āma goes into rasa dhātu and creates fever, these symptoms appear. Even if the predominant dosha is vāta, the symptoms will be mainly kapha, although in that case, the rasa dhātu pulse will show a vāta spike. Rasa dhātu has kapha characteristics, so any dosha that goes into rasa dhātu during a fever creates kapha symptoms. However, in a vāta type fever there will be less congestion, in a pitta type more inflammation, and in kapha more congestion.

Palpitations and swelling in the heart or lungs are also common when fever goes into rasa dhātu. If it is vāta fever, there will be more palpitations. Pitta fever will create inflammation of the heart. If it is kapha fever, there will be pericardial effusion.

***Rakta Dhātu.*** When rasa is strong, it will not allow āma or a dosha to enter. Then the āma and dosha will go to rakta, the next dhātu. If rakta dhātu agni is low, the āma will enter rakta and create the following symptoms: bleeding of the nose, mouth, stomach or lungs, vomiting with blood, dizziness, delirium, or hemorrhage under the skin. When fever goes into rakta vaha srotas, it creates bleeding. But in vāta, the bleeding is scanty and will be accompanied by clots and more palpitations, in pitta there is more bleeding and in kapha there is bleeding with mucus.

***Māmsa Dhātu.*** If rakta dhātu agni is strong, then āma will go to māmsa dhātu. If māmsa dhātu agni is low, āma will lodge in māmsa and create *māmsa gata jvara,* which means fever in māmsa dhātu. This fever produces symptoms of bursitis, tendonitis, or fibromyocitis. Many people today have a form of fibromyocitis called fibromyalgia, inflammation of the muscle sheath. Individuals who take synthetic estrogen disturb their māmsa dhātu agni and may develop māmsa gata jvara or fibromyalgia. These people can also have acne, hives, rash, and boils.

***Meda Dhātu.*** In *meda gata jvara* there is profuse, foul smelling sweat, dehydration, and pain in the kidneys or omentum, the fatty protective layer around the abdomen. This condition can create peritonitis, which indicates the fever has gone into meda dhātu.

***Asthi Dhātu.*** If fever has gone into asthi dhātu, there will be pain in the joints and bones as well as hair loss. The nails become brittle and the person may lose teeth.

***Majjā Dhātu.*** *Majjā gata jvara* leads to rigidity in the neck. Meningitis and encephalitis are serious problems of majjā gata jvara. The person gets headache, meningeal irritation, stiff jaw, and tightness in the neck; he or she may become irritable or even lose consciousness.

***Shukra/Ārtava Dhātu.*** When fever goes into shukra dhātu, the person burns ojas and death is sure. Any fever can go into any of the dhātus and create serious complications. Therefore, don't take fever lightly, as it can become serious.

If a patient of fever comes to you, read the pulse and examine the patient. If the person shivers with cold, it is a vāta fever. The subject may subsequently have light bleeding of the nose, but with a little bit of clotting. At that point, the vāta fever has gone into rakta dhātu. If within three days, the subject gets pain in the muscles, the fever has gone into māmsa dhātu. If the person comes to you within the next four days with pain in the joints, the vāta fever has gone into asthi dhātu. This is the logical progression of an untreated vāta fever through the dhātus.

## The Role of Bacteria, Viruses, and Āma

The modern scientific approach says that bacteria or viruses induce disease. Ayurveda says if you eat incompatible foods until your tongue becomes heavily coated, then depending on your level of immunity, you may get a fever. If you really want to have a fever, eat banana milkshakes or fish with yogurt for a couple of weeks. The results depend upon your gastric fire, agni. Ayurveda also thinks along the same lines as Western medicine in this way. Western medicine posits that a bacteria or virus creates an infection, subsequently causing a fever. Ayurveda says that one cause of fever is bacteria and viruses, which create āma on the cellular level. That āma is circulated through rasa dhātu and creates fever.

If tubercular bacteria are introduced into a person's system, that person may not get pulmonary tuberculosis, but rather bone TB or some other type of TB. This is explained by the Ayurvedic concept of khavaigunya, defective space. If there is khavaigunya in the lungs, the person will get tuberculosis in the lungs. If it is in the knee joint, that person will get TB of the knee joint. What Ayurveda wants to convey is that fever is the entry of āma into the dhātu, not the direct result of bacteria or viruses.

# General Management

Whenever an individual has fever, the first treatment is fasting, *langhana*. If the person eats, that food will not be digested but will instead produce more āma and toxins. Whenever there is fever, starve it. The kapha person should take nothing by mouth. This is difficult for vāta and pitta people, who may become dehydrated. There is an herbal tea that induces swedana (sweating) and it can be drunk during langhana. Use equal proportions of ginger, lemongrass, tulsi, and fennel and steep this mixture in hot water for 10 to 15 minutes. The ginger will burn āma and kindle agni; lemongrass is diaphoretic and will promote sweating; tulsi is decongestant and anti-pyretic; and fennel stimulates pāchana, the burning of āma. Just by kindling agni and burning āma, the fever will come back to normal. This is a simple home remedy.

When a person has fever, it takes time to make the body work and regain balance. One should not just take aspirin to bring down the temperature. A person with fever should wait, rest, sleep, and bundle up with blankets. Give the above tea. There should be no reading, watching TV, or talking on the telephone.

Once the person passes an entire day without fever, give softly cooked rice water. Use two cups of water and only a handful of rice. Make a soft gruel, which will be easy to digest. That should be given when the person regains the urge to eat. Generally, a person with a kapha fever has no appetite. Pitta people may become hungry, because pitta is hot, sharp, and penetrating. Because of those qualities, pitta people have strong fever. They may also feel dizziness, nausea, and vomiting, and if these symptoms are present there is no urge to eat. Vāta people with fever have variable appetites.

### Specific Doshic Management

*Vāta Jvara.* For a vāta person you can use this herbal tea:

| | |
|---|---|
| Dashamūla | 500 mg |
| Sudarshan | 400 mg |
| Tagara | 300 mg (for headache) |

Put 1 teaspoon of this mixture in a cup of hot water, let it steep for 10 minutes and then drink it. For headache, put ginger or calamus root paste on the forehead. A nutmeg powder paste on the forehead is also helpful. Never do oleation (snehana) during fever.

A vāta type of fever subsides simply with rest. Cover the patient with two or three blankets and keep the room warm. Give hot herbal tea. For vāta fever, svedana can be more intense. Even under two or three blankets, a vāta person tends to shiver and feel cold.

These treatments are effective, but your diagnosis must be accurate. If you use the wrong tea, it could increase the temperature. Be cautious. Ayurveda is not simplistic; it requires understanding and knowledge of basic principles.

**Pitta Jvara.** For pitta jvara give:

| | |
|---|---|
| Gulvel Sattva | 400 mg |
| Mahāsudarshan | 400 mg |
| Kāma Dudhā | 200 mg |

Take 1 teaspoon, two or three times a day, with warm water, to pacify pitta. In a pitta fever, svedana should be gentle. The pitta subject should be in a closed warm room with dimmed lights, because a bright light will create a headache. Pitta people throw off the blankets because they are hot, but they should cover the body with something light, such as a cotton sheet. If pitta people have too high a fever, they can become delirious or have convulsions. To bring down temperature, sponge them with tepid rose or khus water. Or take white sandalwood powder, add a little cool water, make a paste and apply it to the forehead. Camphor can also be used if the person is not sensitive to it. Mix the camphor with some cool water, dip a cloth into that camphor water and put it on the forehead to bring down the temperature.

**Kapha Jvara.** In the kapha type of jvara, there is a cold, congestion, cough, runny nose, postnasal drip and bronchial secretions with bronchitis or pneumonitis. For kapha fever, svedana can be more intense. For this condition you can use:

| | |
|---|---|
| Sitopalādi | 500 mg |
| Mahāsudarshan | 300 mg |
| Abrak Bhasma | 200 mg |

Take ½ to 1 teaspoon of this mixture two or TID. When a person has bronchial congestion and secretion with a cough, you can use vāsaka, which acts like codeine, to sedate irritation of the cough center. Give ½ teaspoon TID.

Give the above treatments for four or five days. Fever from flu will come down within three days. If it is bronchitis, it must be treated for five to eight days. Pneumonia will take 10 days. It is a potentially serious condition and this formula should be used with the approval of your physician. For a child, use the same treatments, but with a smaller dose.

Influenza is a vāta and kapha disorder. You can use:

| | |
|---|---|
| Sitopalādi | 500 mg |
| Mahāsudarshan | 400 mg |
| Tagara | 300 mg |

This combination brings down temperature and soothes body aches. Ideally, a person should not take a bath during a fever or flu. Taking a bath may make the lungs damp and cold, potentially causing pneumonia. Once the fever has been gone for a couple of days, then take a shower. Similarly, when a baby has high fever, sponge the baby with tepid water but don't give him a bath. For high fever in children, grate an onion and divide the pulp into two parts. Put one part of the onion pulp in a cloth soaked in hot water, then fold the cloth and place it on the belly button. Wrap the other half of the onion pulp in another hot, wet cloth and place it on the forehead. Onion pulp on the forehead and the belly button can bring down temperature within 20 minutes. This can be used with children as well as with adults.

When a person has extreme thirst, make an herbal tea out of equal parts of cumin, coriander, and fennel. This tea relieves thirst, stimulates agni and digestion, burns āma, and improves the taste in the mouth. Another combination for extreme thirst during fever is tea made of mustā, khus, sandalwood, and ginger in equal parts. This tea will relieve dehydration, especially in a pitta type of fever. The same mixture is good in a kapha type of fever, if there is nausea and vomiting. Kapha nausea and vomiting is mucous type, whereas in pitta it is bilious.

There are certain fruits that bring down temperature. For pitta and vāta, use pomegranate, cranberry, or purple grape juice, or sugarcane juice. Give a light diet with no cheese, yogurt, ice cream, or heavy meat. Never eat animal flesh during a fever. It will not be digested and will produce āma.

A cup of lemongrass and cilantro tea with a teaspoon of honey is anti-pyretic and also tridoshic. The lemongrass is good for vāta, the cilantro acts on pitta and kapha, and honey is a good anupāna.

If a person with pitta fever has diarrhea, use ½ teaspoon of kutaja. If you don't have kutaja, then cook an apple and mash it. Add a pinch of nutmeg and cardamom and a teaspoon of ghee. Cooked apple is a good source of pectin, which will help to control diarrhea.

In fever, don't use lemon, lime, or any sour juice. They increase pitta and kapha and will create congestion, cold, and cough.

Chronic fever continues because of the debility of the body and dhātus. Hence, one should maintain a diet that will promote the strength of the dhātus. If the tissues are weak, give:

| | |
|---|---|
| Shatāvarī | 500 mg |
| Balā | 400 mg |
| Ashvagandhā | 300 mg |

This is used as a rasāyana (rejuvenative) to strengthen the dhātus. If the weakness is still there, the person may get *dhātu jvara* related to tissue deficiency. In all types of chronic fever, it is beneficial to give a teaspoon of tikta ghrita (bitter ghee) TID, followed by ½ cup of warm water. This will protect ojas and promote the strength of the dhātus.

*Please Note:* Although fever results from the entry of tridosha into rasa dhātu, there may be a serious viral or bacterial infection. One should always consult with one's physician to rule out these possibilities.

## Chapter 14

# An Ayurvedic Perspective on Hypertension

## Sirābhinodhana and Dhamanī Pratichaya

Summer 1993, Volume 6, Number 1

HYPERTENSION IS A MODERN TERM, but in ancient Vedic literature there is a description of something similar. That condition is called *sirābhinodhana*. Sirā means the blood vessels and *abhinodhana* means tension, which corresponds to the modern concept of hypertension. Sirābhinodhana is a condition where venous blood stagnates and exerts pressure on the blood vessel wall. When pitta is involved, venous hypertension may lead to varicose veins, hematomas, and a tendency to bruise easily. The literature also describes *dhamanī pratichaya,* which means increased intra-arterial pressure. Dhamanī pratichaya corresponds more closely to arterial hypertension, and sirābhinodhana indicates venous hypertension.

When referring to hypertension, modern medicine does not give much importance to the veins, only the arteries. In Ayurveda, venous circulation is related to rasa dhātu and all nutrients enter into the veins. The chyle duct, which carries the end products of digested material from the gastro-intestinal tract, opens into the subclavian vein. The venous system is connected to the arterial system via the heart, which is the junction between venous and arterial circulation. The heart is a most vital organ, not only pumping the oxygenated blood, but also receiving venous blood.

Venous blood that comes into the heart has received food nutrients through the subclavian vein. The blood is then carried through the pulmonary artery from the heart to the lungs, where it is oxygenated, and then through the pulmonary vein back to the heart. The Ayurvedic concept of hypertension includes both venous and arterial circulations. Ayurvedic literature states that dhamanī pratichaya (arterial hypertension), the type most commonly referred to, is a tridoshic disorder.

## Doshic Types of Hypertension

The main site of vāta in the human body is the colon. When there are toxins in the colon, they can be absorbed into the blood and may cause constriction of the blood vessels, especially the arteries. Detoxifying the colon can treat this kind of hypertension. Psychologically, it is often associated with fear, anxiety, stress, and insecurity, which may lead to constriction of the blood vessel walls and produce hypertension.

In Ayurveda, the small intestine is the seat of pitta. Toxins from undigested foodstuff in the intestines produce āma, which moves into the general circulation. Hypertension of this type is due to increased viscosity of the blood. Bile is pitta in nature and this fatty, oily substance makes the blood viscous. Because of its increased viscosity, the blood exerts pressure on the blood vessels. In this pitta type of hypertension, the person may exhibit psychological symptoms of judgment, criticism, anger, hate, envy, and jealousy. These emotions themselves can also trigger an increase in blood pressure.

Kapha type of hypertension originates in the stomach, which is the main site of kapha. Kapha-like gastric mucosal secretions are involved in the digestion of carbohydrates, starch, and glucose. The end products of this phase of digestion are triglycerides. When kledaka kapha from the stomach is disturbed, there is an increase in triglycerides and cholesterol (also kapha molecules). The result is that the blood becomes more viscous. This kapha type of hypertension causes fatty molecules to deposit on the blood vessel walls, which leads to narrowing of the arteries (arterial sclerosis) and possible heart attack.

Another important factor in hypertension is the functioning of the kidneys, which regulate the entire water system in the body. In Ayurveda, the kidneys belong to mūtra vaha srotas, the urinary system. Urine (mūtra) has the important function of carrying excess kledaka kapha out of the body. People who do not sweat sufficiently can also accumulate excess kledaka. There is no equivalent word for kledaka kapha in modern medicine, but it may be responsible for secretion of chemicals known as vasopressins. These stimulate the adrenals and in excess can lead to hypertension. Various urinary dysfunctions may also lead to hypertension. Acute glomerulonephritis is due to excess pitta in the kidney; hydronephrosis is caused by excess kapha in the kidney; and renal failure, which leads to total absence of urinary function, is due to the dryness of vāta dosha. All of these conditions may lead to hypertension.

## Ayurvedic Diagnosis

Ayurvedic texts describe three types of hypertension: vāta, which begins in the colon; pitta, which starts in the small intestine; and kapha, which originates in the stomach. Although there are seven classical types of dhamanī pratichaya, these basic three types can be diagnosed through the clinical barometers of inspection, palpation, and auscultation. For example, the vāta type of hypertension, which begins with toxins in the colon, constricts the musculature of the blood vessels. Pitta usually affects rakta dhātu (blood tissue) and the kapha type generally affects rasa dhātu (plasma).

Traditional Ayurvedic pulse diagnosis assesses blood pressure by feeling the velocity of the blood flow. In vāta hypertension, the radial pulse will be feeble, empty, and superficial, with prominent throbbing felt under the palpating index finger. The person might also have anxiety, nervousness,, and tachycardia. The diastolic blood pressure will be relatively higher than the systolic pressure, which indicates vāta type of hypertension. In addition, the tongue may become dry and the person might have insomnia. The lower eyelids may also be swollen and there will be constipation. If you give dashamūla basti, all of these symptoms will likely subside. This vāta type of hypertension is often temporary.

In pitta type of hypertension, the radial pulse will be felt most predominantly under the middle palpating finger, and it has a collapsing nature, with high volume and low tension, along with full, bounding, hot qualities. Both the systolic and diastolic blood pressures are high. As a general rule, a person's age plus 100 is the optimal systolic blood pressure. Hence, if a person's age is 30, the systolic pressure should be approximately 130 and if a person is 50, the pressure should be around 150. The diastolic pressure should normally be around 90. In this pitta type of hypertension, the person might get hot flashes, a red nose, and prominent blood vessels. Sometimes the person bruises easily and has headaches, dizziness, nausea, vomiting, or nosebleeds. These people are also prone to bloodshot eyes, retinal hemorrhage or cerebral hemorrhage. Pitta hypertension can be a dangerous acute situation needing prompt medical treatment, or it may cause serious cerebral vascular accidents (CVA).

In kapha type of hypertension, the person is often overweight or obese and may have an underactive thyroid gland. In this kapha condition the pulse is best felt under the ring finger, and it is slow, deep, full and wavy or watery in quality. In kapha type of hypertension, both the diastolic and systolic blood pressures increase somewhat, but the diastolic pressure remains steadier. It may be between 85 to 90. The person may also be diabetic, because hypertension with diabetes is a kapha condition. People with this condition tend to get edema and frequency of urination and there may also be diabetic retinopathy, cardiopathy, renopathy, or cerebropathy. Kapha type of hypertension is as serious as vāta type and this condition may even become what is called malignant hypertension.

Vāta-kapha type of hypertension is another form. It causes blood clots (thrombosis). This can be very serious, as it may cause a sudden cerebral or pulmonary embolism or heart attack.

Ayurveda has also explained some of the complications of dhamanī pratichaya and sirābhinodhana. These disorders may lead to cardiac complications (*hridrogam*) or, if they affect the higher cerebral blood vessels, can lead to paralysis, Bell's palsy, stroke paralysis or, in pitta conditions, cerebral hemorrhage. The Ayurvedic concept of hypertension understands the condition as a whole. Not every hypertensive case should be treated with diuretics, which are effective only in some kapha types of hypertension.

## Ayurvedic Recommendations

Ayurvedic literature has specific recommendations for each type of hypertension and its corresponding samprāpti (etiology). In general, a person with hypertension should follow a lifestyle and diet that reduces the primary dosha. In addition to this there should be no consumption of caffeine, salt, sugar, or fatty, fried foods. Deep breathing, daily walks of three miles, and meditation are all beneficial as well.

*Vāta Remedies.* The samprāpti of vāta hypertension begins in the colon and the second chakra due to repressed fear, anxiety and insecurity. Ayurvedic literature says that one should treat the colon, the main seat of vāta, using dashamūla basti, which is an enema made of dashamūla tea. Herbs like kaishore guggulu, yogarāja guggulu, or sarpagandha may help to reduce hypertension and regulate blood pressure, while pañchakarma is also useful, followed by a vāta pacifying diet and lifestyle. In addition, the following herbal program is suggested.

1. An herbal mixture of:

| | |
|---|---|
| Dashamūla | 500 mg |
| Ashvagandhā | 500 mg |
| Shatāvarī | 200 mg |
| Tagara | 200 mg |

¼ teaspoon of this mixture taken after lunch and dinner, with warm water.

2. Triphalā, ½ teaspoon at night. Or one to three teaspoons of castor oil, mixed with one cup of ginger tea, taken at night. This helps to clean the colon.
3. In certain toxic colon conditions one should take dashamūla tea basti three times a week.
4. Rub warm sesame oil on the feet and scalp at bedtime to help relieve stress and normalize blood pressure.
5. Practice the following yogāsanas: camel, cobra, cow, cat, spinal twist, palm tree, and corpse pose, with deep, quiet breathing into the belly button. This will help to relax the blood vessels and therefore lower the blood pressure.

***Pitta Remedies.*** The samprāpti of pitta type of hypertension begins in the small intestine and liver, and may be accompanied by gallbladder toxicity and unresolved anger in the solar plexus. Job responsibilities, stressful relationships, and the combined action of hot, spicy, and salty foods act as precipitating causes. Here one should detoxify the small intestine, liver, gall bladder, and solar plexus with pañchakarma. The person should follow a pitta-soothing diet and take pitta-soothing herbs like shatāvarī, gulvel sattva, and jatamāmsi, which help to regulate pitta in the blood, thereby decreasing its viscosity and the arterial tension.

Generally, the following program would be suggested.

1. An herbal mixture of

| | |
|---|---|
| Shatāvarī | 500 mg |
| Shankha pushpī | 300 mg |
| Brahmī | 200 mg |
| Sarasvatī | 100 mg |

¼ teaspoon of this mixture taken after lunch and dinner, with warm water.

2. Virechana (adminstration of intestinal purgatives) with āmalakī, nishottara, or sat isabgol at night with warm water.
3. Brahmī ghee nasya: three to five drops in each nostril on an empty stomach, morning and afternoon.
4. Practice these yogāsanas: hidden lotus, boat, bow, fish, and the cooling shītalī prānāyāma.
5. No one with high blood pressure should do headstands, the breath of fire (bhastrikā prānāyāma), heavy weight lifting or vigorous exercise. One should sleep on the right side and rub brahmī oil on the soles of the feet and scalp at bedtime.

***Kapha Remedies.*** The samprāpti of kapha hypertension begins in the stomach and spleen, with associated lymphatic congestion and sometimes an underactive thyroid. Since kapha's main sites are the stomach, lungs, and lymphatic tissue, one should cleanse these organs to eliminate the root cause of kapha hypertension. Undigested and unutilized kapha molecules from the plasma cause an increase in cholesterol or triglycerides, which leads to increased viscosity of the blood, causing hypertension, diabetes, obesity, and renal dysfunction. According to Ayurvedic literature, these can be managed by pañchakarma, herbs, and the correct diet and lifestyle.

1. One can take the following herbal formula:

| | |
|---|---|
| Shilājit | 200 mg |
| Punarnavā | 500 mg |
| Mūtrala | 200 mg |
| Kutki | 200 mg |
| Sarasvatī | 100 mg |

¼ teaspoon after lunch and dinner, with warm water.

2. Bibhītakī, ½ teaspoon in a glass of hot water, taken before bedtime.
3. Cumin, coriander, and fennel tea (equal parts of each) drunk throughout the day.
4. The yogāsanas: palm tree, turtle, spinal twist, lion, half bridge, and modified peacock pose. Alternate nostril breathing with outer retention is also beneficial.

## Summary

In Ayurvedic literature, hypertension is not a disease, but rather a symptom of doshic changes, and/or toxicity within the gastro-intestinal tract, and/or emotional or stressful conditions. One should understand the doshas involved and whether it is a sirābhinodhana or dhamanī pratichaya condition. Each type of doshic hypertension should be treated individually, by understanding the particular samprāpti (pathological process) as well as the person's prakruti and vikruti. Then and then only can perfect healing of these particular conditions be achieved.

Please note that hypertension is a serious condition, possibly involving or leading to complications. One should not try to treat oneself using this article as a substitute for consultation with a qualified medical doctor.

# Chapter 15

# Cholesterol and Excess Kapha

## An Integrated Approach

Winter 1989, Volume 2, Number 3

AYURVEDA SAYS THAT cellular metabolism is governed by agni, the fire principle, which is present in pitta dosha. Through metabolic, biochemical reactions that occur within the cells, we utilize carbohydrates, proteins, and fats to release energy and produce new structural cellular material. Agni also maintains and regulates the life span of cells. Organic catalytic agents called the three doshas also control these metabolic reactions. The production of these doshas (vāta, pitta and kapha) is controlled by the genetic code, called prakruti (constitution) in Sanskrit, which is held within the molecules of the cells. This genetic code instructs the cells to behave in a certain way to synthesize specific kinds of food molecules.

Metabolic processes can be divided into two major types: The first is anabolic, which stores energy and involves the build-up of larger molecules from smaller ones. This type of change is governed by kapha dosha. The other type, catabolic, involves energy loss and the breakdown of larger molecules into smaller ones. That type of change is governed by vāta dosha.

Kapha, which contains earth and water elements, is heavy, thick, oily, cool, and cloudy, and it moves slowly in the plasma. It has a tendency to deposit on the vessel walls, causing thickening and narrowing of arteries, and increasing the viscosity of the blood. This results in hypertension and ischemic or congestive heart disease. Kapha molecules comprise a group of organic compounds that include fats, lipids, triglycerides, lipoproteins, and other fat-like substances that are used to supply energy and lubricate the cell membranes. Triglycerides are present in foods of both plant and animal origin. They are found in meats, eggs, milk, and lard as well as in various nuts and plant oils such as corn, peanut, and olive. Cholesterol is present in relatively high concentrations in shrimp, liver, egg yolks, and fatty meat. It is present in lower concentrations in whole milk, butter, cheese, and dark meats. These animal and plant food products also increase kapha, so a kapha-increasing diet also increases cholesterol.

During digestion, triglycerides are broken down into fatty acids and glycerol. The metabolism of these substances is mainly controlled by the bhūta agni (digestive fire of the five elements) in the liver and indirectly by the jāthara agni in the stomach. The liver, with the help of bhūta agni, breaks down triglycerides and lipoproteins, which may then be released into the blood.

The liver is the root of rakta vaha srotas (the blood-carrying channel) and is largely responsible for controlling the circulation of lipids. The liver regulates the total amount of cholesterol in the body, either by synthesizing cholesterol and releasing it into the blood, or by removing excess cholesterol from the blood and converting it into bile and bile salts. Bhūta agni in the liver further uses cholesterol to lubricate cell membranes, provide structural material for the nerve cells (majjā dhātu) and synthesize various hormones.

Due to low agni in the liver, triglycerides and fatty molecules may not be utilized properly. They then begin to accumulate in the adipose tissue, resulting in obesity. Low agni is also responsible for an under-active thyroid gland, slow metabolism, and the release of excess kapha molecules into the bloodstream, which increases the cholesterol level in the blood. As a rule, an individual below the age of 50 years whose cholesterol concentration exceeds 240 mg per 100 ml, or whose triglycerides exceed 200 mg per 1 ml, is considered to have high cholesterol.

Primary hyperlipidemia, or high cholesterol, is classified in Ayurveda as a kapha disorder. This condition is uncommonly common in those individuals with a kapha-predominant constitution, liver or kidney dysfunction, low agni (low metabolism) and/or a diet high in saturated fat and kapha-producing foods. These individuals may also be at risk for ischemic heart disease.

Among the signs of high cholesterol are multiple hairs in the ear passage, a crease on the ear lobule, white rings around the irises of the eyes, and hypertension. Another indication is a broad, deep, slow, wavy and thickened pulse that shows low liver, kidney, and stomach energy. The serum looks cloudy due to excessive kapha molecules in the rasa dhātu (plasma tissue) and there is an accumulation of water in the adipose tissue, resulting in excess weight or obesity and hypertension. There is also clogging of the arteries (atherosclerosis).

### Causes of High Cholesterol
* Low agni
* Low metabolism
* Hypothyroidism
* Lack of regular exercise
* Sedentary job
* Kapha producing diet: fatty meat, dairy, fried food
* Kapha prakruti
* Heredity

### Possible Results of High Cholesterol
* Liver dysfunction
* Pancreatitis

- Gallstones
- Diabetes mellitus
- Low kidney energy

## Management of a Case of High Cholesterol

Those whose cholesterol count exceeds 200 mg should:

- Avoid fatty fried foods.
- Follow a cholesterol free diet. See the kapha-soothing diet in *Ayurveda, the Science of Self-Healing,* page 82.
- Walk three miles daily at a brisk pace.
- Use garlic and onion in cooking.
- Drink "copper water." (*Ayurveda, the Science of Self Healing,* pages 142-143).
- Use the herbs and compounds chitrak, chandraprabhā, ārogya vardhini, and lasunadi vati.
- Drink a cup of madhudaka, which is hot water with a teaspoon of honey, every morning before breakfast.
- Yoga poses: sun salute, shoulder stand, peacock, cobra, spinal twist, locust, and lotus as well as breath of fire (bhastrikā) prānāyāma.
- Meditation.

## Chapter 16

# Chronic Lyme Disease

Fall 2008, Volume 21, Number 2

LYME DISEASE IS a multi-systemic disorder caused by a spirochete, called borrelia burgdorferi, which enters the skin through a tick bite. It is a common disorder in spring and summer seasons, when the deer tick vectors are most active. This is the time when more people go camping and hiking in the mountains.

Lyme disease is epidemic in certain parts of the United States, such as the New England states (especially Connecticut, Rhode Island Massachusetts), New York, New Jersey, Pennsylvania, Delaware and Maryland as well as Wisconsin, Minnesota and the Pacific Northwest.

When the tick bite occurs, if the tick is promptly removed and the area is washed, the toxin will not gain access to the blood stream. This will prevent the occurrence of long-term symptoms. It is still important to see your health care professional at this time, especially if symptoms occur at this early stage.

If the tick is not quickly removed, a characteristic rash develops at the site of the bite, within 12 to 24 hours. It begins as a red ring and then gradually expands to leave a typical "bull's eye" pattern. Not all bites have this bull's eye pattern, but most produce a large rash that is circular in shape. This is caused by the localized reaction of *bhrājaka pitta* under the skin, which produces a rash called erythema chronicum migrans.

There are three stages to Lyme disease:

1. Localized infection at the site of the tick bite. The incubation period is 7 to 14 days. Erythema (redness of the skin) develops during this period as well as headache, stiff neck, muscle spasms and joint pain. It is easy to forget the tick bite occurred if it is only a small injury. Some or all these signs and symptoms can develop within a couple of weeks of being bitten. Many times, stage one of Lyme disease is misdiagnosed as arthritis, muscular pain, migraine or (because of the stiff neck) meningitis. It is not any of these diseases. It is the entry of pitta into rasa, rakta, and māmsa dhātus.

2.  This second stage occurs after the initial one to two weeks of stage one. The spirochete produces non-protective antibodies, which spread throughout rakta vaha srotas (the blood system). This further disturbs rañjaka pitta, moving into the muscles and joints and producing muscular pain and arthritis. It can also result in cardiac arrhythmia or pericarditis due to *avalambaka dushti*.
    Entry of the spirochete into the lymphatic system produces lymphadenopathy. The lymph nodes become enlarged, tender and painful. If majjā dhātu is involved, meningoencephalitis symptoms can be produced. These antibodies are pitta-genic āma (toxins), which produce inflammatory changes in the muscles, pericardium and the joints.
3.  The long-lingering pitta āma stays in the deep connective tissue, where it can produce chronic infections over a period of several years. In this third stage of Lyme disease, the patient may develop severe arthritis or encephalitis. However, these diseases are rarely fatal. Examination of the blood serum typically shows the presence of antibodies. Many times, chronic Lyme disease is misdiagnosed a rheumatoid arthritis, fibromyalgia or fibromyositis. Hence, it is important for the patient to remember the incident of the tick bite.

In addition to seeing their health care professional, the person can be given the following herbal remedies to promote healing and a full recovery from this debilitating disease.

## Herbal Treatment

In general, one needs to use Ayurvedic herbal antibiotics, such as:

| | |
|---|---|
| Neem | 200 mg. |
| Turmeric | 200 mg. |
| Echinacea | 200 mg. |
| Goldenseal | 200 mg. |
| Vidanga | 200 mg. |

These herbs help to control the development of the illness, preventing it from moving from stage one to stages two and three. They can be used separately, or can be mixed together to create a broad-spectrum antibacterial formula.

The pratyanika (specific to) herbal remedy for pitta dosha:

| | |
|---|---|
| Shatāvarī | 500 mg. |
| Gudūchī | 300 mg. |
| Mahāsudarshan | 200 mg. |
| Kāma Dudhā | 10 mg. |

This mixture can be given ½ teaspoon TID. These herbs are all anti-inflammatory and help to balance pitta dosha.

## Topical Treatments for Erythema

1.  Make a paste from a teaspoon of sandalwood powder,[24] a pinch of edible camphor, and a pinch of moti bhasma (pearl powder). An alternative to this combination is red sandalwood and turmeric. Apply this to the site of the erythema.
2.  Drink 2 tablespoons of cilantro juice TID. Also, apply the cilantro pulp topically to the erythema.

---

24. Sandalwood is considered an endangered species by CITES. The Ayurvedic Institute does sell some sandalwood but only in limited quantities.

3. Apply equal parts of coconut oil and neem oil topically to the site of the erythema.
4. Eat ½ cantaloupe and rub the inner white portion (found near the skin of the fruit) onto the erythema.

## Treatment of Specific Complications

T.I.D. = from the Latin means *ter in diem*, three times a day

### For Pericardisis or Cardiac Symptoms

Punarnavā          500 mg.
Pushkaramūla       300 mg.
Arjuna             300 mg.
Shringa Bhasma     10 mg. (or Shanka Bhasma)
Give ½ teaspoon of this herbal mixture TID.

Topically, apply shringa shunti lepa, which is a paste made from equals of ginger powder and shringa bhasma (deer horn ash).

### For Muscle Pain or Spasms

Ashvagandhā        500 mg.
Balā               300 mg. (or Ātmaguptā)
Vidārī             200 mg.
Give ½ teaspoon of this herbal mixture TID.

Topically, apply mahānārāyana oil onto the site of the pain.

### For Arthritis

Lyme arthritis is an intermittent pauciarticular inflammatory arthritis that is due to tick-borne viral disease. It can appear to be rheumatoid arthritis, as it is found in only a few joints. To treat it, one can use:

Amrita Guggula     300 mg. (or Kaishore Guggulu 200 mg.)
Gulvel Sattva      200 mg.
Mahāsudarshan      200 mg.
Kāma Dudhā         10 mg.
Take ½ teaspoon of this mix TID with aloe vera gel. The person should also take half to one teaspoon of bhumi āmalakī nightly.

Topically, apply mahānārāyana oil at the site of the pain. Also, apply sandalwood and edible camphor paste, made from 1 teaspoon of sandalwood powder mixed with a pinch of camphor and some water.

## Treatment of Chronic Lyme Disease

This line of treatment will help to control the Lyme disease. However, in reality, chronic Lyme disease is a long-lingering multi-systemic disorder that needs periodic pañchakarma (detoxification) treatments and a rasāyana (rejuvenation) program.

### Pañchakarma

First, do snehana with sunflower oil and svedana (steam therapy) using sandalwood essential oil or nirgundī essential oil added to the steam box or bath. You can also use ginger or eucalyptus oil instead of the nirgundī. Then the patient undergoes gentle virechana (purgation) with nishottara or bhumi āmalakī. Rakta moksha is also done whenever possible, to cleanse the blood.

### Rasāyana

The following remedies are used to rejuvenate the tissues affected by Lyme disease:

◆ Mahārasnādi kvath, as a rasāyana for the joints, or kumārī āsava.
◆ Mahā sudarshan kvath, as a rasāyana for erythema and pyrexia, or kumārī āsava.
◆ Ashvagandhā arishta, as a rasāyana for māmsa dhātu, or drākshā.
◆ Arjuna arishta, as a rasāyana for the heart, or drākshā.

In general, the person should eat a pitta pacifying diet and avoid foods that are vāta aggravating. He or she should also follow a pitta pacifying lifestyle and avoid aggravating vāta dosha.

# Chapter 17

# Chronic Fatigue Syndrome

Spring 2000, Volume 12, Number 4 and Summer 2000, Volume 13, Number 1

CHRONIC FATIGUE SYNDROME is a complex illness now commonly found in this society. The condition called chronic fatigue syndrome (CFS) is not a new disease. In modern medicine, this illness is associated with an acute viral infection and is often called myalgic encephalomyelitis (ME). Chronic fatigue syndrome is similar to the Gulf War syndrome and it is closely associated with fibromyalgia, myasthenia, neurasthenia, or atypical encephalitis. Its latest name is "Chronic Fatigue Immune Dysfunction Syndrome" or CFIDS. It has been given many names, but I will refer to the condition as chronic fatigue syndrome or CFS.

## The Role of Digestion and Cellular Metabolism

We will begin by studying the important role that digestion plays in health. This is a key to understanding the reasons someone develops CFS. Ayurvedic concepts of digestion, nutrition, and metabolic functions are quite different from western understanding and we will review some of those basic tenets here.

The end product of digested food, called āhāra rasa, is carried to the various tissues. Bodily tissues are called dhātus in Sanskrit. For instance, rasa dhātu is the blood plasma and the lymphatic system. Rakta dhātu is the red blood cells. Māmsa dhātu is the muscles, meda the fatty tissue, asthi the skeletal system, majjā the nervous system and bone marrow. Finally, shukra is the male reproductive system and ārtava the female reproductive system. We will consider these different tissues as we discuss the various manifestations of chronic fatigue syndrome (CFS).

The digestive fire is called agni in Sanskrit. The functions of agni include transformation of food, thoughts, and emotions into the substance of the body and mind. Its strength and capacity determine how well nutrients are utilized by the body. Each stage of digestion has its own agni and the various organs important to the digestive process all have their own digestive capability. The central digestive fire is called jāthara agni. It manifests as hydrochloric acid (HCl) and the various enzymes that are present in the stomach and small intestine. Bhūta agni can be defined as the digestive enzymes and hormones in the

129

liver. Each tissue has dhātu agni, which further transforms the raw materials from food and water into the tissues and their by-products. Bhūta agni in the liver is a bridge between jāthara agni and the dhātu agni and utilizes the end products of digested food to nourish every tissue, organ, and system. Bhūta agni is often affected in CFS.

The smallest unit of the human body is a single cell. Cellular metabolism is related to the fire component of all cells, called *pīlu agni* and *pithara agni*. Pīlu agni is the digestive fire in the cell membrane, which converts the āhāra rasa into cellular plasma. Then pithara agni transforms this subtle essence of the food into consciousness. The pure essence of pīlu agni and pithara agni is tejas. Tejas maintains the cellular metabolic activity and is responsible for cellular intelligence. Every cell has this intelligence, which manifests in pīlu agni as selectivity.

There is a constant flow of communication between cells. That flow of communication is prāna. The mitochondria, genes, RNA and DNA molecules, and even the movement of cytoplasm are all governed by prāna. Prāna is responsible for the flow of cellular intelligence and cellular respiration (oxygen exchange). Because of prāna, every cell is a conscious living being. Ojas is the end product of cellular digestion and the pure essence of all bodily tissues, and it is responsible for maintaining the immune response. It governs cellular and systemic immunity. Ojas corresponds to the pure essence of kapha dosha; tejas to the essence of pitta dosha; and prāna to the essence of vāta.

The Ayurvedic concept of CFS is that it is primarily a disorder of imbalanced agni and depletion of ojas. CFS is called *bala kshaya* in Sanskrit, which means depleted strength. One's biological strength is the integration and functional synchronization of jāthara agni, bhūta agni and dhātu agni. Jāthara agni is responsible for digestive strength and capacity in the gastrointestinal tract. The strength of each dhātu is maintained by dhātu agni. Dhātu strength is defined as the tone of the tissue, the resistance of the tissue and its capacity for self-repair. If there is wear and tear of the tissue, it heals itself because of dhātu agni.

Any imbalance in agni causes problems with digestion and disturbance of ojas, tejas, and prāna. In CFS, ojas becomes depleted, but there is also disturbance of tejas and prāna.

## Causes of Chronic Fatigue Syndrome

If we look at the etiological factors of CFS, an important one is incompatible food combining. An example is eating dairy products and fruit together, such as banana milk shakes, banana splits, yogurt with fruit, and so on. Because of incompatible food combining, we develop cellular toxins (āma). These undigested food particles then float through the system, unable to be further digested. Āma is one of the factors involved in the onset of parasites, bacteria, viruses, or repeated allergies.

Incompatible food combining or eating foods that are unsuitable for one's constitution put an undue strain on agni and cause it to become imbalanced. When the agni system (jāthara, dhātu, and bhūta agni) is adversely affected, production of toxins (āma) results. Āma is a toxic, morbid substance that circulates throughout the body and invades the dhātus. Undue production of āma—systemic āma, dhātu āma, or cellular āma—can be a primary cause of CFS. There are some cardinal signs and symptoms of āma:

- *Sroto rodha* – clogging of the channels
- *Bala bhramsha* – profuse fatigue
- *Gaurava* – physical and mental heaviness, or depression, or mental dullness
- *Anila mūdhatā* – mental confusion
- *Ālasya* – malaise
- *Apakti* – indecision
- *Sangha* – stagnation of tissue, of toxins
- *Klama* – extreme fatigue

These toxins, along with aggravated doshas (vāta, pitta, or kapha), can create disease by invading any cell or dhātu that has a weakness in its cellular (pīlu) agni or dhātu agni. These weaknesses are called khavaigunya. They can be caused by genetic factors, accident or trauma, or chronic factors that imbalance the agni. If there is a khavaigunya in the dhātu agni, something like a short exposure to chemicals can aggravate a dosha and then fatigue can set in. Hence, environmental and food allergies are often present with CFS.

Endocrine imbalance or emotional stress can affect cellular metabolism and produce a profusion of microcytes (abnormally small red blood cells), resulting in anemia. This is common in CFS. Impaired metabolism can also be a factor, including thyroid dysfunctions such as hypothyroidism, which is a kapha disorder; or hyperthyroidism, which is a pitta or vāta disorder. Hepatitis, which is high pitta in the liver, is another disease that can lead to CFS. Other causative factors include acute stress or psychological causes. Feeling unloved, childhood abuse, or rejection can all affect dhātu agni, pīlu agni and pithara agni, causing us to carry these unprocessed cellular memories in our connective tissue. How we are brought up and the events of the first seven years of life stay with us.

Multiple pregnancies can induce CFS in a woman, because she loses ojas in the gestation of the fetus. Between pregnancies, there is a need to recover. Before planning a future pregnancy, the prospective mother should undergo pañchakarma, rejuvenation, and a rasāyana program.

This multi-faceted etiology shows us that CFS is a complex illness. The modern medical system believes that a virus may be the most immediate cause. The Epstein-Barr virus (EBV) creates mononucleosis, which is an undue production of mononuclei or pitta-type of molecules. The latent form of this virus is found in the majority of people with CFS. Another virus involved in CFS may be the herpes virus, which causes a person to get repeated outbreaks of oral or genital herpes.

In Ayurvedic terms, these viruses increase pitta and tejas, which burns ojas. When tejas is burning ojas, the cellular immune mechanism is affected and the person feels exhausted. This increased tejas can create a mild inflammation in the central nervous system and may even create atypical multiple sclerosis (MS).

Before a person develops CFS, they have subtle weaknesses at the cellular level. Something like a virus or cellular toxins can cause further doshic imbalance and create the symptomology of CFS. Some individuals show pitta symptoms, some show kapha symptoms, and others may show vāta symptoms. Let's look at the different signs and symptoms.

### Signs and Symptoms of CFS

Chronic fatigue syndrome is the journey of āma from the GI tract into different dhātus. *Rasa dushti* (disorder of rasa) creates lymphatic node congestion and the lymph nodes become tender. Other common symptoms are mild fever, sore throat, muscle weakness, and generalized fatigue, which means that āma is moving in the rasa dhātu. Rakta dushti can result in anemia or hepatitis; the person looks pale and tired. Then the āma can move into māmsa dhātu. This creates symptoms similar to fibromyalgia such as muscle pain, pain around the joints, headache, insomnia, and depression. A person may have CFS and be treated for fibromyalgia, in which case other symptoms will probably remain.

Muscle pains, headaches, and fatigue are pitta symptoms that commonly happen in the māmsa dhātu. This fatigue may remain for a few weeks, months or even years, and it is not relieved by rest, massage, or any external means. The person has restricted activities, mild fever, and a sore throat. Āma and dosha dushti (imbalance) can create these symptoms of CFS. *Meda dushti* makes the person extremely sensitive to fatty food, to the point that even a small amount of ghee creates a headache. *Asthi dushti* creates pain in the joints and migraine headaches. *Majjā dushti* creates MS-type symptoms (it looks like MS but it is not typical MS), while *shukra* or *ārtava dushti* can create sexual debility.

Symptoms can also be examined according to the various subtypes of the doshas. For instance, if āma goes into the eyes it creates photophobia, which is *ālochaka pitta dushti.* If it affects sādhaka pitta, the person has difficulty concentrating, mental confusion, forgetfulness, and irritability for no reason. Tarpaka kapha disorder creates insomnia and depression. So, if you look at the symptomatology, it is a multi-factorial, multi-dhātu manifestation.

### Chronic Fatigue Symptoms

* Malnutrition due to low agni
* Psychogenic emotional factors
* Circulatory disturbances
* Low ojas
* Excess pitta in the liver
* Excessive activity
* Anemia
* Viral infection
* Accumulation of metabolic waste (ama) in the muscle(s)
* Menopausal hormonal changes
* Lack of prana to the tissues

### Assessment of CFS

Whenever you see a patient with CFS, look for the signs and symptoms she or he has. The patient knows all the symptoms, but you know the signs. Symptoms are subjective; signs are objective. In front of every sign and symptom put a V for vāta, P for pitta, or K for kapha. That means you are alocating all the signs and symptoms according to vāta, pitta, kapha. We also have to find out the person's prakruti (constitution), their vikruti (current imbalance), and how CFS manifests in this individual. That is the unique approach of Ayurveda. If you see ten people with CFS, they will each have a different disease process that created the illness.

During the physical examination, the patient will explain and convey to you his or her symptomatology. Then you can touch their skin and find out if the person is running a fever. Look into the throat and find out whether there is a sore throat. Examine the lymph nodes—anterior, posterior, mandibular, sublingual, and supraclavicular—to see whether any are tender, swollen, or enlarged. Then check the liver and spleen. Are they enlarged? Many times a person with CFS has a history of Epstein-Barr virus (mononucleosis) in high school and the liver is often enlarged and tender. Just make a note of each thing.

You can inquire if there is a family history of MS, or of optic or auditory neuritis, which suggests MS. In an MS patient, there is muscle fatigue even from checking the reflexes. Muscle power and coordination may be slightly affected, but neurological motor system examinations (and in some patients' sensory system examinations) will show extreme muscle fatigue. This is the book picture of MS. In CFS, there can be extreme muscle fatigue but not the severe demyelination found in MS.

Then try to find out whether there is any tumor, checking for tremors in the outstretched hands. Check the reflexes; listen to the heart for tachycardia or palpitations; look at each conjunctiva to see if it is pale or anemic. Look at the fingernails and see if they show calcium, magnesium, or zinc deficiency (white spots). If the patient brings a lab report, you will often see low hemoglobin, increase of white blood cell (WBC) count, and / or erythrocyte sedimentation rate (ESR), or there may be lymphocytosis, an excess of lymph cells in the blood. If the patient has had a magnetic resonance imaging (MRI) test, it may show swelling in the brain and even demyelinating changes, but it is still not MS.

We can use the help of a lab report and MRI to confirm what is going on, since we live in a high tech society, but our diagnosis cannot depend on those tools. We must read the patient's pulse, to determine his/her prakruti and vikruti and which dhātus show a vāta, pitta, or kapha spike. You can find the dhātu pulse at the fifth level. Then inquire about past history, present symptoms, and other personal issues, so we can come to the right understanding regarding the patient's problem.

If you view the CFS patient's tongue, it looks coated, white, and indented around the edges, which indicates malabsorption. Ask the person to swallow and see if there is a lump or impulse on swallowing, indicating that the thyroid gland is enlarged. To rule out thyroid dysfunction, you can listen to the thyroid gland. In such cases, the blood vessels of the thyroid become dilated and there is a 'bruit' or murmur. This physical examination will help you to understand if the patient has CFS.

Modern food is missing vitamins, minerals, and amino acids because of the use of additives and preservatives in the processing of foods. People go to the health food store and buy amino acids and vitamins, but they still show a deficiency of these things. That means that their cellular systems are clogged with āma; their pīlu and pithara agnis are suppressed by āma. There is malabsorption and āma is clogging the channels.

Some individuals with CFS show the characteristics of parasites. If you look at the tongue there are shaved patches. This means that these people have giardia, which can release āma. Parasites, bacteria, candidiasis, or amoebiasis can also be factors involved with CFS.

A person with CFS may have a history of hepatitis B, herpes, EBV, or other virus. These viruses can be related to unprotected sex with an infected partner or drug use involving shared needles. The CFS patient's partner may even be a carrier of herpes or the Epstein-Barr virus.

Some people get CFS after a blood transfusion. Mercury fillings can also be one of the factors of CFS. While eating hot food, molecules of mercury vapor enter into the nervous system. Even social isolation can cause CFS. Here, the person's relationships are the main issue. If relationships are stressful, the cause becomes the effect and the effect becomes the cause. Depression can also develop with CFS. Many times psychiatric doctors treat patients for depression, but they really have CFS. Every neurologist, psychiatrist, and physician should pay more attention to CFS. It may be that the depression is just a symptom, not the disease. The cause is elsewhere.

## Treatment of CFS

The important issue behind any kind of CFS is the long-standing, lingering systemic āma. The root cause of āma is impaired agni. The aim of Ayurvedic treatment is to balance the doshas, balance agni, and eliminate āma. Depending upon the strength of the person and the strength of the disease, there are various options to cleanse the body and mind. The two main approaches are called shodana and shamana.

If the person with CFS has some underlying strength, shodana is recommended. This is commonly called pañchakarma, which means "the five cleansing actions." Pañchakarma is a wonderful detoxifying program that eliminates toxins through one or more of the five methods. Shodana also includes oil massages, steam treatments, eating a mono-diet of easily digested food, and other treatments that help the toxins to loosen their grip, so they can be eliminated by the pañchakarma. For a person with CFS, five to seven days of pañchakarma may not be enough. They often have to do 2 to 3 weeks.

However, pañchakarma is not recommended for an extremely tired and weak person; only if the person has the strength to bear the strain of pañchakarma. For many people with CFS, the best treatment is shamana. Shamana means seven palliative measures that help a person to regain balance. They are:

+ Kindling agni (digestive fire)
+ Detoxifying āma (toxins)
+ Fasting, mono-diet, or eating easily digested food
+ Limiting fluid intake
+ Exposure to the sun or moonlight
+ Appropriate exercise
+ Prāṇāyāma

The important point is that these need to be undertaken according to an individual's needs. For example, one person with CFS may need to increase agni, eat a mono-diet and lie in the sun, but should not limit their fluids or do exercise. Another may need to do exercise and prāṇāyāma, but keep out of the sunlight. Shamana is useful for anyone, but particularly for someone with CFS who is too weak to undergo strenuous cleansing.

After pañchakarma or shamana, the person needs to do rasāyana (rejuvenation). For CFS patients, this would include an immune system booster. Generally an herbal mixture is given to balance the doshas and treat the CFS. Then we have to suggest a proper ongoing diet and lifestyle. If it is vāta type of CFS, we have to give a vāta pacifying diet and lifestyle; and the same is true for pitta and kapha.

Whenever we are dealing with CFS, we will try to create a balance between prakruti and vikruti, based upon the history of the patient and his or her prakruti and vikruti. Our treatment will be directed to agni and the doshas involved, the particular kind of āma, and which dhātus are affected. With knowledge of the prakruti and vikruti, we will understand which dosha is out of balance. It is the skill of the clinician that will find out where this disease is heading and the treatment will vary according to that.

In Ayurveda, we always treat according to vyādhi pratyanika (specific to disease), dosha pratyanika (specific to dosha), dhātu pratyanika (specific to dhātu) and *ubhaya pratyanika* (specific to agni as well as dosha and disease). This is the basis of Ayurvedic herbology. We will use balā as the vyādhi pratyanika for CFS. CFS is called bala kshaya, or depletion of strength, and the very name of this herb means strength, so it is a great herb to build strength and energy. I am just giving you a direction on how to think. You must have a deep understanding of gunas, doshas, and dhātus; then you'll know what you're doing. We cannot treat every syndrome with one medicine; that is not scientific at all.

Ayurveda treats every case of CFS based upon the individual's prakruti/vikruti paradigm. So, forget the label CFS. It is not going to help us understand exactly what that person's problem is. I can use the words CFS just as a broad window through which I am looking, but there are many different shades of the disease process. Any dhātu depletion can manifest as CFS, so it depends upon each person's prakruti, vikruti, lifestyle, and level of stress.

## Vāta Type of CFS

We know the main site of vāta is the colon and that vāta has an affinity to the asthi dhātu, thighs, pelvic girdle, ears, and skin. If the person has more vāta aggravation, we'll definitely find symptoms that are related to vāta, such as dry, rough, or scaly skin, ringing in the ears, constipation, or bloating. Which symptoms manifest depends upon whether this vāta type of CFS is moving in the colon or going into any of the other dhātus. That is why it is so complex.

When vāta dosha creates manda (slow) agni or vishama (imbalanced) agni, the person's digestion is affected. Manda agni means that appetite and digestion are low. Vishama agni means sometimes the appetite is good and sometimes not; sometimes the digestion is ok and other times it isn't; sometimes there is constipation, bloating and distension, while other times there is not.

If vāta goes into the rasa dhātu, the person will have a rise of temperature in the evening, lymphatic congestion, cold (shivering), and fatigue. Fatigue here is due to a defficiency in the functioning of rasa dhātu, which has the function of nutrition. If rasa (and hence, nutrition) is lacking, the person will have progressive fatigue and weakness. This is a vāta type of CFS samprāpti associated with the rasa dhātu.

If vāta goes into the rakta dhātu, the person will feel anemic. This means that the disease process is creeping from one dhātu to another dhātu. If it goes into the māmsa dhātu there will be muscle tics, spasms, twitching, tremors, and fatigue. If it goes into the meda dhātu, the person will have a severe loss of meda (adipose tissue). The person loses fat, the muscles lose their bulk, his/her cholesterol goes extremely low, and the joints crack. When vāta type of CFS goes into the asthi dhātu, the person will get osteoporosis or osteoarthritis. When it goes into the majjā dhātu, there will be neurological symptoms such as neuralgia, tingling and numbness, or loss of sensation. And when vāta goes into the shukra dhātu, the person will have sexual debility and premature ejaculation.

I am just sharing with you a mono-doshic vāta type CFS. We give balā as the vyādhi pratyanika. If we are dealing with vāta dosha, we need one herb that is vāta pratyanika, another that is specific for agni (*agni pratyanika*) and one specific for the dhātu involved (dhātu pratyanika). For vāta pratyanika, we often use purified guggulu. But for vāta type of CFS, since āma is moving into the deep tissue, I'd use yogarāja guggulu. An alternative in cases where there is less āma is ashvagandhā.

But now I have to kindle the agni, otherwise the yogarāja guggulu is not going to work. Here I can use chitrak, which kindles and balances agni. Next, I have to pay attention to the dhātu. If it is rasa dhātu, I'll use tulsi or fresh ginger, or sudarshan if there is fever. So, the first herb deals with the fatigue and weakness, the second with the dosha, the third herb deals with the agni and the fourth deals with the dhātu. This formula of balā, yogarāja guggulu, chitrak, and tulsi will work for a vāta type of CFS only if it is in the rasa dhātu.

If CFS goes into the rakta dhātu, we would use something to pacify vāta in the rakta dhātu, such as loha bhasma or abhrak bhasma. Either one will be good for CFS associated with rakta dhātu. If it goes into the māmsa dhātu, we can use ashvagandhā. Yasthi madhu and vidārī are good for meda. Kāma dudhā (a great source of calcium) is good for asthi. Jatamāmsi, brahmī, shankha pushpī, and sarasvatī are good for majjā dhātu; ashvagandhā, vidārī, or ātmaguptā (kapikacchū) for shukra dhātu.

## Pitta Type of CFS

When systemic pitta is increased, it becomes like hot water. Pitta is liquid, hot, sharp, light, and oily. When it increases, it disturbs agni and that agni creates āma with a pitta quality. Agni becomes tīkshna—strong appetite, but poor digestion. That āma moves and creates diarrhea, then malabsorption, and slowly it will create fatigue. So in pitta type CFS, if pitta goes into the liver, the person will often get a viral infection of the liver. If it goes into the rasa dhātu, the person will have a sore throat and pyrexia, and the lymph nodes will be tender. Since we are dealing with CFS, the first herb to think of is again balā, to give energy. We will use shatāvarī because it is a dosha pratyanika for pitta. Agni is tīkshna (sharp but weak), so we need gulvel sattva or gudūchī to balance it. If pitta is in the rasa dhātu, we use neem or mahāsudarshan, which will take care of fever without aggravating pitta. If the pitta goes into the rakta dhātu, we still give balā (vyādhi pratyanika), shatāvarī (dosha pratyanika), and gudūchī (agni pratyanika), and we can add manjishthā or āmalakī to work specifically on the rakta dhātu (dhātu pratyanika).

If pitta enters māmsa dhātu, there will be fibromyalgia or fibromyositis, so we need an anti-inflammatory herb for māmsa, such as kaishore guggulu. When pitta moves into the meda dhātu, there is profuse sweating and the person cannot digest fat. A good herb for pitta in meda is shankha pushpī. If it goes into the asthi dhātu, the person gets periostitis or osteoarthritis. For this we can use pravāl pañchāmrit. If pitta goes into majjā, it can create irritability and pitta type of depression. We use jatamāmsi or brahmī, which is a great formula for pitta in the majjā dhātu. Finally, for pitta in shukra/ārtava dhātu, one can use shankha pushpī.

## Kapha Type of CFS

Now we will switch our attention to kapha dosha. We will keep balā, since it is vyādhi pratyanika. A great herb for kapha dosha is punarnavā, so we can use this as the dosha pratyanika. We can again use chitrak or trikatu for agni. CFS of kapha type will create dullness. When the kapha goes into the rasa dhātu there will be a generalized swelling of the lymph nodes. To remove kapha from rasa dhātu, we can use kāñcanāra. If it goes into the rakta dhātu, it will slow down the erythrogenesis process and create megaloblastic anemia. For this we can use manjishthā, which will reduce leukopenia. If kapha enters the māmsa dhātu, we have to protect māmsa with karaskara or vidārī. These herbs will increase and maintain the muscle tone.

If kapha CFS goes into meda dhātu, we can use kutki or shilājit. Kapha in the meda dhātu will create lipoma and fatty degenerative changes in the liver, and then the person can get CFS. For kapha in the asthi dhātu, we can use punarnavā guggulu if there is swelling of the joints, or even triphalā guggulu if there is systemic āma. If kapha CFS enters majjā dhātu, the person gets depression. We can use brahmī, jatamāmsi, or sarasvatī. For shukra and ārtava dhātus, use shilājit or ātma guptā. Kapha in the shukra/ārtava dhātu will create premature ejaculation, sexual debility, or benign prostatic hypertrophy.

## Summary

We have the discussed the causes, signs, and symptoms of chronic fatigue syndrome as well as the assessment of this condition in Ayurvedic terms. We have also covered the treatment of CFS according to the doshas, dhātus, and the condition of the patient's agni. In Part Two, we will talk about the use of supplements, treating the causes of CFS, and working with balancing the mental and emotional states of the client to fully recover one's strength and health. We will also consider the subtle aspects of healing this multi-faceted condition.

**Table 4: Herbs for Specific Dhātu Dushti**

| Dhātu | Vāta | Pitta | Kapha |
|---|---|---|---|
| Rasa | Adrak (fresh ginger)<br>Tulsi<br>Sudarshan | Mahāsudarshan<br>Neem | Kāñcanāra<br>Ginger<br>Mahāsudarshan |
| Rakta | Loha (iron) Bhasma<br>Abhrak Bhasma | Manjishtha<br>Gudūchī<br>Āmalakī | Manjishtha<br>Katukā |
| Māmsa | Ashvagandhā<br>Balā<br>Vidārī | Kaishore Guggulu<br>Gulvel Sattva | Karaskara<br>Shringa Bhasma<br>Vidārī |
| Meda | Yashthi Madhu (licorice)<br>Vidārī | Shankha pushpī<br>Neem | Kutki<br>Chitrak<br>Shilājit |
| Asthi | Yogarāja Guggulu, etc.<br>Kāma Dudhā | Kaishore Guggulu<br>Pravāl Pañchāmrit | Punarnavā Guggulu<br>Gokshurādi Guggulu |
| Majjā | Jatamāmsi<br>Sarasvatī | Brahmī<br>Jatamāmsi | Brahmī<br>Vacha<br>Sarasvatī |
| Ārtava | Ashoka<br>Vidārī | Shatāvarī<br>Ashoka<br>Aloe Vera Gel | Shilājit<br>Ātmaguptā |
| Rasa | Adrak (fresh ginger)<br>Tulsi<br>Sudarshan | Mahāsudarshan<br>Neem | Kāñcanāra<br>Ginger<br>Mahāsudarshan |

## Part Two: The Ayurvedic Concept of Chronic Fatigue Syndrome

In the first part of this article, we saw that chronic fatigue syndrome (CFS) is primarily a disorder of imbalanced agni and depletion of ojas. CFS is called bala kshaya in Ayurveda, which means depleted strength. Strength depends upon balanced agni (digestive fire). Any imbalance in agni causes problems with digestion and disturbance of ojas, tejas, and prāna. In CFS, ojas becomes depleted but there is also disturbance of tejas and prāna. The typical patient of CFS has low prāna and high tejas of poor quality.

The most common manifestation of CFS is in pitta predominant people with high pitta in the liver. Epstein-Barr Virus, hepatitis, and other viruses directly affect the liver, and these viruses and other pitta-aggravating causes can disturb the five bhūta agnis in the liver. When the bhūta agnis are increased, the digested food does not retain enough nutrients to optimally nourish the tissues. Rasa, rakta, and māmsa dhātus are most commonly affected, but pitta can move into any of the tissues. This can lead to extreme fatigue and all the other symptoms we discussed as being typical of CFS.

Pitta-type of CFS is most common but, as noted earlier, any of the doshas can disturb any of the dhātus and create a condition of chronic fatigue. We will consider some treatments for specific causes, such as the viruses mentioned above, but first we will consider the use of supplements from an Ayurvedic perspective.

***The Use of Supplements.*** CFS is a complex condition. We have discussed the different types of formulas for CFS according to the specific dhātu. Modern medicine does not have a drug for CFS. They often use antiviral, anti-bacterial, and anti-parasitic drugs. In some therapies, they give certain amino acids that may enkindle the agni, such as tyrosine, phenylalanine, tryptophan, or glutamine. You can buy these at the health food store. Melatonin is now a popular supplement. Although it has been said that melatonin boosts the immune system, excessive amounts can create depression.

Some practitioners prescribe chelation and multi-vitamin and mineral therapies, but when agni is low and the dhātus are clogged with āma those vitamins and minerals will just create more āma. There is also a condition called hypervitaminosis, which is the result of taking high quantities of vitamins. Some people take 3000 mg of vitamin C at a time. That is too intense; more than 1000 mg at one time can become toxic to the liver. If the person shows a deficiency of vitamins, Ayurveda says that before putting any vitamins into the body we must cleanse the body through pañchakarma or one of the cleansing methods mentioned in the first part of this article.

The aim of Ayurvedic treatment is to address the underlying cause and balance the doshas. By kindling agni, the person with CFS can better absorb the nutrients from food and eliminate unwanted toxins. However there are sometimes additional factors that contribute to CFS and these too need to be treated.

## Treating a Specific Cause

CFS is called bala kshaya, or depletion of strength. When we talked about herbal formulas, we used balā as a common herb to promote strength. Other herbs were chosen according to the specific dosha and dhātu involved, because the disease can take different paths. However in some cases, there is a specific cause of CFS that also needs to be addressed. Then we need to add one further herb to our original formula that is *hetu pratyanika* (specific to the cause), because to treat the cause is to treat the effect.

For instance, if we have detected that the cause is parasites (krumi), we need to know what type of krumi (pinworm, tapeworm, roundworm, amoebae, giardia, etc.). We have different herbs for the different parasites. Vidanga is good for pinworm, roundworm, and threadworm. For giardia, we can use neem, while for candidiasis, use shardunikā or hingvastak chūrna.

Herpes virus is a long lingering virus in the neuromuscular cleft that tends to flare up when the person becomes stressed or engages in sexual activity. If the cause of CFS is herpes, we can use kāma dudhā, moti bhasma, or indra and also tikta ghrita topically. In India we also use raupya bhasma or chandrakalaras. Other viruses may also need specific treatment.

If hepatitis is a complication of CFS, we have to treat the hepatitis. If CFS is associated with diabetes, treat the diabetes according to dosha. There is a sūtra that states that one disease can become the cause of another disease. Diabetes itself is a multi-syndrome disorder that can affect the immune system, and therefore we need to treat it first. Our treatment is against the cause: if the cause is a virus, we treat the virus; if the cause is parasites, we treat the parasites; if it is hepatitis, we treat the hepatitis.

If the cause is sensitivity to chemical exposure, the best treatment is to do pañcha-karma and then use a rejuvenative tonic such as chyavānaprāsh, Shakti Prāna®, or tikta ghrita. So although the general cause of CFS is cellular weakness (khavaigunya) in one or more tissues, the specific cause or causes also need to be addressed.

Effect can also become cause. For instance, CFS can create a number of psychological symptoms that can in turn exacerbate the CFS. When a person has severe depression, we have to use anti-depressive herbs. If anxiety and tachycardia are present, we have to take care of them along with the main line of treatment. If muscle pain and muscle fatigue are the main symptoms, then we have to use a painkiller for the māmsa dhātu. If there are arthritic changes, we have to take care of the asthi dhātu. If fever is a persistent problem, we have to use antipyretic herbs. People develop drug dependencies, using narcotics, tran-quilizers, or painkillers, because of CFS, so we have to deal with that, too. The treatment plan is multi-factorial.

## Treating According to Physical and Mental Constitutional Imbalances

According to the Ayurvedic system of medicine, every individual has a unique consti-tution, called prakruti. Constitution is of two types: *dosha prakruti* and *manas prakruti,* respectively meaning the physical and psychological constitutions. Dosha prakruti is also called *deha prakruti* and is governed by vāta, pitta, and kapha with their unique permuta-tions and combinations. For example, in one person a ratio of the doshas may be $vata_3$, $pitta_2$, and $kapha_1$, while in another it might be $vata_1$, $pitta_3$ and $kapha_2$. Manas prakruti, or the psychological constitution, is governed by *sattva, rajas,* and *tamas*.

Our constitution is the unique genetic code that we are born with. This genetic code of the individual is present in every cell; in every RNA and DNA molecule; in every system and organ. That genetic code can be studied clinically through the ancient Ayurvedic art of *darshana, sparshana,* and *prashna,* which are inspection, palpation, and questioning and auscultation, respectively. Through clinical observation, you can determine the individ-ual's genetic code, or prakruti.

Dosha prakruti is always subject to change, and the altered state of the doshas is called vikruti. The doshas are like protective barriers that are constantly acting and reacting to diet, lifestyle, and environmental changes. When the doshas become overwhelmed and can no longer adapt to these changes, they go out of balance. The dosha that is predomi-nant almost always goes out of balance first. A vāta prakruti has an inclination to vāta vikruti (imbalance) and to vāta disorders. However, if the cause is extremely pitta aggra-vating, even a vāta person can get a pitta type of disorder, but it can be easily controlled because pitta does not have favorable conditions to stay in that particular body. In other words, prakruti is disease proneness. This applies to both physical and mental prakruti.

Manas prakruti can be, for example, $sattva_3$, $rajas_2$, and $tamas_1$. Sattva is clarity, purity, the capacity to understand, comprehend, and realize; it is love, compassion, and care. These are the expressions of sattva. Rajas is activity, movement, planning, aggres-siveness, and competitiveness. Success-oriented individuals are rajasic. They want to be famous, political, and influential people in society. That can also be due to high pitta. Unfortunately, sattvic people typically do not want to become leaders and are not inter-ested in politics. Tamas is darkness, inertia, ignorance, and confusion. Diet, lifestyle, and environmental changes will also affect these psychological qualities. An enlightened person will have $sattva_3$, $rajas_3$, and $tamas_3$ because they counterbalance each other. Such a person is free from the gunas.

CFS can begin with changes to the psychological qualities (gunas) of sattva, rajas, and tamas. Because of high sattva quality, a person may do too much fasting or intense meditations. Intense spiritual practices can deplete the person's ojas and strength. Similarly, if the rajas quality increases, the person becomes hyperactive and does not eat properly, this may disturb vāta dosha and bring on CFS. Or high rajas can cause someone to push one's self to the point of exhaustion, which severely deranges pitta and vāta. If tamas is increased, it slows agni (which is sattvic and light) and the metabolism becomes slow. As a result, the person can become depressed, heavy, and possibly anorexic. Whether the anorexia is physiological or psychological in manifestation, imbalanced agni is the cause.

The sattva, rajas and tamas qualities should be balanced. There must be a balance between the material and the spiritual life. Everything must be in its right place. Any quality that becomes overpowering is bound to affect ojas. Ojas can be depleted by the imbalance of these gunas and by *prajnāparādha,* which means not listening to one's natural bodily intelligence.

In cases of CFS, we should pay attention to these qualities. If kapha is increased, it will induce a tamasic quality. If pitta is high, it may enhance rajasic and sattvic qualities. When vāta is increased, it induces more rajasic quality. The problem of qualitative sattva, rajas, and tamas imbalances can be corrected by treating the dosha. If you understand the doshic changes in CFS, i.e., which dosha is involved, and follow that doshic line of management, you will be a successful healer. CFS is an immune dysfunction condition and immunity can be affected by not only dysfunction of ojas, tejas, and prāna, but also by a chronic disorder of vāta, pitta, or kapha, which may lead to a sattva, rajas, or tamas imbalance. The reverse may also be true, whereby an imbalance of the three gunas can lead to disorders of ojas, tejas, and prāna and the three doshas. So, the most important factor in treatment is dosha, although we also treat according to vyādhi pratyanika (specific to disease) and dhātu pratyanika (specific to dhātu) as well as agni pratyanika (specific to agni) and hetu pratyanika (specific to cause).

## Balancing the Chakras

Along these lines, we can now talk about chakra imbalances, which can go together with endocrine disorders or *kundalinī* syndrome. Anatomically speaking, every chakra is surrounded by a nerve plexus. Physiologically, every chakra is connected to the neighboring organs. Psychologically, it is connected to certain emotions. The chakra system is a complex system of neuro-physiology, neuro-psychology, and endocrinology that is related to the immune system. Any chakra that is working under stress is bound to affect the neighboring organs.

Chakra imbalance, kundalinī syndrome, and endocrine disorders may lead to CFS, which has a psychogenic factor. We may take and do everything so seriously that we burn our ojas. As a result, we may become aggressive, competitive, and success-oriented. We may follow a system or method and take it very seriously, but if we take it to an extreme,

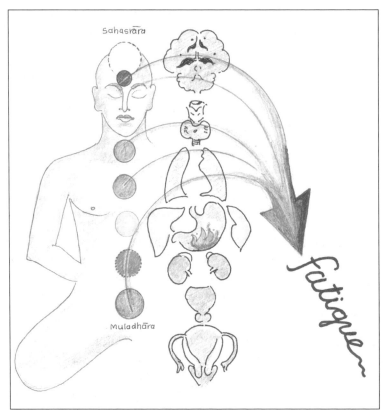

we can deplete our ojas. In life, we have relationships with the world and the chakras are these different relationships with the world.

*Mūlādhāra* is the chakra of survival. We need food, water, and air to survive. Food is energy and the end product of digested food is eliminated through the workings of the root chakra, which is mūlādhāra. Mūlādhāra is the chakra of our basic needs. In this root chakra, there is sex energy. Sex is the highest form of the lowest energy. This is the chakra of material existence.

*Svādhishthāna* is the chakra of procreation. Sva (pronounced swa) means self. The lover meets the beloved on the physical plane. Sex without desire is the highest form of love and sex with desire is the lowest form of love. Sex can transcend into blissful love and become samādhi. In the second chakra is sex in action, that is, procreation. This is also a biological need. When these basic needs are satisfied, then another factor appears in the third chakra, *manipūra,* which is power. In the lowest chakra, matter meets with matter. In the second chakra, man meets with woman. In the third, the leader meets with the follower.

In the fourth chakra, or *anāhata,* devotion meets with the devotee. The lowest three chakras are animal chakras: food, sex, and power. The fourth chakra is the center between the lower three and the higher three. It is the chakra of devotion, love, and trust. If you look into the heart chakra there is a small window and if you enter there, you'll see a staircase that will lead you to the throat chakra, or *vishuddha,* the chakra of communication. In communication, the inner meets with the outer. You communicate with your wife, your husband, your boyfriend, or your girlfriend. This is a very important chakra. Here love becomes song and compassion becomes speech.

Then comes the third eye, or *ājñā* chakra, where *īdā, pingalā,* and *sushumnā* meet. That is why it is called trikūta. Whether kundalinī travels through the right, left, or center channel—īdā, pingalā, sushumnā—she has to come here. Trikūta means three roads meeting together. This is the place to meditate; this is where alpha meets with omega. Alpha is the individual soul, your unique individual atman; omega is the higher self. So, this is the meeting point of alpha with omega, of Shiva with Shakti, Purusha with Prakruti, *jīva* with Shiva. This is the place of the *guru,* the master.

Chakras are reservoirs of consciousness that contain the neuroelectrical and spiritual energies moving along the ascending and descending tracts of the spinal cord. They also convey the stimuli coming from the higher centers to the lower organs through the sympathetic and parasympathetic systems. The chakra system is connected to the endocrine system. The endocrine system is composed of ductless glands, like the pituitary, pineal, thyroid, parathyroid, thymus, pancreas, adrenals, gonads, and Bartholin's glands in women. This glandular system is under the control of the chakra system and not the other way around. Therefore, endocrine imbalance happens as a result of chakra imbalance.

*Sahasrāra,* the crown chakra, is in the area of the pineal gland. The pineal gland secretes a very superfine essence of tarpaka kapha called *soma.* Inhibition of soma secretion creates extreme fatigue in the crown chakra, leading to indecisiveness, inability to concentrate, depression, migraine type of headache, and insomnia. This kind of CFS also creates forgetfulness, irritability, confusion, and foggy thinking. Before tarpaka kapha, sādhaka pitta and prāna vāta are disturbed, the electrical potential of sahasrāra, the cerebral cortical area, is affected and the energy from the right hemisphere does not flow freely to the left hemisphere. We have seen that these two sides of the brain are bridged together by a primordial brain called the diencephalon. When that bridge becomes blocked, your intuition goes against your intelligence, or your intelligence goes against your intuition. Intelligence and intuition should go hand in hand. Sometimes CFS happens when logic goes against intuition. Logic is beautiful but it has no wisdom. Intuition has great wisdom and wisdom is the application of logic and intuition simultaneously. Even scientists use intuition.

So, if you take a case history of CFS with depression carefully, you'll see that either their logic goes against their own intuition, or vice versa. This is tarpaka kapha encroaching sādhaka pitta and the best herbs for this are brahmī and sarasvatī. Brahmī ghee nasya can be used, or shirodhāra can be done. Cranial-sacral therapy can help, too. Crown chakra disorders of CFS can be managed this way.

Ājñā chakra is connected to the pituitary gland. This gland plays a very important role in the immune system. It is the conductor of the gland orchestra. It secretes and controls thyroid stimulating hormone (TSH), adrenocorticotrophic hormone (ACTH), growth hormone (GH), and the gonadotrophic hormones. So, pituitary dysfunction can be related to CFS and lead to hormonal imbalance. The herbs that act on the third eye are saffron, red sandalwood, jyotishmatī, and sarasvatī to some extent. The third eye is the eye of wisdom, of insight. What the other two eyes cannot see, the third eye sees. Jyotishmatī opens the third eye, so it may help to balance the pituitary functions and maintain the immune response.

The vishuddha chakra is functionally related to the thyroid and parathyroid. If the thyroid gland is overactive, the metabolism becomes fast and in the long term, this can cause the person to feel tired and fatigued. Similarly, the thyroid also plays an important role in metabolic activity and indirectly maintains the immune response. Thyroid dysfunction may be an indirect cause of CFS. The herbs that act on the thyroid are shilājit, gulvel sattva, vacha, and sarasvatī. These herbs are used when CFS is associated with the throat chakra. The cardinal signs of CFS affecting this chakra are repeated sore throats, pharyngitis, and flu symptoms. For flu, we can also use mahāsudarshan and sitopalādi. The herb sarasvatī can be used in a formula for any of the three higher chakras. Sarasvatī is also the name for the goddess of speech, intelligence, and wisdom.

Above the heart is the thymus gland. The thymus produces ojas and T lymphocytes, and plays an important role in the immune mechanism. In children, the thymus is quite large but it shrinks as we mature. In patients with tuberculosis or a chronic illness, the thymus is almost absent, totally consumed by the disease. The thymus gland is under the control of the heart chakra. Generally, when the energy of the heart chakra gets stuck, the person becomes intensely emotional, with a lot of grief and sadness. The chest and lungs are the seat of grief and sadness. For example, when a woman loses her loved one, she may hold intense grief and sadness in her breast tissue, and she is more likely to get breast cancer.

Because of heart chakra imbalances, the thymus does not produce optimal numbers of T lymphocytes, which include the scavenger and killer cells. Naturally, the lymph glands become congested; the axillary and the cervical lymph nodes become tender and swollen, and the person gets a low fever. The lymphatic system, the chyle and the thymus are all linked to rasa dhātu. The job of rasa is to produce white blood cells. In cases of thymus inhibition and CFS, we use yashthi madhu (licorice), neem, golden seal, osha, or echinacea to promote thymus gland activity and produce white blood cells to fight infections.

Manipūra chakra is related to the pancreas. The pancreas can go out of balance because the person is holding anger, judgment, and criticism in the solar plexus. The solar plexus becomes tight, which may build up stress in the pancreas, and slowly inhibit pancreatic secretions. This can lead to diabetes mellitus, or diabetes mellitus may lead to CFS as a secondary complication. The diabetes mellitus patient may get myalgia and sleep disturbance, fluctuation of blood sugar, and extreme fatigue. In this case, we can use chitrak for agni, kutki for lekhana (scraping fat), and/or neem and turmeric to regulate blood sugar.

Svādhishthāna chakra is related to the adrenal glands. The adrenals play quite an important role in CFS. There is a term called professional adrenal burnout. It means people work hard and experience job and emotional stress, and their adrenal secretions become insufficient, causing adrenal fatigue. This could be one of the factors involved with CFS. Herbs that help to normalize adrenal secretions include yashthi madhu, gokshura, punarnavā, ashvagandhā, or ginseng.

Mūlādhāra chakra governs the activities of the gluteal muscles, prostate, testicles, epididymis, ovaries, fallopian tubes, and endometrium. Some women get extreme CFS in their premenstrual period, because there is an endocrine disorder causing fluctuations and imbalance between estrogen and progesterone hormones. Even genital and vaginal herpes can cause CFS. In these cases, we have to give supportive therapy to the mūlādhāra chakra. The herbs that act on this chakra are vidārī, ātmaguptā, shatāvarī, ashoka, and triphalā. In women, the herbs that work on the fallopian tubes are gudūchī, ashoka, and bilva. In men, the herbs that work on the testicles and epididymis are vidārī and ashvagandhā. These herbs will be effective in CFS with special reference to chakra and endocrine disorders.

## Summary of Treatments for CFS

We have seen how to treat CFS using herbal therapy. Take care of the dosha with dosha pratyanika, the dhātu with dhātu pratyanika, the specific disease symptoms with vyādhi pratyanika, and treat the cause with hetu pratyanika. Amino acids, such as tyrosine, phenylalanine, tryptophan, and glutamine as well as various minerals may also be helpful. However you can also recommend natural food sources of these amino acids and minerals. For instance, cow's milk and almond milk are great sources of tryptophan.

In fact, there are a few useful food remedies for CFS. You can soak almonds overnight, then in the morning peel them and blend them with milk, ghee, and date sugar. This is a great drink for CFS. Fresh dates are also good. Wash the dates, dry them, remove the seed, and soak them in ghee for a couple of weeks or more. For a one month supply, you can put about 30 dates in 1 lb. of ghee and eat one every day in the morning. You can also chop a banana, put it in a bowl and add warm ghee, date sugar, and a pinch of cardamom. Eat it between meals and it will give you energy. Since bananas are a good source of potassium, this will help muscle fatigue. At bedtime, you can drink a warm cup of milk with a teaspoon of ghee and a pinch of turmeric. Ghee, milk, and turmeric at bedtime is a general tonic.

The CFS patient should reduce sexual activity, avoid strenuous exercise and work under the hot sun, and minimize anything that causes stress. The person needs a daily regime to avoid burnout. There needs to be a balance of plenty of rest and gentle exercise when energy permits. CFS is a complex syndrome, but Ayurveda can help people with CFS to find balance and health in their life.

# Chapter 18

# Breast Self-Exam

Spring 2006, Volume 18, Number 4

AT THE SAME TIME each month or when your monthly period has ended, check for any change in the normal look or feel of your breasts. If you notice any changes, report them to your doctor or nurse. Have regular breast exams and ask about a mammogram.

- FEEL for any Changes, Standing or Lying Down
- Lie down on your back with a pillow under your left shoulder
- Use the pads of the three middle fingers on your right hand to check the left breast
- Press—using light, medium, and firm pressure—in a circle without lifting your fingers off the skin
- Then press, using an up and down pattern, laterally across the breast
- Feel for changes in your breast, in your armpit, and above and below your collarbone. Gently squeeze the nipple to check for discharge. Discharge during lactation is normal.
- Repeat on the right breast using your left hand
- You can also follow these steps while bathing or showering, using soapy hands.
- Stand and LOOK for Any Changes
- Visually inspect your breasts in four steps:
- Hold your arms at your side
- Bend forward with your hands on your hips
- Hold your arms over your head
- Press your hands on your hips and tighten your chest muscles
- TELL a Doctor or Nurse about Any Changes from Normal
- See your doctor or nurse if you notice any of the following in your breasts:
- A lump, hard knot, or thickening
- Any swelling, warmth, redness, or darkening
- A change in the size or shape
- Dimpling or puckering of the skin
- An itchy, scaly sore or rash on the nipple
- A pulling in of your nipple or other parts

- Any nipple discharge that starts suddenly
- New pain in one spot that does not go away

## Breast Self-Exam Methods

# Chapter 19

# Obesity

## Staulya

Winter 1988, Volume 1, Number 3

IN AYURVEDA, OBESITY is defined as a metabolic disorder that produces an increase in weight and gradual pendular development of the breasts, abdomen, and hips, later spreading to the extremities. Generally, it occurs in an individual where the caloric intake is more than the physical activity. As a result, there is an accumulation of fat stored as adipose tissue (meda dhātu). The excessive deposition of adipose tissue is commonly in the breast, abdomen, and hip areas. However it may be distributed predominantly in the lower part of the trunk and thighs, which is more common for females, or in the upper part of the trunk and extremities, which is usual for males.

There are certain conditions in which the individual's weight gain is not due to obesity, such as fluid retention in edema, ascites, kidney diseases, and pregnancy. Physiologically, the weight that body builders and weight lifters gain cannot be considered obesity. Similarly, idiopathic (cyclic) edema in females, which is characterized by periodic swelling during the pre-menstrual period, is also not obesity.

According to Ayurveda, obesity is an excess kapha disorder causing low metabolism and low agni. There is a progressive fall in the basal metabolic rate (BMR) due to low agni that accompanies weight gain. There is also lethargy, decreased physical activity, excessive sleep, breathlessness on exertion, and sweating even with minimal physical activity, which results in excessive thirst. Obesity is also associated with serious disorders such as hypertension, diabetes mellitus, cardiovascular disease, and pulmonary insufficiency.

There are seven basic individual constitutions:

- Three mono types: vāta, pitta, or kapha predominant
- Three dual types: vāta-pitta, pitta-kapha, or vāta-kapha predominant
- One triple type: vāta-pitta-kapha, equally distributed, very rare

Through different permutations and combinations of each dosha, there are many variations on these basic seven types of constitution. In all body types, when kapha dosha is increased, the imbalance may become obesity.

Kapha has the following qualities that are present in a person's diet, lifestyle and habits: heavy, slow or dull, cold, oily, slimy, soft, dense, liquid, static, gross, sticky, cloudy, and/or sweet. Heavy, slow, cold, oily and gross qualities are observed in foods such as cheese, meat, and fatty fried foods, while cold, cloudy, and dense qualities are found in ice cream, chocolate, yogurt, and other dairy products. Kapha qualities are also aggravated by constantly snacking, not doing much exercise, sleeping on too soft a bed, prolonged sleeping and napping during the daytime, and drinking alcohol and cold water.

The biological attributes of kapha are similar to those of meda dhātu (adipose tissue). The food products, lifestyle, and habits that have the same attributes as kapha also have the attributes of meda, and are responsible for the pathogenesis of obesity.

A kapha-producing diet, lifestyle and habits that increase the heavy, cold, and slow attributes in the body will in turn reduce the light, hot, sharp attributes of agni, causing slow metabolism, weight gain, and increased deposition of adipose tissue on the breasts, belly, and hips. The same phenomenon occurs in hypothyroidism, anterior pituitary deficiency, Cushing's syndrome, and diabetes mellitus type 2, which are all excess kapha disorders according to Ayurveda.

Obesity may be due to steroid toxicity. Patients who have undergone surgical treatment may have to carry out a prolonged period of steroid therapy. According to Ayurveda, steroids have similar properties to those of kapha, containing the heavy, slow, liquid, and gross properties. The patient retains water, becomes moon-faced, and puts on weight, which results in obesity. Obesity is frequently associated with gonadal deficiency, both in males and females, due to excess kapha dosha and psychological factors. It is also common in females during menopause, when psychological factors can be responsible for increased appetite. Under these circumstances, food is used as a substitute for satisfaction or as an escape from problems. These persons may even become alcoholic.

Depression, anxiety, fear, and insecurity are frequently responsible for increased food intake resulting in obesity. Just controlling the person's diet and food intake under these circumstances is not going to work. The underlying emotional disturbance must also be dealt with. Stopping the use of alcohol and tobacco also results in increased appetite and therefore may produce obesity. Obese subjects do not leave food on their plates. They generally eat a lot and love to drink excessive amounts of chilled water or soda drinks. Over-eating may be a familial and cultural habit. These habits are firmly implanted from generation to generation, beginning at an early age. The mother often compels the child to eat more, out of love. However, watching television and drinking cold drinks can cause obesity even in children under the age of ten.

## Management of Obesity

One must determine the exact cause of obesity in an individual; whether it is due to hypothyroidism, diabetes mellitus, menopause, emotional factors, hormonal imbalances or some other reason. The condition can then be managed accordingly.

According to Ayurveda, obesity is due to excess kapha in the system and low agni. In particular, it occurs when there is a slow fat-dissolving metabolism, which is low meda agni. Hence, we must eliminate kapha-producing foods from the diet and increase the person's meda agni. Herbs that help to increase meda agni and thereby improve the fat metabolism are kutki, chitrak, and shilājit. Herbal compounds include trikatu, ārogya vardhini, chandraprabhā, and triphalā guggulu.

An obese person tends to accumulate fat over the diaphragm and around the heart and lung tissue. There is diminished air entry, pulmonary insufficiency, and breathlessness on exertion. To improve the vital capacity of the lungs, use an herbal compound called trikatu. This contains equal amounts of dried ginger, black pepper, and pippalī (long pepper). Take 300 mg of this twice daily after food with warm water.

Kutki improves liver function, stimulates metabolism, and helps to scrape the adipose tissue. Taking 200 mg of kutki about fifteen minutes before a meal will help to regulate the appetite. An obese person tends to become excessively hungry due to emotional factors and this can be controlled by kutki, thus helping the person lose weight. One teaspoon of honey with one cup of warm to hot water taken early in the morning also does scraping of adipose tissue in an obese person.

Due to an accumulation of fat in the connective tissue, prāna (chi) becomes blocked and this results in palpitations, breathlessness, and low sex drive. This condition can be corrected by using 200 mg of the compound triphalā guggulu, twice daily on an empty stomach. Chandraprabhā is an ancient, authentic herbal formula that is effectively used in obesity due to diabetes mellitus. The dosage is 250 mg twice daily after meals.

Ayurveda recommends that obese people undertake a special cleansing program with oil massage and medicated steam treatments as well as eating a special diet. Fasting also helps to improve the metabolism. Similarly, water intake should be regulated, because excessive consumption of water lowers the perosn's metabolism by inhibiting agni. Four to six glasses of liquids a day is sufficient for most obese people. These may be taken in the form of herbal teas such as tea made from equal parts of cumin, coriander, and fennel. In order to regulate thirst, one should do shītalī prānāyāma, which involves inhaling through the mouth when making a tube of the tongue and then exhaling through the nose, and the lion pose, which is done by sticking the tongue out as far as possible and roaring like a lion. These exercises strengthen the thyroid and help to regulate metabolic activity, which helps to regulate the deposition of adipose tissue. The sun salutation and other yoga exercises, such as spinal twist, are also of great value in controlling obesity. These should all be practiced on a regular basis.

To deal with the underlying causes of obesity, one must deal with the emotional aspects. However, regular yoga exercise, prānāyāma and medical treatment help the emotional body as well as the physical body. In the old Ayurvedic texts, it says it is easier to manage a thin person than an overweight person.

### Dietary Guidelines for Excess Kapha

*Fruits to Enjoy.* Apples, apricots, berries, cherries, cranberries, dry figs, lemons, mango, peaches, pears, persimmon, pomegranate, prunes, raisins

*Fruits to Avoid.* Most sweet and sour fruits, avocado, bananas, coconut, fresh figs, grapefruit, grapes, oranges, papaya, pineapples, plums

*Vegetables to Enjoy.* Pungent and bitter vegetables, asparagus, beets, broccoli, Brussels sprouts, cabbage, carrots, cauliflower, celery, eggplant, garlic, leafy greens, lettuce, mushrooms, okra, onions, parsley, peas, peppers, white potatoes, radishes, spinach, sprouts

*Vegetables to Avoid.* Sweet and juicy vegetables, cucumber, sweet potatoes, tomatoes, zucchini

*Grains to Enjoy.* Barley, basmati rice, corn, millet, dry oats, rye

*Grains to Avoid.* Cooked oats, brown or white rice, wheat

*Meats and Eggs that are Permissible.* Dark meat of chicken or turkey, rabbit, eggs (not fried or scrambled), venison, shrimp

*Meats to Avoid.* Beef, lamb, pork, seafood (with the exception of shrimp), fried or scrambled eggs

*Legumes.* All except kidney beans, soy, mung beans, and black lentils

*Nuts.* There should be no nuts or seeds except small amounts of sunflower seeds and pumpkin seeds

*Sweeteners.* None except raw honey

*Spices.* All are good except sea salt.

*Dairy Products.* None should be consumed except for ghee and goat milk.

*Oils.* No oils except small amounts of almond, corn, or sunflower oil.

# Chapter 20

# Backache and Sciatica
## Kati Shūla and Grighrasī

Summer 1997, Volume 10, Number 1

*VĀTA VYĀDHI* (VĀTA DISORDERS) include neuromuscular and neuroskeletal problems, such as lumbago and sciatica. *Kati shūla* is the Sanskrit term for lumbago or lower back ache. Kati means lower back and shūla means pain. *Grighrasī* means sciatica.

The entire pelvic cavity, including all of its organs and bones, is under the control of apāna vāyu. If apāna vāyu enters into asthi dhātu (the bone tissue), majjā dhātu (nerve tissue), or māmsa dhātu (the muscles and ligaments) during the spreading stage of pathogenesis, it can, depending upon the site of the khavaigunya (weakness), cause either of these two conditions related to the lower half of the body.

Lumbago (kati shūla) is pain in the lower part of the back, in the lumbosacral joint or sacro-iliac joint, while sciatica (grighrasī) is pain along the pathway of the sciatic nerve. Pain from sciatica is felt in the buttock. From there it radiates down to the posterior aspect of the thigh, then it goes to the calf, following the lateral aspect of the lower leg to the outer border of the toe. The pain starts in the buttock area and it follows the track of the nerve. Lumbago and sciatica are closely associated and can exist together. Aggravation of vāta is responsible for both these conditions.

## Etiological Factors
In the ancient Ayurvedic literature the causes of these two conditions were given in beautiful Sanskrit poetry. The etiological factors include:

***Trauma, such as a car accident, lifting heavy objects, or twisting the spine.*** Exerting oneself beyond capacity will pull the muscle, ligament, or connective tissue and manifest as pain. At times, individuals do yoga without sufficient knowledge and beyond their capacity, twisting the spine. Twisting of the spine can also happen in a car accident, or from lifting a heavy weight with flexion of the spine. While lifting a heavy weight, one should bend the knees and ankles, and then lift, using the support of the muscles of the thighs, gluteus, and calf. If people just bend and then try to lift, at that moment the spine becomes twisted.

Wrong way of
lifting heavy object

Right way of
lifting heavy object

*Constipation with gases in the rectum.* These gases exert pressure on the lumbosacral area and can cause pain. Constipation is a vāta disorder.

*Cystitis.* Any problem in the bladder, such as cystitis, may create referred pain in the lower back.

*Vaginitis, cervicitis, or even colitis.* In these conditions, vāta is pushing pitta in the bladder, vagina, cervix area, or colon, as well as the rectum.

*Congestive dysmenorrhea.* Congestive dysmenorrhea (congestion in the myometrium) will refer pain to the back. That kind of pain is usually associated with the premenstrual period.

*Herniation of an intervertebral disc.* Anterior and posterior ligaments weaken and lose their tone because of aggravation of vāta. This condition can also be the cause of lumbago.

*Gulma.* Spinal tumors, such as neurofibroma or meningioma, are caused by apāna vāyu pushing prāna vāyu pushing tarpaka kapha in the majjā dhātu.

*Ankylosing spondylitis.* Vāta pushing pitta in the majjā dhātu and asthi dhātu can create ankylosing spondylitis, leading to lower back pain.

*Cancer.* Lumbago is also present in malignant diseases of the pelvic cavity. Cancer of the prostate, cervix, or rectum can create pain in the lower back.

*Koch's spine.* In common terms, this condition is called bone tuberculosis (TB). Bone TB is secondary to pulmonary tuberculosis.

People who have open tuberculosis with cavitation, caseation,[25] and infiltration are less likely to develop lumbago. In closed tuberculosis or tubercular lymphadenopathy, where the cervical glands are matted in a chain, the abdomen becomes shaped like a boat. The person has a low-grade fever, nocturnal perspiration, evening rise of temperature, and loses weight. That person is prone to Koch's spine, which is tuberculosis of the intervertebral disc, and can create fusion of the vertebrae L4 and L5, or L5 and S1. When these vertebrae are fused, due to deposition of calcium, there is restricted movement to the lower back that can create kati shūla.

25. Transformation of tissue into a soft, cheese-like mass.

***Osteoarthritis.*** In osteoarthritis (asthi gata vāta) of the sacroiliac joint, vāta has gone into asthi dhātu. Degenerative changes of the joint, resulting in osteoporosis, are called *asthi saushīrya*. I have even seen a young boy of 20 with degenerative changes. That patient had an underactive parathyroid gland, which governs calcium metabolism, causing the bones to lose calcium.

***Āma.*** Metabolic toxins, created by improper digestion, incompatible food combining, or environmental poisons.

***Infection.*** Local bacterial infection can produce either lumbago or sciatica.

These are the etiological factors of the lumbago-sciatica syndrome. Sometimes they go together and the patient doesn't know if it is sciatica or lumbago. There can be vāta, pitta, and/or kapha causes. There may be vāta pushing pitta, creating inflammation; or vāta pushing kapha, creating spinal tumor, meningeal tumor, or neurofibroma.

Whenever considering lower back pain, bear in mind all of these etiological factors. Don't jump too quickly to a conclusion. Understand the complete history, including the family history. In some families there is a genetic disposition for lumbago, sciatica, or obesity, which may lead to backache.

| OTHER CAUSES OF BACKACHE |
|---|
| • Strain and stress |
| • Overwork |
| • Under-exercised back muscle |
| • Sudden jerking movements |
| • Reflex actions, e.g., sneezing |
| • Obesity |
| • Pregnancy and childbirth |
| • Dysmenorrhea |
| • Scoliosis |
| • Anxiety, fear, insecurity |
| • Kidney disease |
| • Heart, lung, bone or reproductive organ disease |
| • Malformation due to congenital anomaly |
| • Tilted pelvis — if one leg is shorter than the other |

## Signs and Symptoms

The onset of lumbago pain or sciatica may be sudden or gradual. There can be attacks of lumbago that precede sciatica by a month or year. It is variable. Just a month ago, someone may have been suffering from lumbago, then today that person has sciatica. Lumbago also may be a complication of sciatica and vice versa. These complications may appear within a short or long period of time. Lumbago may also appear as sudden, severe, low back pain.

***Vāta.*** First, you must classify whether the type of pain is vāta, pitta, or kapha. Vāta pain is a shooting, throbbing, and pulsating type of pain. It is increased by movement of the lumbosacral and sacroileac joints. The pain can be so severe that the person is prevented from straightening or can do so only with difficulty. If you ask the person to stand straight, he or she stands slightly bent. The rough quality of vāta creates this stiffness. Vāta type of pain is more severe during vāta times: dawn and dusk, fall season, whenever there is cold or damp weather, a cloudy day, or a storm.

In severe vāta pain, there is parasthesia, loss of sense of touch, with numbness and tingling and sometimes wasting of the calf muscle. Vāta is dry, light, and rough. These qualities create *māmsa dhātu kshaya,* which shows as wasting or weakness of the calf muscle. This may cause foot drop. In *vāta grighrasī,* the quality of pain is shooting, cutting, throbbing, radiating, fluctuating, and migrating. It runs along the track of the nerve. Vāta pain is relieved by support and touch, such as massage.

***Pitta.*** In pitta type of grighrasī, the pain is burning, sharp, sucking, and pulling. There is pain and tenderness on pressure. This pain is exacerabated by coughing or sneezing, which increases pressure in the vein and in the subarachnoid space in the spinal area. Because pitta is sharp and burning, there is a tender spot. If you press the midpoint of the gluteal fold, the patient will jump. Another test is to have the patient lie on his back, with flexion of the leg and extension of the knee, and perform dorsiflexion of the ankle. This action stretches the sciatic nerve and will cause severe pain in the sciatic patient. That indicates pitta type of grighrasī, which is often provoked by vāta.

In grighrasī, if vāta is pushing pitta, there will be inflammatory changes. If vāta is pushing kapha, there will be dull and static pain. Therefore, to bring radical healing, we must clinically distinguish between these three types of grighrasī—vāta, pitta, kapha. There is no pain without vāta, no inflammation without pitta, and no congestion without kapha. It is vāta that causes the pain to move or radiate. When the grighrasī is secondarily pitta, there is inflammation as well as pain. If the secondary dosha is kapha, there is congestion along with pain.

Prolapse of an intervertebral disc may create inflammation. In a prolapsed vertabrae, vāta is involved first and then pitta. Then the person may get lumbar scoliosis and tenderness. If you look at the tongue, there will be a zig-zag line at the back of the midline of the tongue and then a straight line will come forward.

Symptoms may vary in intervertebral disc prolapse, depending upon which root nerve is affected. If the first sacral root nerve (S1) is involved, there will be loss of ankle jerk. Every reflex has a root value. We must know these root values, so that we can know exactly where the lesion is. When the lesion is at S1, there is also weakness of eversion[26] and weakness of the plantar reflex. If L5 is affected, there may be sensory loss, dorsiflexion of the toe, and foot drop. In some patients of prolapsed disc, because of involvement of apāna vāyu, the patient may have incontinence of urine, which is associated with L4, L5, S1 and S2.

Don't treat lumbago lightly. It can create serious problems, such as foot drop, incontinence, parasthesia, numbness, muscle weakness, and wasting.

To understand kati shūla and grighrasī syndrome, first read the person's pulse. Find the prakruti and vikruti. Then go to the fifth level and find asthi dhātu. What kind of spike is present—vāta, pitta, or kapha? Pulse diagnosis is the key to this ancient Vedic wisdom. Then ask the person to stand and observe how he or she stands. Then have the patient lie on the table and observe. Find out if both ankles are equidistant. If the pelvis is twisted, it indicates that one leg is a little longer than the other, which occurs if there are scoliotic changes. Measure the distance on the right and left sides to make this clear. Then touch the dorsum of your hand to the thighs, calves, and foot to determine temperature. If the

---

26. The condition of being turned outward.

temperature is dry and cold on the affected side, it indicates vāta. If the temperature is hot, it is pitta. If the skin is damp and cold, it is kapha.

This differential diagnosis will increase your diagnostic skill. Don't just jump to an herbal solution without developing this knowledge. There are a thousand herbs, but knowing which herb should be used in each condition is a skill we have to develop. When you have knowledge, there is a great deal of security, because you know what you are doing.

### Management

Now we will move to the management of the lumbago and sciatica syndrome. First, find out whether the condition is vāta, pitta, or kapha type, through study, symptoms, and your clinical observation. A thorough examination must be done before you can proceed further.

> T.I.D. = from the Latin means *ter in diem,* three times a day

## Treatment with Āma

If it is vāta type, find out if it is with āma (sama) or without āma (nirāma). With āma, the person will have coating of the tongue, bad breath, and constipation. In that case, don't do snehana (a specialized Ayurvedic oil massage) or svedana (an herbalized steam bath) because pañchakarma is not recommended during a toxic (āma) condition. Instead, use āma pachan with trikatu—ginger, black pepper, and pippalī—¼ teaspoon with honey TID. Also use triphalā guggulu, 200 mg TID. Give gandharva harītakī, one teaspoon at night with warm water. Keep the colon clean and remove āma, but do not suggest oil massage. Doing oil massage during a severe āma condition will actually push the āma into the deep tissues. Even the most expert massage therapist may commit such a mistake in treating a person with an āma condition, if this knowledge of Ayurveda is lacking.

If it is pitta type with āma, use kaishore guggulu, 200 mg TID. Also give trikatu 200 mg with aloe vera juice TID, and bhumi āmalakī, one teaspoon at night with warm water.

For kapha type with āma, use punarnavā guggulu, 200 mg TID, and include trikatu, 200 mg TID, taken with hot water and/or honey. Punarnavā guggulu reduces swelling and congestion. The above program is preliminary therapy to help to move the āma out of the system.

Examine the etiological factors. If constipation is present, triphalā will take care of it. If there is cystitis, cervicitis or colitis, then treat those causes. In these cases, the sciatica or lumbago is a symptom, not the disease. If it is cystitis, cervicitis, or colitis, you have to treat vāta pushing pitta. If it is a spinal tumor, treat vāta pushing kapha and use kāñcanāra guggulu, 200 mg TID. Ayurveda does not treat symptomatically; it deals with the root cause.

If the cause of lumbago and sciatica is ankylosing spondilitis, use anti-inflammatory herbs. The best anti-inflammatory herbs in Ayurveda are kaishore guggulu, gulvel satva, and kāma dudhā. If TB is the root cause, then treat the TB. Laghu mālinī vasanta—a traditional Ayurvedic medicine—is used in India, but not approved in the U.S. One tablet twice a day is the recommended dosage. Trauma, childbirth, and toxic infection also need special treatment.

We have discussed treating the doshas, with attention to vāta, pitta, or kapha with āma. Now we will shift to vyādhi pratyanika, treatment of the disease itself.

### Rest

In vyādhi pratyanika, rest for at least four weeks is essential in severe pain from a slipped disc. Sleeping on a firm mattress supported by boards is helpful for kapha type. Immobilization is important, resting the involved part of the body. A water bed or a soft bed is not good for lumbago. Soft beds are uneven and sleeping on an uneven bed is also a cause of lumbago or sciatica syndrome. Sitting for a long time is also aggravating, because it exerts pressure. Likewise, lifting heavy objects should be avoided. This may seem obvious, but some people continue to do heavy lifting because their job requires it.

### Exercise

Back stretching exercises are quite helpful. Yoga is a good accessory therapy but it is important to guide the patient properly. Beneficial postures include modified camel pose, modified cobra pose, and *mahā mudrā*. Include passive yoga exercises. The person lies on their back and you gently lift their legs, supported with a pillow. The person should learn the squatting pose, which is relaxing. When a woman has recently delivered a child and has a backache, she should sit in a squatting pose. The person should sit with pillow support behind the lower back, which relaxes the lumbosacral joint. Sitting flat on the floor is stressful to the back. When sitting in an armchair, using pillow support is quite effective.

Certain yoga prānāyāma (breathing techniques) are effective for lower backache. For example, use alternate nostril breathing with inner retention.

### Additional Management

* Raise your fitness level and increase aerobic capacity
* Wear special shock-absorbing inserts in your shoes
* Find your most restful position to sleep and do so in a horizontal position
* Stop overdoing things
* Try kaishore guggulu, mustā, and mahānārāyana oil massage
* Get a posture check
* Warm up your muscles before exercise
* Try water exercises and yoga
* Marma point, acupressure, or trigger point therapies
* Give up smoking
* Take it easy on sexual activity
* Warm up your lower back by applying external heat

## Treatment without Āma

*Snehana.* When āma is removed, treatment should include snehana and svedana. For a vāta person, use mahānārāyana or sesame oil for abhyanga. For a pitta person, use sunflower oil. For a kapha person, corn oil with vacha oil is effective. But never do snehana when there is āma.

*Svedana.* For svedana, put nirgundī or eucalyptus powder in the sweat box. A ginger and baking soda bath will also help pacify the pain. For a pitta person, give a short svedana, only 5 to 10 minutes in duration, because prolonged svedana is not good for pitta. For a kapha person, give a long svedana, 20 minutes to half an hour. Care should be taken in treating vāta to monitor the person during the svedana.

*Diet.* The person should follow the right kind of diet—vāta-pacifying food in a vāta condition; pitta-pacifying diet in a pitta condition; kapha-reducing food in a kapha disorder.

*Basti (Therapeutic enema).* For vāta, use dashamūla tea basti. Boil 2 tablespoons of dashamūla in one pint of water for 10 minutes. Cool and strain. If there is no āma, add ½ cup of sesame oil. That is called anuvāsana basti. If the person has muscle wasting, numbness, and tingling, use balā tea. Boil 2 tablespoons of balā powder in a pint of water for 10 minutes. Cool it, strain it, and then add ½ cup of sesame oil.

If there is severe tenderness, indicating pitta type pain, use gudūchī basti. Boil 2 tablespoons of gudūchī with a pint of water for 10 minutes. Cool and strain this, then add ½ cup of coconut oil. Coconut oil is anti-inflammatory and this basti will relieve inflammation.

To treat sciatica and lower back pain, you should do a basti every day for the first week, every other day the next week, every third day the third week, then once a week for the next six months.

For slipped disc, use a madhu tailam basti, which is one cup of sesame oil and ½ cup of honey mixed together. First, give a regular water enema and clean the colon. After a good bowel movement, wait for one hour. Then inject one cup of warm sesame oil and ½ cup honey mixed together. Give this once a day during vāta time, either in the early morning or very early evening. Ask the patient to retain it as long as he or she can. In some people it will not be passed, as it will be absorbed into the colon. This basti prevents muscle wasting. It will strengthen the ligament and help the disc to return to normal. It is also effective in treating urinary incontinence, because it enhances the strength of the sphincter muscle. If the nerve is affected in the segment of L4, L5, or S1, it may cause incontinence. Madhu tailam basti improves nerve conduction and is helpful in bringing back sphincter control in a slipped disc condition.

## Herbs

If you do not know the type of sciatica or lumbago, use the following formula:

| | |
|---|---|
| Dashamūla | 500 mg |
| Vidārī | 300 mg |
| Tagara | 300 mg |
| Mustā | 300 mg |
| Kaishore guggulu | 300 mg |

This mixture should be given ½ teaspoon TID with warm water, before food, to work on the lower part of the body.

For specific vyādhi pratyanika use:

| | |
|---|---|
| Yogarāja guggulu | 300 mg for vāta type |
| Kaishore guggulu | 300 mg for vāta pushing pitta type |
| Punarnavā guggulu | 300 mg for vāta pushing kapha type |

159

There are various guggulus, so choose the guggulu according to prakruti and vikruti.

Sometimes a kidney stone can create lower backache. In that case,use:
Gokshurādi guggulu300 mg

At the time of pain, give lemon juice and potassium carbonate.
1 cup of lemon juice
pinch of potassium carbonate

The following combination is effective for kapha and vāta type of pain.
Deodara          300 mg
Dashamūla        300 mg
Ginger powder    300 mg
Garlic powder    300 mg
Give ½ teaspoon TID to relieve pain of sciatica and lumbago.

Ayurveda says that even a fractured vertebra can be healed by mahāyogaraja guggulu, but it contains mercury and so its use is prohibited in the United States.

Rub the lower back with Maha Ganesh® oil and mahānārāyana oil before a bath.

There are also psychological causes for lumbago and sciatica. The sacrum supports the lumbar vertebrae. Whenever there is insecurity and fear, the sacrum moves slightly downward and creates a gap in the lumbosacral area, where vāta is easily aggravated and can cause pain. For a psychological cause, we treat the problem with Tranquility Tea© and support. Psychological counseling is also effective.

## Marma Chikitsā
*Trik, Ūrū, Sakthi Ūrvī, Jānu, Gulpha,* and *Pārshni* are marma points that are specific for treatment of this syndrome. *Pārshni marma* is a point at the central part of the heel that will relieve sciatica pain when it is pressed.[27]

Ayurveda is a fascinating medicine. It gives wonderful information to help the patient of lumbago and sciatica.

---

27. Illustrations are shown in the appendix on page 235.

# Chapter 21

# Diseases of Bones, Joints, and Connective Tissues

## Asthi, Sandhi, and Majjā Roga

Fall 1991, Volume 4, Number 2

AYURVEDA, THE SCIENCE OF LIFE, is an ancient art of healing that deals with all rheumato-logical diseases, which are called in Sanskrit *asthi, sandhi,* and *majjā roga.* These names indicate disorders of the connective tissue (majjā dhātu) that also involve joints (sandhi) and bones (asthi dhātu). In these rheumatic diseases, the presence of pain, stiffness, and swelling of parts of the musculo-skeletal system are the prominent feature.

According to Ayurveda, vāta dosha and asthi dhātu (bone tissue) are intimately associ-ated, due to the porous nature of the bones. They have a container-content relationship. The large intestine is the main site of vāta, and its mucous membrane nourishes the bones by absorbing minerals. Agni (digestive fire) and apāna vāyu govern this function in the colon. If agni is low, there will be production of āma (toxins) in the colon. Eventually this toxic material will be carried by vāta into the musculo-skeletal system, where it clogs the channels by producing congestion in the connective tissue. Depending upon which of the other doshas are involved, this āma may create various pathological conditions in the connective tissues, bones, and joints. These conditions may be of three types: inflamma-tory/infective, metabolic, and degenerative.

*Inflammatory/Infective Types.* Inflammatory or infective type of rheumatism is caused by pitta. Systemic pitta dosha and āma can linger in the asthi dhātu and produce acute rheumatic fever and rheumatoid arthritis, or make one vulnerable to infective ailments such as gonococcal or syphilitic arthritis.

*Metabolic Types.* Dhātu agni can undergo metabolic changes when āma is present in the blood. This can cause deposition of crystals in the joints, which, in turn, can manifest as gout and chondrocalcinosis.

*Degenerative Types.* When āma blocks asthi vaha srotas and aggravates vāta dosha, degenerative disorders can result, including osteoarthritis, spondylosis, and other painful syndromes of the connective tissues.

# Rheumatism

Rheumatism is a broad term as used in modern medicine. It embraces a diversity of symptoms and diseases of the connective tissue. Rheumatic diseases affect people of both genders and all ages and ethnic groups. The frequency of rheumatic disorders increases with age. One can observe that about 35% of people over the age of 60 have rheumatic complaints of one sort or the other. These ailments may severely disable a person or even shorten the span of life due to cardiac complications.

## Rheumatic Fever (Acute stage of Āma Vāta)

When an individual has low agni and eats incompatible food combinations, such as milk with fish or banana or meat with dairy), frequent tonsillitis or pharyngitis may result. Eating ice cream and drinking cold liquids may also reduce natural resistance and slow down the digestive fire (agni), which will result in production of āma in the gastrointestinal tract. Āma is then carried by vāta into the general circulation. When āma enters rasa dhātu, it results in further disturbance of agni. This imbalance of the fire principle, together with the invading āma in the rasa and rakta dhātus, causes a systemic inflammatory condition. It is called rheumatic fever, and it comes as a sequel to pharyngitis or tonsilitis. Rheumatic fever principally involves the joints, heart, central nervous system, and subcutaneous tissues. During the acute stage of the condition, vāta dosha carries āma throughout the body; then pain and swelling may migrate from joint to joint, affecting several large joints at once. This can lead to polyarthritis, fever, carditis or rheumatic valvular heart disease with a specific type of murmur. All these symptoms are the manifestations of toxic āma circulating throughout the body. Not everyone who has this kind of infection will develop rheumatic fever, but a subject having low agni, poor resistance, and systemic āma could develop rheumatic fever several days after an acute infection.

## Etiology and Pathogenesis (Nidāna and Samprāpti)

The ancient Ayurvedic literature says a great deal about the wrong kind of diet and lifestyle being important etiological factors in rheumatic fever. Over-active individuals and those who eat incompatible foods and chilled drinks are particularly susceptible. In addition to food-induced āma, other causes include bacteria, chronic constipation, and repressed emotions. Constant exposure to a cold draft, being in a chilly and damp climate, and low natural resistance are among the vāta-aggravating and agni-diminishing components that play a major role in the pathogenesis of this malady. Rheumatic fever can occur at any age, but because kapha and āma are similar in attribute, it is more common in childhood up to the age of 15, which is during the kapha stage of life.

Rheumatic carditis is the result of āma affecting avalambaka kapha and usually manifests first as a heart murmur of either mitral or aortic incompetence. In extreme cases, āma may be responsible for pericarditis and congestive heart failure leading to death. Carditis manifests as increased, irregular heartbeats and enlargement of the heart. This complication needs prompt medical supervision.

Āma can also create painless swellings (subcutaneous nodules) over bony prominences on the muscle tendons of hands and feet, elbow and patella, scalp and scapula.

Vāta pushing āma in the central nervous system can lead to prāna disorders, by creating irregular chorea-form movements. Chorea is a delayed manifestation of rheumatic fever, because it takes time for the āma to enter the nervous system. This vāta condition is associated with emotional instability, ungroundedness, and anxiety. In a pitta individual, rheumatic fever will likely manifest with high fever, abdominal pain, and nosebleeds. A kapha person will exhibit low-grade fever, swelling and loss of appetite.

The duration of rheumatic fever varies according to prakruti. In a vāta person it may last 6 weeks, in a pitta individual about 12 weeks, while in a kapha person it can remain present for 6 months. The chronic nature of the kapha type rheumatic fever may cause *dhātu kshaya* (degeneration of the tissues), which may lead to vāta disorders and rheumatoid arthritis.

## Chikitsā Sūtra of Āma Vāta (The Management of Āma Vāta)

The ancient Ayurvedic skills used to deal with āma vāta (rheumatic fever) are unique. The following are the basic principles of management of this disorder:

*Langhana.* Langhana is a therapy that involves fasting or eating light foods, which will indirectly bring down the person's temperature by breaking the chain of toxemia. In this case, Ayurveda suggests rice broth, very softly cooked rice, or tapioca as the best foods. All these should be spiced with cumin, mustard and ginger powder. This helps to kindle agni, burn the toxins lodged in the tissues and clear up the clogged channels. After langhana therapy, the tongue will become clean, the pulse will slow and the toxic pyrexia (elevated temperature) will be reduced. Langhana should be continued until positive indications of detoxification appear.

*Svedana.* Svedana means the application of heat. Methods include using a hot sauna, steam bath or shower, or applying a hot sand bag to the inflamed joint or joints. An herbal paste can also be applied directly to the affected joints, followed by application of heat. One such preparation can be made with powders of bachan, dhattūra, and vacha, along with with sufficient water to form a paste. These herbs should not be used internally. After applying the paste to the painful joints, one should sit near a fire or heater. This will dry the paste, pull toxic āma from the synovial membranes, and reduce pain, swelling and inflammation.

In the case of rheumatic fever, svedana should be done using dry heat, not wet heat such as a steam bath or shower. Āma is itself wet, so the dry quality of such heat helps to reduce āma. Dry heat will also help to detoxify the connective tissue and will clear the channels, thereby preventing further pathogenesis.

*Tikta Herbs.* Tikta means bitter taste, and bitter herbs are related to the elements Ether (ākāsha) and Air (vāyu). Thus they spread quickly into the subtle channels of the tissues. While overall the bitter taste is cooling, in this instance we use herbs that are both bitter and heating, such as rāsna, guggulu and parijata. These bitter, heating herbs will do āma pāchana (detoxify āma), clear blocked channels, and have an anti-pyretic and anti-inflammatory action. A few compounds containing these herbs include yogarāja guggulu, kaishore guggulu, mahārasnādi kvath, and parijatak guti.[28]

*Katu Herbs. Katu* means pungent. *Dīpana katu* are pungent herbs that enkindle agni and do āma pāchana (detoxification). Some pungent dīpana herbs include ginger, black pepper, and pippalī. These can also be combined and used as a compound called trikatu. They improve the immune system, circulation and appetite, and clear the tissues. They are also carminative, which means they dispel gas.

## Pañchakarma and Rasāyana

Once the fever and toxic manifestation of āma are under control, it is good to do pañchakarma therapy for at least seven days. Pañchakarma should not be done during the toxic, acute stage of pyrexia (fever), as it could then push āma into the vital organs. Once detoxification has progressed through use of the previously mentioned herbs, it will often be helpful to perform vamana (vomiting therapy), which will cleanse the stomach of āma. To induce vomiting one may drink licorice or calamus tea. Three days after vamana therapy, Ayurveda advises taking a dashamūla tea basti (herbal enema). For a total of five days, perform this basti daily, made of one pint of dashamūla tea, to remove residual āma from the colon.

Once the āma is totally removed from the GI tract, one should follow a rasāyana therapy suitable for the individual's prakruti. For vāta prakruti, ashvagandhā rasāyana is effective; for pitta, shatāvarī rasāyana is good; for kapha, punarnavā rasāyana is best. All constitutions may take balā rasāyana.

If there are cardiac complications with a heart murmur, Ayurveda recommends the use of suvarna bhasma (gold ash), arjuna, punarnavā, and deer horn ash at this stage of the treatment. All of these are helpful in cases of carditis.

Two teaspoons of castor oil can be taken along with ginger tea at bedtime when fever is absent, as it is highly effective as an anti-rheumatic. This remedy contains natural steroids and detoxifies the skeleto-muscular system and the connective tissue of the joints.

Garlic, ginger, mustard, and mint chutney can be included in the diet. If vāta dosha is elevated, herbal wines such as mahārasnādi kvath, drākshā, and dashamūla arishta are effective.

Through the use of vamana, basti, and rasāyana as well as proper diet and lifestyle, one can prevent the recurrence of rheumatic fever and rheumatoid arthritis. These disorders are generally complicated cases to manage, so it is advisable to consult an Ayurvedic physician who can offer expert advice on how best to proceed.

---

28. Guti is a round tablet as compared to a vati, which is a flattened tablet.

# Chapter 22

# Headache

Summer 1998, Volume 11, Number 1

AYURVEDIC ANATOMY DIVIDES the body into six parts: the head, trunk and four extremities. *Shira* means head, *shākhā* means extremity, and *madhyama* means the trunk. The head is also called *uttamānga*. *Uttama* means noble or great, while *anga* means a part of the body. The greatest part of the body is the head, because a person is identified by it: if the head is covered, we don't know who the person is.

The head is the seat of the four of the five doors of perception: eyes, ears, nose, tongue, and mouth. It is also the seat of the brain and it is connected to the trunk by the spinal vertebrae. The head and the face together express emotions and most of the srotāmsi (bodily channels), are related to the head.

Shira shūla means headache and it is a complex disorder. Ayurveda classifies shira shūla according to the dosha involved: vāta, pitta, or kapha type. Although headaches are quite common, this disorder can be distressing and may have serious significations. A headache is also classified according to whether it relates to majjā or asthi dhātu (nervous or bone tissues) and is considered to be a disorder of mano vaha srotas, the pathway of the mind. The gastrointestinal and respiratory tracts may also be involved.

***Doshic Headache.*** The three doshic types of headache are discerned by the nature and structure of the pain. A vāta headache is throbbing, shooting, and vague. It comes during the vāta times of day, which are dawn and dusk, and it is more common during fall (vāta season). A vāta headache is associated with constipation, indigestion, and abdominal discomfort. It is usually present in the occipital area at the base of the skull. Muscular pain in the neck and misalignment of the cervical spine can also cause an occipital headache. Stagnation of chronic āma in the colon is another cause, and traumatic accident and injury, such as whiplash or cerebral concussion, can also create a vāta type of headache. A vāta headache may also be due to too much exercise or insufficient sleep, or even a change in one's pillow or bed.

A pitta type of headache is due to excessive exposure to sunlight. It is usually located in the temporal area and is usually caused by hyper-acidity and acid indigestion. A pitta headache is associated with nausea, so vomiting can relieve that type of pain. The pain of a pitta headache is intense, sharp and penetrating and it makes the person irritable. This type of headache is more common during midday and midnight and during the summer season.

A kapha headache is slow, dull, and aching. It is located in the front of the head. It may be associated with kapha type of allergies, a cold, or congestion. A kapha headache often occurs during kapha times, which are mid-morning and mid-evening as well as spring season. Gravity plays an important role in a kapha headache. If you bend down, the headache is more intense.

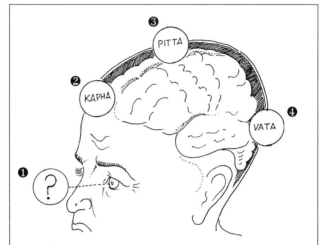

### Emotional Headache.
Emotional headaches are often located in the frontal areas of the head: the superior, middle and inferior frontal gyrus. Vāta emotions, such as fear, anxiety, and insecurity create a headache in the superior frontal gyrus. The middle frontal gyrus area is

❶ OBSERVATION of difficult situation or unpleasant sight.
❷ KAPHA aggravation has tamasic quality and can lead to sinus congestion.
❸ PITTA aggravation has excess sattva, producing acid indigestion or righteous indignation.
❹ VĀTA aggravation has rajasic quality and can generate anxiety or constipation.

related to pitta and associated with anger, hate, envy, judgment, and intense stress. Pain in the inferior frontal gyrus is related to kapha and associated with depression, attachment, greed, and possessiveness.

***Pathological Headache.*** The central top of the head is called the vertex. When this area is aching, it might be due to high blood pressure, cerebral vascular accident, or a space-occupying tumor of the pineal or pituitary gland.

***Referred Headache.*** A referred headache may be due to a tooth or gum infection. This type of headache will go from the cheeks to the temple to the parietal area. Trigeminal neuralgia is a typical pain along the track of the trigeminal nerve. It also goes from the cheeks to the temple to the parietal area. Rhinitis or an infection in the throat, nose, or tonsils can also create a headache in the parietal area. A person who has influenza and fever may get a bitemporal headache.

***Allergy and Chemical Toxicity and Sensitivity.*** Exposure to toxic chemical substances, such as insecticides or disinfectants, or even to certain pollens, may produce a pitta headache. Foul air, poor ventilation, carbon monoxide poisoning and some drugs, including tobacco and alcohol, can also create a headache. Some people are sensitive to wine, chocolate, or hard cheeses and these substances may cause a headache.

*Eye Problems.* Increased intraocular pressure, which is associated with glaucoma, and refractory errors may result in an intraorbital headache. Toxins in the liver (rañjaka pitta) can disturb allochaka pitta in the eyes and create photosensitivity and pain when the eyes are moving. This kind of headache falls under the pitta category.

*Ear Infection.* Ear infection and mastoiditis can create both temporal and parietal headaches.

*Osteoporosis.* Asthi dhātu is a seat of vāta dosha. When vāta is increased and asthi dhātu is decreased, this leads to osteoporosis, which may be responsible for ringing in the ears. This is a vāta disorder and can cause headaches in the supramastoidal area.

*Metabolic Disorders.* Headaches can also be produced by poor digestion, absorption and assimilation. These may be due to a deficiency of B12 or other vitamins or minerals, such as calcium, magnesium, and zinc, which will create changes in the plates of the skull and cause muscle stiffness, creating a headache. Metabolic disorders that can induce headaches also include hypoglycemia or hyperglycemia, sprue syndrome (chronic malabsorption), and obesity.

*Systemic Headache.* When there is a dysfunction in a srotas or system, it can create a headache. Nephritis, uremia, biliary tract disease, liver diseases such as hepatitis, rheumatism, diabetes, and severe anemia are systemic conditions that are all connected to mūtra vaha srotas (the urinary channel). Gastrointestinal tract disorders include hyper-acidity, pyloric stenosis, chronic constipation, acidosis, and alkalinosis. These conditions are associated with anna vaha srotas (the food channel) and are due to metabolic disorders of the digestive fire. Cardiovascular disease, such as congestive heart failure, myocardial infarction and edema, may increase pressure in the vascular system and cause a headache, while endocrine and pituitary tumors can create increased intracranial pressure. Hormonal dysfunction, leading to amenorrhea, polycystic ovary, increased prolactin secretions and pituitary adenoma, can also create headaches.

*Migraine Headache.* A migraine headache is caused by vāta pushing pitta in the hematopoietic system. This imbalance is responsible for disorders of the cranial blood vessels. It will create either artitis (inflammation of the arteries) or dilation of the carotid artery, along with visible pulsations in the temporal artery, leading to a migraine. There is alternation of the pain of a migraine headache. It often intensifies during pitta time (10 to 2 AM and PM) and then gradually subsides. Migraine headaches can create pitta type of depression, which can be serious. This kind of headache is also quite common in meningeal diseases, encephalitis, arteriosclerosis, and intracranial vascular disease.

*Miscellaneous Causes of Headache.* Headache may be due to fatigue, exhaustion, sunstroke, misalignment of the spine, prolonged strain of the neck muscles, or even cerebral metastasis of cancer. Withdrawal from any addictive substance, histamine toxicity, carbon dioxide retention, hypertensive encephalopathy, meningeal irritation or a history of posterior cranial fossa fracture can also create a headache. Headaches may also be due to a local skull lesion and the involvement of the trigeminal, glossopharyngeal, and vagus cranial nerves; the fifth, ninth, and tenth respectively.

***Sattva, Rajas, and Tamas.*** Intense sattva is characterized by righteous indignation and being unnecessarily discriminatory, judgmental, and fanatical. This can lead to temporal headache and is best treated with tagara. Rajas makes the mind hyperactive and nervous, inducing insomnia and leading to occipital headaches. Shankha pushpī will help in this condition. Overindulgence in tamasic activities, such as eating meat, sleeping for several hours during the day, and having a dull and monotonous lifestyle, can all create a sinus headache. The best remedy in this case is the herb brahmī.

## Management of Headaches

With such a vast picture of headaches, one must find the underlying causes and then treat accordingly. During an attack, use essential oils, pastes, nasya, and marma point therapy to alleviate the pain. Then follow up with more long-term management, using the herbs and procedures suggested in "Doshic Management of Headaches" on page 169.

***Essential Oils and Pastes.*** For a vāta headache, gently apply nutmeg paste or oil to the temples and frontal area. Hina, musk, cinnamon, garlic, and sesame oils are also effective.

| GUIDELINES FOR KNOWING THE SOURCE OF HEADACHES |
|---|
| • Temporal headache — TMJ, migraine, hyperacidity and cerebral vascular accident. |
| • Facial pain — dental infection, nerve involvement and electrical pain. |
| • Instant onset of pain may be due to ruptured aneurysm and is a severe condition. |
| • Cluster headache — peaks over three to five minutes, migraine. |
| • Pain during lifting heavy load or coughing or sneezing may be due to fractured posterial cranial fossa or skull injury. |
| • Accentuation of pain by environment. If pain is increased by head bending back or from side to side, it may be due to meningitis, which is serious. |
| • Pain during ovulation — PMS, hormonal imbalance. |
| • Pressure headache: increased intracranial tension, consider a tumor. This headache wakes the person at midnight. |
| • Local pain and tenderness — frontal and paranasal sinusitis. |
| • When the person sleeps with no pain, but gets a headache the moment he wakens, that is emotional. |
| • When headache is increased by movement of the eyeball, there is involvement of the meninges, which may lead to meningitis. |

For pitta, apply sandalwood paste or oil to the site of the pain. Jatamāmsi, jasmine, khus. and coconut oils are helpful as well.

For kapha, apply ginger or vacha paste. Camphor, eucalyptus, clove, cinnamon, or cardamom oils can also help to relieve kapha headache.

***Nasya.*** For vāta, use plain ghee or Sidha Soma® oil. For pitta, use brahmī ghee. For kapha, use vacha oil or dry vacha powder.

***Marma.*** Apply the appropriate doshic oil to the marma points shown in the illustration on page 169. Other points for headache include *Ūrdhva Skandha* (mid-point along top of shoulders, between neck and arm) and *Hasta Kshipra* and *Pāda Kshipra*.[29]

*Yoga.* Someone with a headache should not do inverted yoga poses. Simple āsanas, such as camel, cobra, cow, boat, bow, bridge, and spinal twist are helpful, as is ujjāyi prāṇāyāma. Empty Bowl meditation is also effective.

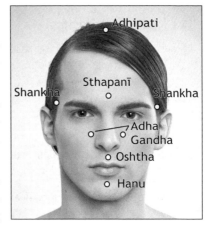

*Diet.* If headaches are caused by food allergies, one should generally avoid sour foods, peanuts, mushrooms, tomatoes, cheese, chocolate, fermented foods, and leftover food.

If the cause of the headache is emotional, try to resolve the issues triggering the headache. Use meditation and non-judgmental watchfulness. Counseling may also be useful in helping to determine the root cause.

One should be aware of the time when the headache is present and its relationship to food, emotions, and environmental or emotional stress. These simple Ayurvedic recipes, although not a quick fix, will eradicate the doshic cause and make the person's life free from headache. One should always consult with experts and have proper medical treatment if the problem persists.

## Doshic Management of Headaches

The herbal treatments that follow are for simple conditions. Other conditions we have mentioned, such as tumors or aneurysm, are more serious and require medical intervention.

### For Vāta Headaches

1) Use ½ teaspoon of the following mixture three times a day (TID) after food, with warm water:

| | |
|---|---|
| Dashamūla | 500 mg |
| Ashvagandhā | 400 mg |
| Balā | 300 mg |
| Tagara | 200 mg |

2) Take 1 teaspoon of harītakī an hour before sleep, with warm water.

3) Massage neck and shoulders with Mahānārāyana Oil.

### For Pitta Headaches

1) Use ½ teaspoon of the following mixture TID after food, with warm water:

| | |
|---|---|
| Shatāvarī | 500 mg |
| Gulvel Sattva | 400 mg |
| Shanka Bhasma | 200 mg |
| Kāma Dudhā | 200 mg |

2) Take 1 teaspoon of āmalakī an hour before sleep, with warm water.

3) Massage with coconut oil at the site of pain.

---

29. Illustrations shown in the appendix on page 236.

## For Kapha Headaches

1) Use ½ teaspoon of the following mixture TID after food, with warm water:

Sitopalādi          500 mg
Mahāsudarshan    300 mg
Trikatu             200 mg
Abrak Bhasma      200 mg

2) Take 1 teaspoon of bibhītakī an hour before sleep, with warm water.

3) Massage with eucalyptus oil or Tiger Balm® at the site of pain.

## For Headaches Caused By Allergies

Use bee pollen, which helps build immunity.

## For Toothache

Apply clove oil to the affected tooth, or swish warm sesame oil in the mouth.

## For Tonsillitis or Sore Throat

1) Use ½ teaspoon of the following mixture TID after food, with warm water:

Tālīsādi            500 mg
Mahāsudarshan    400 mg
Tikta               200 mg
Goldenseal         200 mg

2) Gargle with salt and turmeric at bedtime and in the morning.

## For Ear Infection

1) Use ½ teaspoon of the following mixture TID after food:

Goldenseal   200 mg
Echinacea    200 mg
Osha         200 mg
Turmeric     300 mg
Neem         300 mg

If ear infection persists, see your doctor.

## For Emotional Headaches

Use ½ teaspoon of the following mixture TID after food:

Jatamāmsi        300 mg
Brahmī           300 mg
Shankha Pushpī   300 mg

## For Sunstroke

1) Rub Bhringarāja Oil® onto the soles of the feet and the scalp at bedtime.

2) Use Brahmī Ghee® nasya, five drops in each nostril, twice daily.

3) Take sarasvatī, ½ teaspoon TID with water.

4) Avoid the sun.

## For Eye Problems

1) Use ½ teaspoon of the following mixture TID after food:

Punarnavā    500 mg
Brahmī       300 mg
Jatamāmsi    300 mg

2) Put 1 drop of castor oil in each eye at bedtime.

3) Rub soles of feet with castor oil at night.

## For Migraines from Vāta Pushing Pitta in the Majjā Dhātu

1) Use ½ teaspoon of the following mixture TID after food:

Ashvagandhā   500 mg
Gudūchī       400 mg
Jatamāmsi     300 mg
Tagara        300 mg

2) Use Brahmī Ghee® nasya, five drops in each nostril, twice daily.

3) Have an early breakfast. Then an hour after breakfast, eat a banana with one teaspoon of ghee, a pinch of cardamom and half a teaspoon of sugar.

# Chapter 23

# Migraine Headaches
## An Ayurvedic Perspective

Summer 1991, Volume 3, Number 1

MIGRAINE HEADACHES FALL into one of three categories: vāta, pitta, or kapha type. Kapha headaches are congestive and, strictly speaking, do not fall in the category of migraine. Vāta types of migraine headaches are more common at vāta time, which is 2 to 6 AM and PM, or pre-dawn and dusk. A vāta-increasing diet and incompatible food combinations such as milk with yogurt, bananas, or fish aggravate vāta migraines. Such headaches commonly occur on the left side of the head and are associated with light-headedness, constipation, gas, and tightness in the neck and shoulder area.

Pitta type of migraine headaches is associated with the sun. The moment the sun rises, with its heat and light, the headache starts. When the sun moves to its zenith at noon the headache is greatest, and at sunset the headache subsides. This type of headache is commonly on the right side and is sometimes diagnosed as sinusitis. Associated symptoms may include nausea, vomiting, heartburn, and sensitivity to light.

Kapha type headaches are due congestion in the system. The pain of this type of headache usually increases when the person bends over, while a more upright posture is found to relieve this pain.

To remedy vāta-type migraines, it is necessary to follow a vāta-pacifying diet. Basti (enema) is also indicated. In this case, five ounces of warm sesame oil, followed by one pint of strained dashamūla tea, is injected into the rectum and retained for thirty minutes, before being expelled. Then apply warm oil and heat to the temporal area of the forehead. Finally, nasya (nasal administration) of vacha, balā, or ashvagandhā oil is usually effective.

To deal with a pitta migraine, use virechana (purgation therapy). For this, ½ to 1 teaspoon of triphalā should be given at night with warm water. It is also important to follow a pitta-pacifying diet, with no sour food, citrus fruits, or acid-producing foods. Nasya is also good for pitta migraines. The best substances are brahmī or jatamāmsi ghee or even plain ghee.

Kapha headaches respond well to vamana (therapeutic vomiting). First apply warm sesame oil to the chest and back, and then drink a cup of licorice tea. Next, rub the tongue to stimulate the gag reflex. The resultant vomiting helps to relieve congestion from the chest, bronchi, lymphatics, and sinuses. Nasya is effective here too, using vacha powder or a combination of vacha, brahmī, and jatamāmsi. This will help to improve clarity of perception and relieve the congestion associated with a kapha type of headache.

During the period of most intense pain for vāta and kapha headaches, take one teaspoon of ginger powder, make it into a paste using warm water and apply it to the forehead. Kapha headaches can also be relieved by applying a paste made from calamus root powder (vacha). For intense pitta headaches, make a paste of sandalwood powder and apply this to the forehead.

Super Nasya Oil® is a nasya that contains sandalwood, eucalyptus, rose, and basil oils. Even when it is uncertain which dosha is causing the migraine, this balanced nasya oil is frequently effective. Administration consists of three to five drops in each nostril, followed by vigorous sniffing.

Gemstones can be of some help in relieving headaches. They work principally on the astral level and the electromagnetic field of the physical body. For pitta type of migraine, a red coral necklace with a pearl at the center can be effective. A pearl necklace is also excellent. Vāta headaches may be reduced by the use of pink or blue quartz, whereas a darker quartz or medium quality ruby, both of which are heating, is indicated for kapha headaches. Rudrāksha is effective for vāta and kapha headaches. Soak the rudrāksha beads in a cup of water overnight and in the morning drink the water. This will help to relieve an emotional migraine. During the pre-menopausal period, hormonal changes in a woman may create a migraine. Rudrāksha water is also useful in this case, as is wearing tulsi beads.

According to Ayurveda, there is no disorder without disturbance of the doshas. Hence, by balancing these energetic elements, the body can maintain a state of health.

# Chapter 24

# Parkinson's Disease
## Vepathu or Kampa Vāta

Spring 1997, Volume 9, Number 4

PARKINSON'S DISEASE IS a condition of disturbed systemic vāta dosha, which has gone into majjā dhātu (the nervous system.) Ayurvedic literature contains a complete description, etiology, symptomatology, pathology, and management of this condition, which is called *vepathu* or *kampa vāta*. *Kampa* means tremors. *Vepathu* means 'to go out of track' and it comes from the Sanskrit word *pātthā,* meaning passage.

James Parkinson, a British physician (1755-1824), studied vepathu and discovered where the pathological lesion takes place. Centuries before Dr. Parkinson's work, Ayurvedic literature described this disease in exactly the same way as Dr. Parkinson and called it kampa vāta. There is currently no satisfactory treatment for Parkinson's disease in western medicine. This article will present the views of both modern science and Ayurveda as they pertain to Parkinson's, in order to provide a complete picture for the reader.

Old medical books describe Parkinson's disease as paralysis agitans or shaking palsy. These names suggest neurological agitation. Ayurveda says that psychologically, the person with Parkinson's tends to be controlling or aggressive. When such a person loses control over a situation, majjā dhātu (the nervous system) becomes tense and performs under stress.

The initial and most debilitating physical feature of Parkinson's disease is absent or slowed movement. This poverty of movement results in the classic, masked-face appearance of a Parkinson's patient. Cogwheel rigidity may accompany this and the Parkinson's tremor is usually the most conspicuous feature of the illness. The tremor has a regular rate and primarily involves the hands and feet. Because the tremor is most evident when the person sits quietly with arms supported, it is called a resting tremor.

Patients of Parkinson's disease often lose their postural reflexes, which are the compensatory mechanisms that alter muscle tone in response to a change in position. This reflex loss, in combination with slowed movement and rigidity, results in a gait impairment characterized by shuffling, short steps and a tendency for the gait to accelerate in an attempt to catch the center of gravity. In addition, the voices of these people often become tremulous and low in volume, lacking normal fluctuations in pitch. Their handwriting also becomes small and tremulous.

As this illness progresses with the patient's age, dementia is a common complication. In addition, some people exhibit psychotic thought and behavior, manifesting as visual hallucinations, delusions, and chronic confusion. The sleep-wake cycle becomes disturbed and depression is also common.

## An Ayurvedic Understanding

How does Ayurveda describe this condition? A khavaigunya (defective space) is present within the area of the basal ganglia, which is in the deep core of majjā dhātu. Vāta dosha from the colon undergoes sanchaya (accumulation), prakopa (aggravation), and prasara (spread) and then in the fourth stage of disease—sthana samsraya (localization)—it lodges in this defective space in the basal ganglia. Vāta, because of its subtle quality, enters the extrapyramidal system and inhibits its functioning, affecting the person's coordination, gait, balance, and maintenance of posture. Prāna vāta, which works with sādhaka pitta in the cerebral cortex and tarpaka kapha through the basal ganglia, has an important function in coordination. Coordination is synchronization between prāna and apāna subtypes, with prāna providing sensory input and apāna providing motor function.

Classically, Parkinson's is found in a pitta-predominant person; a powerful person who has hundreds of people working under him or her, who is controlling and then loses that control. Loss of control creates fear, which causes a desire for control. They go together. A person who is pitta predominant and vāta secondary is most vulnerable. One in every thousand of the population is particularly prone to Parkinson's disease and I have seen hundreds of Parkinson's patients in India. These pitta people have an overpowering and controlling nature, and they always come from the space of confidence, courage, and aggressiveness. Then suddenly they lose something of value, such as a job, and they feel they have lost control. Or there may be some vatagenic factors, such as age. From 55 onward, the person is in the age of vāta and is more prone to Parkinson's. Divorce may also be the precipitating factor. In the first 25 years of marriage, there may have been a good relationship with understanding, sharing, and caring. Then suddenly a mid-life crisis may lead to divorce. A combination of stresses creates a vāta derangement and increased vāta dosha enters into the majjā dhātu, creating movement disturbances and involuntary movements, along with a lack of coordination, rigidity and tremors.

The defective space in the basal ganglia mentioned above is the cause of the Parkinson's lesion. The nuclei are affected and the nucleus itself contains sādhaka pitta. Between two nuclei, the communicating system is affected, which is tarpaka kapha. The neurotransmitter dopamine becomes deficient. Neurotransmitters are the product of sādhaka pitta, which manifests as tryptophan, serotonin, acetylcholine, melatonin, and dopamine. In Parkinson's, there is a deficiency of dopamine, as if sādhaka pitta is unable to perform its function because it is dried out by the excess vāta.

Paralysis agitans also results from a slow viral infection present in other conditions. Many times Parkinsonism comes as a complication of encephalitis, which is a pitta-related disease. In general, encephalitis, which is viral, creates a khavaigunya (defective space) in

174

majjā dhātu. Later, at the age of 55 or 60, in combination with other etiological factors, vāta undergoes sanchaya, prakopa, prasara, and then sthana samsraya (deposition) takes place in the basal ganglia. In that way, encephalitis can lead to Parkinson's disease.

The presence of a brain tumor is another causative factor for Parkinson's. A tumor that is either lodged within the extrapyramidal system or in the meninges (meningioma) can be the innermost cause in this type of Parkinsonism, where vāta is pushing kapha.

Venereal disease—gonorrhea and syphilis—can also be a factor. If not properly treated, the syphilitic bacilli move through the blood and can create a meningovascular syphilitic lesion. This type of lesion creating Parkinson's is from vāta pushing pitta.

Looking at these modern concepts with an Ayurvedic interpretation can give great insight. We have seen that psychological causes are important to consider. A person with pitta predominant and vāta secondary who tends to be aggressive, competitive, successful, and a workaholic can suffer a shock if he or she suddenly loses a job. Similarly, if a person who is quite dominating has a relationship break up during a mid-life crisis, that creates trauma and fear and can affect majjā dhātu. Depression can also be a precipitating cause.

Drug poisoning can also create kampa vāta. Drugs such as LSD, amphetamines, or marijuana affect the nervous system. Copper and lead poisoning is another possible factor, as is exposure to pesticides. Copper, manganese, lead, and carbon monoxide poisoning should also be considered. Carbon monoxide affects the brain, especially the extrapyramidal system, and a person can get Parkinson's from over-exposure to carbon monoxide.

The etiology of Parkinson's involves systemic imbalanced vāta and chronic āma, toxins, circulating in the body. Vāta and āma move throughout the body in the circulatory systems and then go into the rasa, rakta, māmsa, meda, asthi, and majjā dhātus. In majjā dhātu, vāta may push pitta or vāta may push kapha. If vāta pushes kapha, it can create a tumor in the extrapyramidal system of the brain, resulting in Parkinson's disease. If vāta pushes pitta, it may create a syphilitic meningovascular lesion within this area, which can also lead to Parkinsonism.

Within the fifth decade of life, between 50 and 60, the person becomes more prone to vāta disorders. Vāta may enter majjā dhātu by its subtle, dry, and rough qualities and create depigmentation and atrophy of the globus pallidus in the brain, which is involved with muscle movements and motor control. This may lead to depleted majjā dhātu and affect the coordination between prāna and apāna, thus creating tremors.

Generally, the patient comes to the practitioner because of tremors, and many conditions can create tremors. One must take a history and find out if the person has a great deal of anxiety, insecurity, or fear, which can all create tremors. Also, if the person has a toxic thyroid goiter, that will create tremors. Tremors are also present in an alcoholic patient, so one must ask about a history of alcoholism.

However, Parkinson's tremors have certain characteristics. They show up in the hand as fine tremors. If you place a piece of paper on the back of the person's outstretched hand, the tremors become visible. The Parkinson's patient has typically slow, rhythmic tremors, especially noticeable on the thumb. Then the tremors from the thumb move to the proximal parts of the extremity, moving to the wrist and then to the elbow.

In the earlier stages, vāta is mobile and irregular. Because of these qualities, the tremors are more accentuated by stress and embarrassment, although lessened during activity. Yet there is also rigidity, which means tremors with increased tone. Tone is a sustained state of contraction that is maintained by prāna and apāna vayus and coordinated at the spinal cord through the reflex arc. In kampa vāta, tremors are associated with rigidity and jerky sensations and gradually the fine tremors become more coarse. Flexion of the neck, elbow or knee is also a problem and the patient walks in short steps, as if walking downhill. Because of the tremors, most skillful actions are affected. The patient's handwriting becomes disturbed, he or she cannot thread a needle, and even fastening a button becomes challenging. Turning over in bed or rising from a chair is difficult, as if the person becomes like a statue.

In the classic picture of the Parkinson's patient, there is loss of the normal swinging of the arms while walking. The person walks with small steps, as though walking downhill. The face is without expression and even the eyes blink slowly and are without expression. Speech is slurred and talk is heavy and monotonous. The person's body becomes stiff and the gait looks like a statue walking. Ankles and knees are flexed; elbows and wrists are flexed, with the fingers making a pill-rolling movement. To compensate for prāna vāta dushti, bodhaka kapha is over-secreted, resulting in over-salivation, with saliva sometimes drooling down the face. Swallowing is slightly difficult and the facial muscles become rigid and masked, with no emotional expression of sadness, happiness, or joy.

We have discussed how in the sthana samsraya or deposition stage of samprāpti, vāta dosha lodges in a defective space in majjā dhātu. Later, māmsa dhātu is also affected because of the majjā dhātu dushti created by vāta. Rasa and rakta act as carriers for vāta dosha and once māmsa dhātu is affected; muscle tone is increased, leading to hypertonia, rigidity, and stiffness. It is as if patients of Parkinsonism are drowning in their own rigidity, both mental and physical. How we think and how we behave are bound to affect the nervous system. Fear, which is associated with vāta, creates emptiness. Therefore, the muscles become rigid to occupy the space of emptiness. Parkinson's rigidity, tremors, and spasticity frequently have their cause in psychological emotions.

One of my patients in India was bright and brilliant and he used to tease me. I was in Ayurvedic school at the time. He said to me "Come on, tell me my problem." I said to him, "Your problem is high pitta. You are controlling." "How will it manifest?" he asked. I told him that if he didn't drop that old habit, one day he would get Parkinson's disease. When I went to India recently, he saw me and he cried. He said that what I had told him long ago was now true. He had developed Parkinson's. I asked him how it happened. He told me an interesting story.

He had a high position in a governmental office. Under him there were two hundred people, which is a typical position for such a pitta-predominant man. He had some kind of dispute with a higher authority and they transferred him from one state to another. Because of that, he was in a state of shock and then developed Parkinson's. So shock or fear can create the trauma that precipitates Parkinson's—the shock of divorce, losing a job, or losing your residence.

# Treatment

How can Ayurveda help such a patient? Modern medicine uses drugs such as dopamine that can have drastic effects. Most of these drugs create more dryness, which is a vāta symptom. The person gets dry skin, dry mouth, dehydration, and blurred vision. In addition, dopamine is toxic to the liver, so it provokes pitta as well. It may also produce cardiac arrhythmia, so the heartbeat becomes irregular in some patients, and it increases systolic blood pressure. The person requires increasingly higher doses, but the higher the dose, the worse the pitta symptoms, such as nausea, vomiting, high blood pressure. It becomes a vicious circle.

Ayurveda looks at every individual according to his or her prakruti (constitution) and vikruti (current state). First determine the prakruti and vikruti. (see 'Eight Steps of Ayurvedic Healing') There is no doubt that kampa vāta is a vāta disorder, but there are three types—vāta pushing pitta, vāta pushing kapha, and vāta alone. Ayurvedic treatment is different for each of these three types.

## The Eight Steps of Ayurvedic Healing

There are eight components in the traditional Ayurvedic program of healing which distinguishes it from other systems of healing. They are:

- Determine the person's prakruti (constitution)
- Determine the vikruti (the present altered state of the doshas in the body)
- Find out the cause or causes of the illness, such as wrong diet, lifestyle, emotional patterns, quality of relationships, genetic predisposition, etc.
- The first line of treatment: removal of the cause or, if not possible, minimizing the effects, such as putting on a coat in cold weather.
- Provide the proper regimen: diet, exercise, prānāyāma, etc., according to prakruti, vikruti, seasons, climate, etc.
- Detoxification: either shaman (palliation) or shodana (elimination) such as panchakarma
- Provide therapies which are (a) antagonistic to the provoked dosha and (b) antagonistic to the disease, based on the principle that opposite qualities balance
- Rasāyana (rejuvenation) for the body in general, to increase immunity and to strengthen specific organs, tissues, and the mind

In the absolute vāta type of Parkinson's, the patient has cold hands, cold feet, extreme rigidity, the skin becomes rough and dry, and there is difficulty swallowing. The patient looks stiff and has problems with constipation. In my book, *Secrets of the Pulse,* there is a specific pulse described for the Parkinson's patient, in chapter 5, page 85. On the fifth level, when you feel the majjā dhātu pulse, there is a vāta spike that is hard and slender, with a slow rise and fall. If you feel this pulse, you will never forget it.

In the vāta pushing pitta type of kampa vāta, the vāta spike goes to the pitta site and the pulse is full and bounding. The person has profuse sweating of the palms and the skin feels hot and looks flushed. The sclera have a yellowish tinge and the patient has nausea, vomiting or loose stools. There is angular stomatitis, which is inflammation of the oral mucous membrane. Additionally, the systolic blood pressure tends to become high. These are typical characteristics of L-dopa toxicity.

In the vāta pushing kapha type of Parkinsonism, the vāta spike goes to the kapha site under the index finger on the majjā dhātu pulse, which is at the fifth level. The person has a slightly puffy face, anorexia, and low appetite. There is over-salivation, the person looks drowsy, and the skin is cold and clammy. These symptoms indicate a tumor in the extrapyramidal system.

## Pañchakarma

*Snehana.* The first treatment is snehana, which is oil massage. The skin is the door to the internal pharmacy. The application of massage oil aids in healing the doshic imbalance that is present. When we apply oil, it releases certain neuro-peptides within the subcutaneous tissue. These are the same neuro-peptides released in the nervous system that help to create a balance between serotonin, melatonin, and dopamine, thus pacifying vāta dosha and eliminating stiffness and tremors. For the pure vāta type, use sesame oil; for the pitta type, sunflower oil; for kapha type, corn oil. The entire body should be massaged and the oil should be warm.

*Svedana.* Svedana means hot steam therapy and nirgundī svedana is used for vāta. The leaves of nirgundī are boiled and that steam is used for treatment in a steam box. Nirgundī minimizes atherosclerotic changes. It is anticholinergic and relaxes the muscles, relieves spasms, pacifies vāta and eliminates pitta and kapha molecules from the system. For pitta and kapha, use eucalyptus in the steam therapy.

With pañchakarma, snehana and svedana may do half of the job, as they relax the muscles and remove rigidity, so that the tremors begin to minimize.

*Shirodhāra.* Shirodhāra is the continuous flow of warm oil onto the third eye, which stimulates the secretion of serotonin and melatonin. The release of these neurotransmitters helps to relax the muscles. Shirodhāra also stimulates tarpaka kapha and pacifies prāna, udāna, and apāna vāta. It brings tranquillity and relaxation.

*Nasya.* For vāta, the classical prescription is to use a vacha oil nasya. It is an herb that has been used safely in India for thousands of years. Unfortunately, the FDA has placed restrictions on the use of vacha in the US, so it cannot be used internally. However, using vacha aromatically and topically is legal. If there is pitta involvement, use brahmī ghee nasya. For kapha, use dry vacha powder for sniffing, called virechana nasya. Vacha oil is also good for kapha as well as vāta. Super Nasya Oil® nasya is balancing for all three doshas. Use of nasya for the nasal mucous membrane stimulates the basal ganglia, which is involved in the extrapyramidal system and performs the functions of equilibrium, maintenance of posture and proper gait. Hence, these functions may be helped by nasya.

### Ayurvedic Internal Medicine

Hypothyroidism is one causative factor in Parkinson's disease. In this condition, tarpaka kapha is blocking prāna vāta. Sometimes tarpaka kapha blocks both prāna and sādhaka pitta, leading to hot flashes or heat. If the patient of Parkinson's also has hypothyroidism, which is a kapha condition, you can use 300 mg each of shilājit and kukti TID.

*Dashamūla Tea.* Dashamūla tea is used for all three doshas and is literally a combination of the roots of ten herbs. Some roots work on vāta, some on pitta, and others on kapha.

Give dashamūla tea two or three times a day. To make the tea, place one teaspoon of dashamūla in a cup of hot water for 10 to 15 minutes, strain, and then give to drink. As a sweetener, add honey for kapha and vāta, or maple syrup for pitta.

*Garlic Milk.* Lasuna is garlic. Take one clove of garlic, chop it into small pieces, put it in a cup of milk and bring to the boil. This brings tranquility and acts like melatonin. Milk is also an effective source of tryptophan and induces relaxation. Garlic milk is used for kapha and vāta types of kampa vāta.

*Triphalā.* Triphalā is not only a laxative; it also acts as a rasāyana. It is a superfine food that eliminates free radicals from the system and it rejuvenates all seven dhātus. To rejuvenate majjā dhātu, use ½ to one teaspoon of triphalā daily at night. It keeps the colon clean, burns āma, and removes toxicity.

*Basti.* Dashamūla tea basti (enema) with oil removes toxicity and creates negative pressure in the colon, so that vāta in the majjā dhātu starts coming back to the GI tract. This helps to relieve one of the causes of kampa vāta.

*Gold Water.* Gold water or colloidal gold rejuvenates the nerve tissue. To use gold water, take one teaspoon twice a day on an empty stomach, or 10 drops of colloidal gold diluted in one teaspoon of water twice a day. Mahāyogaraja guggulu is a useful remedy that contains gold. If mahāyogaraja guggulu is unavailable, use yogarāja guggulu with gold water as an anupāna for vāta type of Parkinson's. Use kaishore guggulu for pitta type and punarnavā guggulu for kapha type.

*Other Measures.* People with Parkinson's need general supportive measures. Because of rigidity, they may fall and while cooking they may burn themselves. Family support is important to prevent injury.

Dietary restrictions should include no nightshades, such as potato, tomato and eggplant, and no beans. They should strictly follow a vāta-pacifying diet.

Because people with Parkinson's have disturbed vāta, their agni is vishama, so they need small but frequent meals, with sufficient calories and liquids. They tend to become easily dehydrated, so include water, relaxing herbal teas, and fruit juices to combat the dehydration.

Following a daily routine and an Ayurvedic lifestyle is important for patients of Parkinson's. The patient should practice gentle yoga stretching with support as required, including the camel, cobra, cow, boat, bow, and bridge poses. It is my observation that these are effective in relaxing the muscles. Illustrations are on page 181.

The person can also benefit from So'Hum meditation, which is powerful yet relaxing. Breathing and sound have great effect upon the extrapyramidal system. The best mantra in this case is pronounced 'hreem.'

We are fortunate to have the knowledge of both Ayurveda and modern medicine available to us. All medical systems have value. A healer's heart should be open to all systems and all possibilities. Ayurveda is a living system that embraces all life and all medical systems. Ayurveda looks at each individual, disease and imbalance specifically, and then recommends a treatment regimen particular to the cause or causes, the unique individual and the presenting symptoms. The treatment regimen may include components from several medical systems, such as herbology, yoga, meditation, counseling, and even pharmaceutical drugs and surgery when necessary. In this way, we can bring a complete and holistic approach to a patient of Parkinson's.

## For Vāta-type Parkinson's

| | |
|---|---|
| Ashvagandhā | 500 mg |
| Ātma Guptā (Kapikacchū) | 300 mg |
| Vidārī | 300 mg |
| Balā | 300 mg |
| Tagara | 200 mg |

Tagara is a tranquilizer and muscle relaxant. Balā has anticholinergic action, which relieves muscle spasm, gives muscle energy, regulates normal muscle tone, and relieves rigidity. Vidārī inhibits tremors and ātma guptā is a specific remedy for Parkinson's disease. Ashvagandhā helps to heal the lesion in the extrapyramidal system.

## For Pitta-type Parkinson's

| | |
|---|---|
| Shatāvarī | 500 mg |
| Ātma Guptā (Kapikacchū) | 300 mg |
| Gudūchī | 300 mg |
| Balā | 300 mg |
| Vidārī | 300 mg |

Balā and vidārī are specifically antagonistic to the disease. Shatāvarī and gudūchī are used to pacify pitta.

## For Kapha-type Parkinson's

| | |
|---|---|
| Punarnavā | 500 mg |
| Ātma Guptā (Kapikacchū) | 300 mg |
| Gokshura | 400 mg |
| Vidārī | 300 mg |
| Balā | 300 mg |

Punarnavā is a cerebral diuretic. Again we are using vidārī, ātma guptā, and balā to treat the disease.

## Recommended Yoga Poses

Camel
Cobra
Cow (2)
Boat
Bow
Bridge

*Postures, clockwise
from top*

# Chapter 25

# Male Health Issues

Winter 2006, Volume 19, Number 3

IN AYURVEDIC LITERATURE, the prostate gland is called *ashthīlā,* round pebble, for its resemblance in structure. Made of muscular tissue, it secretes an alkaline, soft, liquid and slightly dense seminal fluid, in which sperm floats. The gland is located just below the bladder and surrounds the neck of the bladder and the urethra. Both the *shukra vaha srotas,* male reproductive channel, and mūtra vaha srotas, urinary channel, share the common passage of the urethra and the neck of the bladder.

Ashthīlā's function is to act as a pump and during sexual intercourse it helps to ejaculate semen forcefully to reach its goal. This gland, however, may become inflamed, infected, or enlarged. Predominately during old age, or around age 60, this gland may become enlarged, a condition called benign prostatic hypertrophy. However, nowadays this is also manifesting in younger men in their 40s. Though it is not a serious thing, chronic enlarged prostate can create recurring urinary tract infections.

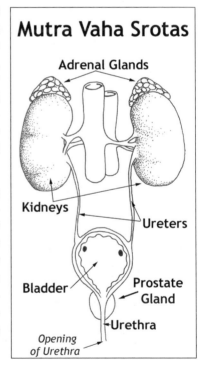

**Mutra Vaha Srotas**

Adrenal Glands

Kidneys

Ureters

Bladder

Prostate Gland

Urethra

Opening of Urethra

## Prostatism and Prostatitis

In old age, the agni of shukra is low and it can lead to undue production of raw shukra dhātu, reproductive tissue, leading to enlarged prostate. The enlarged prostate in turn constricts the urethra and the flow of urine from the bladder; this condition is called prostatism.

Prostatitis is the inflammation of the prostate gland. According to Ayurveda, this is a pitta-type disorder in which the apāna vāyu pushes pitta into either shukra or mūtra vaha srotas and causes inflammation of the prostate gland, generating prostatitis.

Prostatitis can be uncomfortable, irritating, or painful because it disrupts urine flow. Later, the swelling increases with consequent blockage and retention of urine flow. The urine backs up from the urethra to the ureters and ascends, causing inflammation in the kidneys. When chronic prostatitis occurs, it can lead to bladder or kidney damage and marked malaise of these organs.

### Samprāpti (Etiology and Pathogenesis)

Repeated attempts and prolonged effort to start the flow of urine is the pūrva rūpa (prodromal signs and symptoms) for both prostatism and prostatitis. Gradually there is decreased urine flow and the force of flow is weak or may dribble near the end of the act of urination. At this point, the man feels as if the action is completed but leakage may occur afterwards, wetting the underwear. This contributes to the typical urine odor of these conditions. Additionally, some amount of residual urine remains in the bladder, as the bladder never empties itself completely. The residual urine can become a fertile breeding ground for bacteria to grow and be the cause of bladder infections.

### Nidāna (Causes)

Causes for prostatitis and prostatism are sexual transmitted diseases such as gonorrhea, syphilis, herpes, urinary tract infections, or low agni of shukra vaha srotas. In cases of low agni, tejas starts burning ojas and there is excessive production of prostate tissue resulting in a high PSA (prostate specific antigen) count.

### Signs and Symptoms

Trouble starting urine flow or reduced flow with dribbling result in increased frequency of urination causing the person to wake up at night to urinate, thus creating insomnia. Burning urination, fever, and chills, caused by the pitta-type inflammation, are other signs of these conditions.

### Diagnosis/Assessment

A doctor does the assessment through a physical examination and, typically, the examination of the prostate is performed by digital rectal examination (DRE). The physician examines the size, feels the condition of the prostate, and massages the prostate. Further findings of pus in the urine on the same day of examination would be indicative of abnormality. In some cases, a urine culture is collected for bacterial examination; in others, an IVP[30] is recommended and, in obscure cases, a rectal ultrasound and prostate biopsy may be performed. In an Ayurvedic assessment, both the shukra dhātu pulse and the bladder pulse would be weak.

---

30. Intravenous pyelogram, an x-ray for the urinary tract using contrast material by injection in the bloodstream.

One should inquire about weight loss as well. If there has been rapid weight loss, then the prostatic hyperplasia may be malignant. If there has been no significant weight change, the prostatic hyperplasia is generally benign. Additionally, one can observe the flow of urine in passing. If the flow goes more to the right side, that is indicative that the left gland is enlarged.

## Chikitsā (Management)

Asthila belongs to both shukra and mūtra vaha srotas. So, one needs to remember always to include in the herbal formulation substances that address the following: the dosha pratyanika (dosha specific), vyādhi pratyanika (specific to disease), ubhaya pratyanika (specific to dosha and disease), dhātu pratyanika (specific to tissue), and srota pratyanika (specific to bodily channel).

In cases of bacterial infection with burning sensation, in India, one would use sūkshma triphalā (triphalā powder that has been potentized by a triphalā concoction several times) and gandhak rasāyana (compound of purified sulphur), 200 mg of each TID with an anupāna (vehicle) of cumin, coriander, and fennel (CCF) tea. In the USA, one would use 200 mg each of goldenseal, shilājit, echinacea, haridrā, and take ½ teaspoon of this mixture TID for a similar effect.

In cases of fever and chills, have the client take punarnavā 500 mg, gokshura 400 mg, and mahāsudarshan 300 mg with aloe vera gel, ½ teaspoon, TID.

If a person has dribbling urination, they should drink large quantities of water to flush the prostate and gently massage the perineum with castor oil. Also, a bath with 1/3 cup of baking soda (no ginger) would be helpful to relieve dribbling.

In cases of prostatic enlargement, the dosha pratyanika of choice would be ashvagandhā for vāta, shatāvarī for pitta and punarnavā for kapha. Shilājit would be the vyādhi pratyanika, to reduce the enlarged prostate; gokshura, the dhātu pratyanika, to maintain the tone of the prostate tissue; and kutki or gokshurādi guggulu for scraping of the abnormal growth as ubhaya pratyanika.

Other herbal formulas that have been proven to be useful in maintaining health in the area are chandraprabhā vati, gokshurādi guggulu, shilājit, ashvagandhā pills, and the very alkaline ushīra to reduce burning.

When PSA values are high, Ayurveda suggests consumption of a handful of white sesame seeds with jaggery[31] as one's only food for one to two days. Also, take internally a

The PSA count is done by evaluating the nanograms of prostate specific antigen per milliliters of blood.

In the past, most doctors considered PSA values of 4 or below normal. Recent research found prostate cancer in men with PSA levels below 4.0 ng/ml. Many doctors are now using the following ranges, with some variation:

- 0 to 2.5 ng/ml is low
- 2.6 to 10 ng/ml is slightly to moderately elevated
- 10 to 19.9 ng/ml is moderately elevated
- 20 ng/ml or more is significantly elevated.

31. Unrefined brown sugar obtained from the sap of the East Indian jaggery palm.

formula comprising equal parts (300 mg each) of punarnavā, trikatu, shilājit, and gudūchī with hot water. Take this for 90 days as a preventative measure and to maintain proper dhātu agni of the prostate gland.

## Āsanas and Kriyā

The best yoga āsanas for prostate are *kukkutāsana,* cock or rooster pose, *vajrāsana,* thunderbolt pose, and *dhanurāsana,* bow pose.

A *kriyā* (action) that is called *Ganesha dhauti kriyā* can be very helpful. After each bowel movement, wash the anal orifice with warm water and apply castor oil to the anal orifice. The technique then is: with a properly clipped and filed nail, put the castor oil on the left middle finger and insert it into the rectum. Breathing by the mouth to relax the sphincter muscle, gently rotate the finger three times clockwise and three times counter-clockwise while pulling forward in an attempt to massage the top of the prostate. This kriyā is quite effective to reduce the size of the prostate gland. You can wear surgical-type gloves for this, available at any drugstore.

Another practice that can be done for self-healing is the *ashwini mudrā,* which means female horse gesture and is done by contracting the sphincter muscles of the anus. This practice improves the circulation in the prostate gland and maintains its tone. The technique is very similar to *mula bandha* (root lock); however, it does not require the breathing technique. This technique is contraindicated in cases of fissures, fistula, thrombosed piles, and prolapsed piles/hemorrhoids.

Recurring sexual intercourse is considered to help maintain the health of the prostate gland. In cases of prostatic problems, therapeutic sex is often advised. However, frequency of intercourse should be maintained at once or twice a month.

# Impotence

The corpora cavernosum penis[32] normally are filled with blood during sexual excitement. *Klaibya,* impotence, is an inability to achieve and maintain an erection, which is necessary for sexual intercourse. The blood in the prostate is rich in ojas, which causes the penis to become rigid, erect, and firm with tone. Impotence is a lack of blood supply to this gland, often due to high cholesterol, high triglycerides, diabetes, and obesity. Impotence is classified as a partial or total impairment of function.

**BHASMA**

A specialized Ayurvedic preparation alchemically produced by fastidious purification and burning into ash; bhasmas are very potentized, easily absorbable, and release prāna into the system.

There are two types of impotence, primary and secondary. In primary impotence, either kapha is blocking vāta or vāta is pushing kapha in the shukra vaha srotas, creating a block. In this case, the man has never had the ability to have an adequate erection from the onset of puberty. This primary impotence may be due to trauma or intense fear. In secondary impotence, there is an inability to complete the act of intercourse to the fullest satisfaction for both partners, which may be interrupted

32. The two columns of erectile tissue on the dorsum of the penis.

by premature ejaculation. In both cases, impotence can create low self-esteem, put a strain on the marriage, and stress the relationship.

## Nidāna

In primary impotence, causes can be varied ranging from a vāta or kapha-provoking diet and lifestyle to physical trauma, psychological trauma, job-related stress, fear of pregnancy, unresolved deep-seated grief, sadness, and/or childhood sexual trauma or abuse.

Secondary impotence may occur in a person who is recovering from a heart attack or has undergone major surgery. In these cases, the fear of death transfers itself to a fear of sex because during orgasm there is a temporary death. Secondary impotence may also occur as a result of antihypertensive drugs, tranquilizers, diuretics, antidepressants, drugs, pituitary surgeries or tumors, alcohol, marijuana, smoking cigarettes, and excessive masturbation, which depletes shukra dhātu.

Structural abnormalities, obesity, chronic consumptive disease, tuberculosis, diabetes, hypertension, stress, trauma, and sexual trauma in previous relationships can be both primary and secondary causes.

The *asthāyi shukra dhātu,* which is raw or unprocessed reproductive tissue, is generally processed by shukra dhātu agni, creating ojas, vigor, and vitality. If the nutritional fire of shukra dhātu is low, it can create imbalanced hormonal changes and diminished testosterone.

## Signs and Symptoms

First, one can notice a lack of interest in sex; this is followed by an inability to maintain an erection. One should understand that this does not mean infertility or the person's inability to father a child when, in general, the sperm count is good.

Normally the inability to maintain an erection causes irritability and low self-esteem. This sexual anxiety leads to abnormal behaviors ranging from seeking stimulation through pornography to extramarital affairs as a proof of manhood. Using romance as a stimulus to maintain an erection is short-lived for the organ that cannot endure. These behaviors cause further conflict in the man's relationships, thus producing more frustration, irritability, and low self-esteem.

## Assessment

Assessment of this disease can be done by darshana (observation), sparshana (palpation), and prashna (questioning) to find out the cause of impotence. In addition, check the blood pressure and the person's weight. Run blood tests for hormone and cholesterol levels. Rule out diabetes and venereal diseases. Perform a urine examination to assess semen-urea content. Often impotence can be a weight-related problem, even when the man is only twenty or thirty pounds overweight.

Modern medical assessment tests include the nocturnal penile tumescence test (NPT) performed by an electronic monitoring device or a snap gauge fitted around the penis. This test can determine if a man is having normal erections during sleep, their duration and stiffness. If there are no erections in the course of two days then there is a definite physical cause and not an emotional cause. Another test is the intercavernosal injection test, in which a medication is injected into the base of the penis to produce an erection and fullness, stiffness, and duration of the erection are then measured.

## Prevention

To prevent impotence, a man should limit or abstain from the consumption of drugs and alcohol. Another preventative measure is to maintain proper weight and, if necessary, embark upon a weight-reduction program. Ayurveda recommends a regular yoga practice that includes *sūrya namaskāra* (sun salutation) and prāṇāyāma.

The herbal approach to heal this problem would be the use of aphrodisiacs, called *vājīkaranam*. Typical vājīkarana substances are herbs such as ashvagandhā, balā, vidārī, kapikacchū, also called ātma guptā, gokshura, shilājit, pippalī, and spices such as cardamom and bay leaves. Vājīkaranas also encompass the use of almond milk, goat's milk, goat testicle soup, and dates in ghee or date shakes.

> **DATES PRESERVED IN GHEE**
>
> Warm one pound of fresh ghee and pour over 30 unseeded dates in a glass jar. Stir gently to evenly distribute the ghee amongst the dates. Close the container and allow it to sit for at least 15 days. As an aphrodisiac and to promote healthy ojas, consume one date daily for a full month.

A week or two of the cleansing program pañchakarma can be very helpful. Typically, the administration of a basti (enema) containing dashamūla and ashvagandhā milk will follow the snehana (oiling) and svedana (sudation or sweating) treatments. This combination has a very powerful healing and rejuvenation potential.

To help maintain an erection there is an herbal ointment that can be applied to the pubic bone and penis to enhance circulation and tone. Prepared in a ghee base, use a combination of herbs such as ashvagandhā, vidārī, clove, deer musk, nutmeg, gokshura, and ātma guptā. One can substitute ashvagandhā oil for the ghee. In general, Ayurveda recommends the use of garlic milk, ashvagandhā milk, shatāvarī milk, chyavānaprāsh and, in India, mākaradvāja, to enhance and maintain erectile function.

> **DASHAMULA-ASHVAGANDHA MILK BASTI**
>
> 1 pint of water
> 2 Tbs. of dashamūla
> 2 Tbs. of ashvagandhā
> 1 cup of warm milk
>
> **Option One**
> Bring the herbs to a boil in the water for 3 minutes, turn off heat and allow the brew to cool before straining. Once strained add one cup of warm milk to the brew.
>
> **Option Two**
> Bring the herbs to a boil in the milk and water together. Then strain and allow to cool.

## Surgical Solutions

Some patients may require surgical repair of the artery or vein. Various surgical implantation methods can help to produce a functional erection. Many require training to master the techniques and all have some side effects including but not limited to local bruising, scarring, complications, surgical risks, and penile pain. Psychological counseling by a sex therapist is usually advised as well.

## Conclusion

The male reproductive system is important in the life of every man. For some men, disorders of shukra vaha srotas are connected with physical causes such as obesity, diabetes, and hypertension. Trauma and emotional issues can be causative factors as well, leading to low self-esteem that may put a stress on relationships. The clinician must always consider both physical and emotional factors when managing male sexual health. Additionally, Ayurveda offers many non-surgical remedies that can support and enhance male sexual function, leading to greater satisfaction in one's life.

**MAKARADVAJA**

Also called cinnabar-gold and known as the best alchemical drug for longevity, is a renowned of mercurial rejuvenator or bhasma, whose main ingredients are mercury, sulphur, and gold. It regenerates vigour and vitality, improves immunity, and assists in body development by increasing metabolic activity. The best forms of Mākaradvāja have gold leaf on the outer surface of the pill as well as gold within.

# Chapter 26

# Female Health Issues

Winter 2005, Volume 18, Number 3 and Spring 2006, Volume 18, Number 4

IN THE ANCIENT Ayurvedic literature, there are many recommendations about ārtava vaha srotas. This is the female reproductive system and it includes the ovaries, fallopian tubes, fundus of the uterus, uterine wall, cervix, cervical canal, and vaginal cavity.

In the process of tissue nutrition, the end product of digested food, called āhāra rasa, nourishes the seven tissues: rasa, rakta, māmsa, meda, asthi, majjā, and shukra or ārtava dhātus. Rasa dhātu is primordially important, as it carries hormones and nutrients, and is responsible for the gaseous exchange of oxygen and carbon dioxide. In the process of tissue nutrition, the immature (asthāyi) rasa becomes mature (sthāyi) and in that transformation, by-products (upadhātus) of rasa dhātu are formed. These include stanya (the lactating tissue) and raja (menstruation). It takes five days for rasa dhātu to reach maturation, ten days for rakta, fifteen for māmsa, and so on. Hence, it takes ārtava and shukra dhātus up to 35 days to reach maturity.

## The Menstrual Cycle

Menstruation starts at menarche and continues until menopause. Menarche is typically between the ages of nine to 14. In girls with hyperactive pitta, menarche can start at age nine, while in kapha types it usually doesn't begin until age 14, 15, or even 16, because kapha is slow. Menopause is the age of vāta. It may start as early as age 35 in some pitta women, but can occur at age 58 to 60 in kapha types.

Menstruation, one of the by-products of rasa dhātu, is called raja. Poetically, Sushruta describes the menstrual process as 'the weeping cry of the vagina for the deceased ovum.' During the 25 to 30 days of the menstrual cycle, the new ovum or egg is formed and enters the fallopian tubes where it eagerly waits to meet with a sperm. However, if the sperm does not show up, the ovum dies. The menstrual flow is a funeral for this deceased ovum.

According to modern science, the endometrial tissue thickens during the menstrual cycle to prepare the uterus for a possible future pregnancy. According to Ayurveda, this thickening of endometrial tissue is due to poshaka kapha,[33] which is a by-product (mala)

191

of rasa. Approximately midway through a monthly cycle of menstruation, ovulation occurs. Ovulation is a process by which the ovary, which is called *antah phala* or 'inner fruit', ripens and releases an egg (ārtava) by means of *ārtava agni,* which relates to estrogen. This egg travels via the fallopian tube toward the uterus.

If fertilized by a sperm, the egg starts to slowly move from the fallopian tube into the uterine cavity, as it is seeks a place for nutrition. Implantation takes place at the fundus. If the fundus is healthy, with many capillaries, implantation occurs and the fetus grows there. However, if the woman is anemic, weak, undernourished, or has tuberculosis, then the fundus is weak as well. Weakness, in combination with *apāna vāyu dushti* (a disorder of downward vāta), and exacerbated mobility, can lead to implantation in the lower segment of the uterus. This leads to placenta presentation, also called placenta previa, and it is unhealthy, as it can cause hemorrhage prior to or during labor.

If, instead, there is excess kapha, the increased sluggishness can cause the fertilized egg to stay within the fallopian tube, instead of proceeding on its journey to the uterus. If implantation happens there, it gives rise to ectopic gestation. For correct implantation to occur there needs to be poshaka kapha, which relates closely to the role of progesterone in modern science.

If the egg is not fertilized, the thickened endometrial lining tissue starts breaking down. In Ayurveda, it is apāna vāyu that breaks this endometrial wall, due to its dry, hard, and rough qualities. Then those pieces of endometrial wall are passed as part of the menstrual flow.

The menstrual flow contains these broken-down pieces of endometrial wall as well as the unfertilized egg, red blood cells, white blood cells, and mucus. As it is related to rasa dhātu, this monthly cycle is controlled by rasa dhātu agni, ārtava dhātu agni, apāna vāyu, and poshaka kapha.

Modern medicine claims the cycle is controlled by the female hormones secreted by the ovaries and pituitary gland. In Ayurveda, these hormones are nothing other than ārtava agni and they are regulated by prāna vāyu, sādhaka pitta, and tarpaka kapha.

## Dysmenorrhea
Dysmenorrhea, which means painful menstruation, is called *kashthārtava* in Ayurveda. *Prathamik kashthārtava,* meaning primary dysmenorrhea, occurs shortly after the onset of menstruation in young teenagers and in women who have never been pregnant. *Dvitīyak kashthārtava,* which is secondary dysmenorrhea, develops later in life, after the woman has been menstruating for sometime. This can be due to a vāta imbalance leading to narrowing of the blood vessels and cervix, a pitta malfunction leading to endometriosis, or a kapha imbalance leading to a fibroid tumor.

There are two internal causes of vāta dushti (qualitative disturbance of vāta): one is dhātu kshaya (debilitated tissues), which leads to the second, sroto rodha (blockage of the channels). Therefore, dhātu kshaya can bring about a narrowing of the cervix. Generally

---

33. For more information on poshaka kapha, see "Management of Rasa Dhātu Mala," *Ayurveda Today,* Summer 2008, Volume 21, Number 1.

during menstruation, when the uterus contracts, the cervix should dilate. Contraction of the uterus is governed by prāna and dilation of the cervix by apāna vāyu. When this rhythm is disturbed, the cervix remains closed. In this condition, called pinhole os, the woman has severe pain, the blood doesn't flow, and blood clots are held within the uterus. In the passing of these clots, they force a dilatation of the uterus in a type of nature-induced dilatation and curative.

In pitta-type of kashthārtava, rañjaka pitta from the rakta and rasa dhātus goes into the endometrial wall and creates inflammation. This is called endometritis. Due to the hot and sharp qualities of pitta, the mucus lining of the endometrium and cervix become inflamed, causing pitta-type of dysmenorrhea.

In kapha-type of dysmenorrhea, excess poshaka kapha is produced and it accumulates within the uterine wall, leading to fibrotic changes. These too can lead to dysmenorrhea.

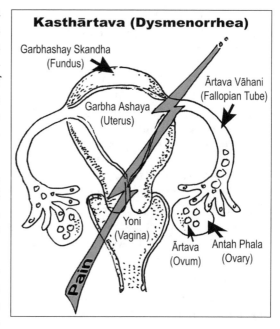

**Kasthārtava (Dysmenorrhea)**

*Etiology (Nidāna).* In vāta-type dysmenorrhea, a vāta-provoking diet is a common etiological factor. This means the consumption of too many raw vegetables, beans, chickpeas, and so forth. Other causes can be too much traveling, excessive physical activities, especially jogging, jumping, and trampolining as well as unresolved fear and anxiety. Also, prostaglandin, which is present in chocolate, provokes vāta.

There is a path of samprāpti (pathogenesis) for each dosha as it accumulates and then spreads through the system. Here we'll talk about the first four stages of samprāpti as it relates to dysmenorrhea. Vāta undergoes sañchaya (accumulation) and prakopa (provocation) in the colon, then prasara (spread) throughout the body. During this time, there is constipation, gas, and bloating. Then *vāta sthana samshraya* (deposition) happens within the capillaries of the uterus, so there is contraction of the blood vessels and that decreases the blood flow. It is this constriction that causes pain during menstruation in vāta-type of dysmenorrhea.

In pitta-type of dysmenorrhea, the woman's diet is typically pitta provoking: hot, spicy foods, sour fruits, and citrus fruits. Working in hot conditions, plus emotionally unresolved anger and frustration are also common. These physiological and psychological factors trigger pitta, which undergoes sañchaya and prakopa in the grahani (small intestines), then prasara and sthana samshraya happens through the walls of the blood vessels, causing inflammation of the uterus and endometrium.

In kapha dysmenorrhea, the causes include eating dairy products such as cheese, yogurt, and ice cream, plus eating gluten (mainly from wheat products) as well as insufficient exercise and excessive emotional attachments. Kapha undergoes sañchaya and prakopa in the stomach, then prasara, and in the fourth stage of disease kapha passes through the rasa dhātu of the uterus and enters the endometrium wall. There it produces thickening, possibly causing a fibroid tumor.

***Signs and Symptoms (Lakshana).*** In vāta-type of dysmenorrhea, there is constipation, bloating, lower backache and severe cramps, and the woman also has insomnia, palpitations, fear, and anxiety. There is scanty menstruation, but more clots than normal. Symptoms appear to be more intense during the earlier part of menstruation. Once the woman passes the clots, they cause dilatation of the cervix, and as a result she feels better.

In pitta-type of dysmenorrhea, there are hives, rashes or urticaria, plus mild attacks of urethritis, cystitis and burning urination. In earlier menses, there is acne on the face, nausea, vomiting, diarrhea or loose stools, headache, and irritability. Pitta dysmenorrhea is experienced more during the mid-menses. Once the excessive heat is released through the menses, the woman feels better.

In kapha dysmenorrhea, there is a thick, watery, curd-like, white discharge. There is more mucus and less blood. The uterus looks or feels bulky, and there is a dull, aching pain. There is also increased frequency of urination (polyuria), water retention, and swelling. The woman's bra and rings on her fingers become tight, and she is lethargic and doesn't feel like going to work. She would rather eat candy, cookies, and chocolate and watch TV at home. There is often depression during this period. Lethargy and excessive sleep take over and some women have excess salivation, a runny or stuffy nose, and sinus congestion. This generally occurs during the earlier part of the period, although it may happen throughout the menses.

***Management (Chikitsā).*** For proper management, one must take the family history and personal history. Sometimes, one can take advantage of the support of modern technology, such as an ultrasound, to find out whether there is a uterine fibroid. In some cases, an x-ray may be required.

In Ayurveda, what is important is pulse diagnosis. As well as assessing the prakruti-vikruti paradigm, one would concentrate on the fifth-level dhātu pulse. At this level, dysmenorrhea would show as a weak ārtava pulse, with vāta pushing pitta, pitta pushing kapha, kapha blocking vāta, or pitta in ārtava dhātu.

Management in vāta dysmenorrhea requires abhyanga (oil massage), with nirgundī oil or mahānārāyana oil applied to the lower abdomen and lower back. This should be followed by svedana (sweating), using local fomentation or a hot bath to ease the pain. Internally, the person can begin taking fifteen days prior to the menses, ½ teaspoon of an herbal combination of:

| | |
|---|---|
| Dashamūla | 500 mg |
| Ashvagandhā | 400 mg |
| Mustā | 300 mg |
| Tagara | 200 mg |
| Yogarāja Guggulu | 200 mg |

This should be taken TID with warm water, before meals. This remedy pacifies vāta dosha and relieves pain. After cessation of menses, one should administer a dashamūla tea basti (enema) containing ½ cup of sesame oil. This is followed by a vāta-pacifying diet. For vāta dysmenorrhea, the best yoga poses are camel, cobra, and cow pose, while best types of prāṇāyāma are nāḍī shodana and anuloma viloma.

Management in pitta dysmenorrhea requires abhyanga with coconut oil or sunflower oil. No svedana is generally needed, because pitta is already hot by nature. However, a baking soda bath is effective during painful periods. To do this, put one-third of a cup of baking soda (not baking powder) into the bathtub and fill with warm water.

Internally, beginning fifteen days prior to the menses, the person can take ½ teaspoon of an herbal combination of:

| | |
|---|---|
| Shatāvarī | 500 mg |
| Gudūchī | 300 mg |
| Kāma Dudhā | 200 mg |
| Ashoka | 300 mg |

This should be taken TID with aloe vera gel, before meals. After the cessation of menstrual bleeding, virechana (purgation) can be performed with one teaspoon of bhumi āmalakī at bedtime. For pitta dysmenorrhea the best yogāsanas are boat, bow, and bridge poses, and the best prāṇāyāma for pitta is shītalī.

Management for kapha type of dysmenorrhea requires snehana with visha garbha tailam or a kapha-pacifying oil medicated with heating herbs, such as trikatu or chitrak. Chitrakadi tailam is a good example. This should be followed by svedana, either using dry heat from the topical application of ginger paste to the lower belly, or wet svedana by means of a ginger bath. This means adding ginger powder to a bathtub of hot water. Internally, fifteen days prior to the menses, ½ teaspoon of an herbal combination of:

| | |
|---|---|
| Punarnavā | 500 mg |
| Kutki | 200 mg |
| Shilājit | 200 mg |
| Trikatu | 200 mg |

This should be taken TID before meals with honey. After the cessation of menses, a kapha-pacifying diet and exercise routine should be followed. For kapha, the best āsanas are lotus, locust, lion, palm tree, and spinal twists, and the best prāṇāyāma are bhastrikā and kapāla bhāti.

# Premenstrual Syndrome

Premenstrual syndrome or PMS is a complex set of physical and emotional symptoms that is experienced a week or so before the menstrual cycle begins. It appears five to fourteen days before the menstrual cycle and usually disappears after menstruation. In the past, PMS was thought to be caused by emotional instability or hysteria. The word *hysterus* is Greek and it means uterus. Uterine dysfunction is called hysteria. However, there is a definite cause and reason for PMS and it is not only an emotional disorder.

*Manifestation.* Like dysmenorrhea, PMS can be a mono-doshic, dual-doshic, or triple-doshic disorder. The etiological factors are also similar to those of dysmenorrhea.

In vāta-type PMS, systemic vāta undergoes sañchaya, prakopa, and prasara and then the sthana samshraya happens in the ārtava vāta srotas, leading to fluctuations of the hormones. In pitta PMS, the pitta accumulates and is then provoked and spreads. In kapha PMS, increased kapha spreads through the body and fluid retention is the result.

*Signs and Symptoms (Lakshana).* In vāta-type of PMS, there is nervousness, anxiety, tachycardia, insomnia, debility, and lower backache. In pitta-type of PMS, there can be hives, rashes, urticaria, acne, cystitis, irritability, and migraine headache. The nipples become sensitive to the touch and the breasts become tender. There may be repeated attacks of cystitis or urethritis, with burning sensations while passing urine. In kapha-type of PMS, there is fluid retention, bloating, enlarged breasts, and ankle swelling. The woman may put on a couple of pounds of excess weight, have white discharge, and a bloated, puffy face.

*Management (Chikitsā).* Before approaching management, one should take the client's history: her personal history and family history. One must also find out the symptomatology and read the pulse, especially the prakruti, vikruti, and ārtava dhātu pulses.

Whenever we are dealing with PMS, it is rare to have a mono-doshic disorder, as this syndrome is almost always a combination of two or three doshas.

When there is anxiety, tachycardia, palpitations, and headaches, the woman should avoid methylxanthine, a group of naturally occurring agents in caffeine. This means avoid coffee, chocolate, tea, and colas.

For headaches, herbs such as tagara and jatamāmsi can be taken in equal proportion: ½ teaspoon of the mixture TID. Also for headaches, nasya with vacha oil is highly recommended.

When a woman has anxiety, tachycardia, or insomnia, tranquilizing herbs such as brahmī, jatamāmsi, and shankha pushpī can be used or she can try my formula, Tranquility Tea©.

For edema, reduce salt intake and avoid pickles, cucumber, watermelon, ice cream, candy, cookies and chocolate. Some diuretic herbs, such as punarnavā and gokshura, can be helpful in the quantity of ½ teaspoon TID.

| Signs and Symptoms of PMS |
| --- |
| **Vāta** |
| Sadness |
| Hopelessness |
| Self-deprecation |
| Tenseness |
| Anxiety |
| Feeling 'on edge' |
| Mood swings |
| Fear |
| Loneliness |
| Insomnia |
| Overwhelm |
| Lower backache |
| **Pitta** |
| Irritability |
| Anger |
| Interpersonal conflict |
| Judgment |
| Criticism |
| Lack of patience |
| Breast tenderness |
| Swelling |
| Suicidal thoughts |
| Cystitis |
| Acne |
| Hot flashes |
| **Kapha** |
| Depression |
| Decreased interest in usual activities |
| Withdrawal from social relationships |
| Difficulty concentrating |
| Fatigue |
| Lethargy |
| Poor appetite |
| Bloating |
| Weight gain |
| Leukorrhea |
| Food cravings |

T.I.D. = from the Latin means *ter in diem*, three times a day

To create emotional balance, one can do alternate nostril breathing, called anuloma viloma prāṇāyāma, and also have an oil massage and take a hot bath. *Marma chikitsā* is also helpful and the best marmas for PMS are *Nābhi, Bhaga,* Sakthi Ūrvī, Jānu, Gulpha, and Trik.[34] Nutmeg essential oil can be applied to these energy points.

If a woman has a hormonal imbalance, Ayurveda suggests the use of food precursors of estrogen, such as shatāvarī, kumārī, ashvagandhā, vidārī, and soy, or precursors of progesterone, including nirgundī, kapikacchū, and balā. Also, primrose oil in a 500 mg capsule daily can help in maintaining hormonal balance.

Uterine tonics to strengthen and tonify the uterus are shatāvarī ghrita (or shatāvarī ghee), yashthi madhu ghrita (licorice ghee), and vidariadi ghrita (vidārī ghee). Note that shatāvarī should not be given if there is pathology involving āma. Ideally, to maintain balance, one would use dashamūla ghee for vāta, shatāvarī ghee for pitta, and tikta ghee for kapha.

For prevention of PMS, daily yoga āsana and prāṇāyāma are beneficial as well as abhyanga (oil massage) and svedana (steam therapy), plus weekly *uttara basti* (see Uttara Basti on page 203) to pacify vāta in the lower uterine passage. For abhyanga, cottonseed oil can be applied topically along with lotus oil.

> **SHATAVARI MEDICATED GHEE**
>
> Shatavari, powdered
> Water, filtered
> Ghee
> Take one part of shatavari to 16 parts of water, stir together in a stainless steel cooking vessel.
>
> Bring this to a boil then turn the heat down until the concoction is simmering. Cook at a simmer until the mixture is reduced to ¼ the original amount. Cool and strain.
>
> Then add ghee that is equal in volume to the volume of the concoction. Cook this mixture over medium heat until all the water evaporates. It is very important that the water is completely eliminated as otherwise the ghee will spoil.
>
> Pour into a glass container with a tight fitting lid. This will keep indefinitely. You can use the same principles of this recipe to make other medicated ghees.

## General Rasāyana and Foods to Favor

Rasāyana (rejuvenation therapies) for dysmenorrhea and PMS include shatāvarī and kumārī (aloe vera). Medicated wines, such as ashok arishta and kumārī arishta, can be taken in the dosage of four teaspoons with an equal amount of water after lunch and dinner.

The best foods to favor in dysmenorrhea and PMS are broths, urud dhal soup, winter squash, zucchini, and pumpkin for vāta. Mung dal soup, red lentil soup, grapes, shatāvarī milk, and coconut milk are good for pitta. Kapha should favor light and easily digested foods.

Avoiding grief and sadness is the rasāyana for vāta, avoiding judgment and argument is that for pitta, while letting go of attachment as well as not sleeping during the daytime is the rasāyana for kapha.

---

34. Illustrations are shown in the appendix on page 236.

**Part Two**

We have discussed the menstrual cycle, managing imbalances, and the role of diet as well as PMS, its symptoms and management. In this next section, we cover disorders of menstrual flow and maintaining vaginal health.

# Menorrhagia

Menorrhagia is a disorder characterized by excessive bleeding at the time of a menstrual period, either in the number of days or the amount of blood passed or both. In Ayurveda, this condition is called *asrugdhārā* or *adhoga rakta pitta*. This pitta disorder is quite common during the pitta time of life, mainly between the ages of thirty to forty. It can lead to iron deficiency anemia.

For a woman with pitta prakruti and/or pitta vikruti, one should look at her diet as well as her lifestyle activities. Physical activities like jogging, jumping on a trampoline, heavy weight lifting, or hiking can provoke vāta dosha and this can lead to menorrhagia.

*Etiology (Nidāna).* The samprāpti (pathogenesis) of menorrhagia varies according to the condition. There is an assortment of ways that pitta becomes aggravated and excessive bleeding is one of the signs of high pitta. In the tissue nutrition of rasa dhātu, its upadhātus (by-products) are stanya (lactating tissue) and raja (menstruation). When vāta dosha is provoked, vyāna vāyu (systemic vāta dosha) will push rañjaka pitta into the rasa and rakta dhātus (blood and plasma tissues). In the case of excessive physical activities, vāta is pushing pitta in the *rajo vaha srotas* (menstruation channel). Surplus pitta in this channel will show up as increased bleeding during menstruation.

Vāta pushing pitta in the ārtava vaha srotas may be also responsible for the disturbance of hormones controlling the overall menstrual cycle. The vāta symptoms of this are lower back ache, lower abdominal pain, distention, palpitation, anxiety, and fear with slight insomnia. The pitta symptoms would manifest as burning sensation in the urethra, cystitis of unknown origin, nipples becoming sensitive to touch, tender breasts with cravings for sweets, irritability, and a judgmental and critical attitude for no apparent reason. In the case of a fibroid tumor, especially the intramural type with increased vascularity, this is also vāta pushing pitta in the blood vessels and it can rupture the capillaries, creating heavy menstrual flow.

As vāta becomes provoked, apāna vāyu in the pelvic cavity also pulls rañjaka pitta into the pelvic area, causing further inflammation of the pelvic organs. There is no inflammation without the ushna (hot) and tīkshna (sharp) qualities of pitta and these are contributing factors in menorrhagia.

Another consideration in prolonged menstrual flow is the strength of agni. When dhātu agni is low (manda or slow agni), there is undue production of raw tissue. This unprocessed tissue from rasa dhātu is eliminated as raw raja (menstruation), producing excessive menstrual bleeding. Low dhātu agni is attributed to hypothyroidism.

The assessment and diagnosis of abnormal menstrual flow is important and should be continued until resolved. Pap smear tests are needed in order to detect serious underlying causes, such as cervical erosion and cervical dysplasia. For some individuals a biopsy of cervix and uterine membrane tissue is done in order to find possible abnormality and to rule out adhoga rakta pitta, a bleeding disorder. A blood profile is also recommended, to find if there is any sign of blood dyscrasia, hemophilia, polycythemia, and/or anemia. Even leukemia can be the cause of severe bleeding.

***General Management (Chikitsā).*** For management of menorrhagia, it is wise to build the health of the client as the loss of blood can be depleting. First, reduce physical activity and get rest. Second, administer sufficient iron to improve the quality of the blood. For iron supplementation in India, we give loha bhasma and abhrak bhasma. In the west, we use foods such as currants, raisins, beet juice, and carrot juice; and we can give kumārī āsava (an herbal fermented wine) and aloe vera. Third, for balancing the hormones, ingest the food precursors of estrogen such as one of the following for a month.

| | |
|---|---|
| Shatāvarī | 500 mg, TID |
| Kumārī Āsava (an herbalized wine) | 4 tablespoons with an equal amount of water, after lunch and dinner |
| Primrose oil capsules | 500 mg at bedtime |

The typical formula for asrugdhārā (menorrhagia) is shatāvarī 500 mg, as dosha pratyanika, then gulvel satwa 300 mg, as an anti-inflammatory, ashoka 300 mg as a hemostatic, and vāsaka 300 mg also as a hemostatic. This formula is given TID, ½ teaspoon with pomegranate, cranberry, or aloe vera juice.

Bhumi āmalakī, is a mild laxative, hemostatic and anti-inflammatory, and a good source of iron. It should be taken in the quantity of one teaspoon at bedtime. Whenever there is a pelvic floor, inflammatory disorder causing profuse bleeding, bhumi āmalakī is the herb of choice. Other very famous hemostatic herbs in Ayurvedic literature are ushīra/khus, dūrvā grass/conch grass, lodhra, ashoka, and vāsaka. Hemostatic minerals are laksha, and pravāl pañchāmrit and kāma dudhā.

Other traditional Ayurvedic compounds used for menorrhagia are shatāvarī ghee, dūrvā ghee, pradarāntak vati and lodhra āsava. In some instances ghee should not be given. For example, if there is āma (toxins) present, then there should be dīpana (kindling of agni) and pañchana (digestion) first.

# Amenorrhea

Amenorrhea is an absence of or abnormal stoppage of the menstrual flow and is called nasthartava or rajah kshaya in Ayurveda. It can be primary (prathamik) or secondary (dvitayak). Prathamik nasthartava, or primary amenorrhea, is lack of menarche or failure to begin the menses by the age of 16. This condition can continue indefinitely. Dvitayak nasthartava, or secondary amenorrhea, is the absence of two, three or more periods in a row in a woman who has been menstruating for some time. Secondary amenorrhea may be a temporary phase.

It is completely normal for menses to be absent during pregnancy, the period of lactation, and after menopause.

***Etiology (Nidāna).*** The samprāpti of amenorrhea creates endocrine gland disorders and hyperthyroidism. When there is hyperthyroidism due to an excess of dhātu agni, the dhātus become depleted, leading to nasthartava. This is usually caused by increased vāta and kapha doshas. In this situation, kapha is blocking vāta or vāta is pushing kapha in ārtava dhātu (female reproductive tissue) as well as in majjā dhātu (bone marrow and nerve tissue).

The occurrence of extreme kapha disorders can also cause primary amenorrhea. This elevated kapha would manifest as hypothyroidism or myxedema, or as a genetic abnormality such as damage to or missing ovaries, the absence of a uterus or vagina, an excessively thick hymen or un-open hymen requiring surgery. Other etiological factors include congenital diabetes, malnutrition, obesity, deep-seated emotional anxiety, extreme stress, or anorexia.

Some things responsible for secondary amenorrhea are activities such as strenuous exercise, aggressive sports, and taking part in marathons, since intense physical training provokes vāta. Also, poor nutrition, fasting, drastic weight loss, jet lag, and traveling can cause dvitayak nasthartava. It may seem surprising but intense spiritual practices—yoga, meditation, and prānāyāma where the goal is enlightenment—can cause secondary amenorrhea as well. These practices cause the energy of the body move up to the higher chakras thereby diminishing the downward movement necessary for menstruation.

Other causative factors for secondary amenorrhea are taking drugs such as corticosteroids and birth control pills, major surgery, severe shock, stress, and loss of body fat.

***Signs and Symtoms (Lakshana).*** Samprāpti differs according to the etiology but common signs and symptoms of primary amenorrhea are general abnormal physical maturation. This includes the young girl failing to develop breasts and an absence of secondary sexual characteristics, i.e., pubic and auxiliary hair. The girl may also exhibit minimal sexual maturity such as at the age of 16 she acts like a little girl or infant and has stunted growth. In secondary amenorrhea there are no symptoms at all other than anemia and weight loss. However, this can be detected by pulse analysis. The 5th level pulse, that is the dhātu pulse, will show either a strong vāta or kapha spike at the ārtava dhātu site.

For assessment and accurate diagnosis, a blood test for genetic hormonal disorder should be done. An x-ray or ultrasound study should be performed to check for the development of the uterus. A complete blood profile for anemia and, if found, discovering the cause of the anemia. One should also check if there is tuberculosis, severe anemia or blood dyscrasia.

***Management (Chikitsā).*** The treatment for primary amenorrhea is a hormonal therapy program including including building therapies such as *brahmana chikitsā* and *tarpana chikitsā*.[35] These are complex programs that should be done with the guidance of an Ayurvedic physician.

Pañchakarma, the Ayurvedic cleansing program, is also helpful. For the pañchakarma procedure of snehana (oil applied by a specific massage), the best oil to use would be a balā tailam (an herbalized oil prepared by a specific sequence of techniques), a vāta-pacifying tailam or almond oil. The svedana (sudation) would be encouraged with nirgundī.

---

35. Refer also to *Textbook of Ayurveda,* Volume 3 for more on these therapies.

Herbs such as shatāvarī, ashvagandhā, balā, vidārī, and ātma guptā would be used to promote *bālya jīvinīya* (strength, life-giving).

For an intact hymen that needs to be opened, a surgical procedure is required. Unfortunately there is nothing that can be done in cases of infantile uterus, the absence of an ovary, or the presence of two small uteri.

If the amenorrhea is due to poor nutrition, then one should undergo a blood nutritive program. If it is from drastic weight loss, then one would help balance meda dhātu (adipose tissue) with meda rasāyana (rejuvenation) herbal combinations like shatāvarī ghee or balā ghee. Take 1 teaspoon TID before meals. When the cause is jetlag-induced amenorrhea, one should have an oil massage and take 1 teaspoon each of balā and trikatu or balā and ginger, mixed together in milk. If the origin is from one's spiritual practices, then reduce or stop these practices entirely. If the patient is taking steroids then they should consider discontinuing the steroidal therapy. Of course they would discuss alternatives with their primary care provider. If amenorrhea is due to stress then one should do less, relax, rub bhringarāja or brahmī oil on the scalp and the soles of the feet, and try So'Hum meditation. You can supplement this with herbs. Take ½ teaspoon TID of a mixture of ashvagandhā 500 mg, jatamāmsi 300 mg, and shankha pushpī 200 mg

If the amenorrhea is a result of major surgery, then one should have rasāyana (rejuvenation) therapy with the herbs shatāvarī 500 mg, balā 300 mg, and vidārī 200 mg. Take ½ teaspoon of this mixture TID. For hormonal imbalance, one can use primrose oil or phytoestrogens like aloe vera, soy, and shatāvarī ghee. For emotional imbalance the ideal herbs are brahmī 200 mg, jatamāmsi 200 mg, and sarasvatī (herbal compound) 200 mg, ½ teaspoon TID. You can also use 10 drops of Deep Love® tincture taken before meals.

### Prevention

Prevention is always better than a cure. So, to prevent amenorrhea and the possibility of amenorrhea, one should seek good nutrition through diet. Be sure to get plenty of iron in the diet and consume food items that are good sources of iron such as papaya, pomegranate, mango, pumpkin, pineapple, currants, raisons, soaked almonds, garlic milk, shatāvarī milk, or shatāvarī kalka with milk at bedtime. Shatāvarī kalka is a compound of shatāvarī roasted with ghee and to which saffron, cardamom, and sugar are added.

For someone who is prone to problems with amenorrhea, maintaining proper body weight by following a healthy, vāta-pacifying diet is important. These women should also avoid excessive strenuous exercise and sports and instead rest, read, and relax!

## Vaginitis

Vaginitis in Ayurveda is called is called *yoni paka*. Yoni means vagina and paka means digestion or inflammation. It is an inflammation of the vagina usually accompanied by burning and itching of the external genital organ.

Flare ups are more likely occur in the summer, due to heat and moisture. Common causes are:

♦   Increased systemic pitta.

- An imbalance in the vagina caused by micro-organisms such as fungus (Candida albicans), bacteria (Gardnerella vaginalis), and protozoa (Trichomonas vaginalis) and by pinworms, roundworms, and threadworms.
- Birth control pills.
- Antibiotics, like tetracycline or erythromycin, which may kill certain flora allowing other to flourish.
- A hot, moist environment or climate.
- Wearing tight pants and synthetic underwear.
- Putting on a wet bathing suit, which is a breeding ground for infectious organisms.
- Sexual intercourse with an infected individual.

Causes of noninfectious vaginitis or vaginitis due to direct irritation are chemical irritation from douches, sprays, bubble bath, talcum powders, poor feminine hygiene, and using scented, colored toilet paper, which will have more chemicals and hence, be more irritating. Vaginitis may also occur during pregnancy, diabetes, and gonorrhea.

***Signs and Symptoms; Management.*** Signs and symptoms vary according to etiological factors. Diagnosis can be complex. It is done by collecting a specimen from the woman and then determining the microorganism involved by microscopic examination of the sample. Once you have a diagnosis, your doctor is likely to prescribe medicines such as metronidazole. However, these can be toxic to the liver. If you would like to try a more natural approach, the following are some suggestions. You can take these herbal formulas for one to two months, along with the medicine prescribed by your physician.

If there is a fungal infection, try licorice tea uttara basti (see instructions below). For bacterial infection, antibacterial herbs like goldenseal, echinacea, haridrā, pushkaramūla, yavānī, and mahāsudarshan and are very effective. Try them alone in tea form or in a base of ghee.

If the woman has an infected sexual partner, she and her partner should be treated for the condition and they should use condoms until the condition has cleared up. Helpful are also chandana āsava, kumārī āsava, and shatāvarī ghee. The ghee can be taken before meals at a dose of one teaspoon. For the herbal wines, take 4 tablespoons mixed with an equal amount of water after lunch and dinner.

In the case of candidal vaginitis, there is more itching, pain during intercourse, and a thick, white discharge resembling cottage cheese with a yeast-like odor. This is quite common during pregnancy and diabetes. The treatment for this is shatāvarī 500 mg, gudūchī 300 mg, shardunikā 200 mg, neem 200 mg, and vidanga 200 mg. This mixture is taken ½ teaspoon TID using aloe vera gel as the anupāna, carrying medium. Also one should do a licorice tea uttara basti (medicated douche) by using one pint of water, two tablespoons of licorice, and one teaspoon of neem, boiled together for three minutes; once cooled, it should be strained before use. This douche should be done at least every other night, until the symptoms disappear.

In the instance of Gardnerella vaginalis vaginitis (formerly called non-specific vaginitis or haemophilus vaginitis), there is itching, burning, with a creamy white, grayish, foul-smelling discharge. It is more common in the summer season. In this case one should do a triphalā tea uttara basti by taking two tablespoons of triphalā and boiling it in pint of water. Once cooled, it should be strained before use. Also take ½ teaspoon of the following formula with pomegranate juice.

| Ashoka | 300 mg |
|---|---|
| Manjishthā | 200 mg |
| Katukā | 200 mg |
| Shilājit | 100 mg |

If the client has Trichomonas vaginalis vaginitis, there is more itching and burning accompanied by a greenish, whitish discharge having a foul odor. This condition usually starts after menstruation. The uttara basti in this case combines two tablespoons each of ashoka and yashthi madhu, boiled together in a pint of water. Cool and strain before use. Take ½ teaspoon of the mixture below TID with gheemadhu, honey and ghee.

| Shatāvarī | 500 mg |
|---|---|
| Ashoka | 200 mg |
| Manjishthā | 200 mg |
| Kāma Dudhā | 200 mg |

In cases of non-infectious vaginitis, there is more dryness of the vaginal mucus membrane and there are red, inflamed patches with irritation but no discharge. This is high pitta in ārtava dhātu. For non-infectious vaginitis where the cause is contact with an external irritant, one should avoid the cause and maintain strict feminine hygiene. To soothe and heal the membranes, coat a tampon with shatāvarī ghee and insert in the vaginal canal. To help the symptoms, take ½ teaspoon of the following mixture TID with aloe vera gel. Be sure to take each dose before food so it will act on the vagina.

| Shatāvarī | 500 mg |
|---|---|
| Gulvel Sattva | 200 mg |
| Kāma Dudhā | 200 mg |
| Motibhasma | 200 mg |

The female reproductive system, ārtava vaha srotas is profoundly important in the life of every woman. In some individuals, ārtava vaha srotas is extremely sensitive to changes in environment, lifestyle, and diet. To help your awareness of your cycle and symptoms, keep a calendar of the dates of onset of menstruation and the cessation of menstruation (the moon cycle) along with a detailed record of the signs and symptoms. In cases of amenorrhea too much physical activity could be responsible, so keeping a balanced yoga, meditation, and exercise practice is important to help maintain healthy biorhythms of the menses. Emotional factors also play an important role in the rhythm of menses. As much as possible one should keep an easy schedule, try not to have sex during menses, and avoid hot, spicy food and alcoholic beverages that can trigger pitta. Any change in the menstrual cycle is a warning sign that the reproductive system may be experiencing detrimental change.

**UTTARA BASTI**

The nine gates of the body (seven openings in the head and two below) are constantly open to outer environmental changes. These are also the main gates of prāna, tejas and ojas into majjā dhātu (in this case, primarily nerve tissue). Through these openings, the external qualities of rough, dry, hot, cold, and others enter directly through majjā dhātu into the mental faculty. These attributes can affect the mind and the functioning of related srotāmsi (channels).

The ancient Ayurvedic literature speaks a great deal about obtaining female health by means of uttara basti (a form of medicated douche). This treatment works on the pelvic space, lumbo-sacral plexus, and mūlādhāra chakra. It has a wide range of actions on the bladder, uterus, ovaries, and sigmoid colon.

In uttara basti, herbal medicated teas are injected into the vagina, working directly on the vaginal mucus membrane, cervix, uterus, fallopian tubes, ovaries, and endometrial tissue. Hence, in Ayurveda, dryness of the vagina, constriction of the cervix, inflammation of the endometrium, fibroid tumors, and several other PMS syndromes can often be effectively managed through the administration of specific herbal teas via uttara basti.

In general, the preferred substance used for uttara basti in vāta predominance is dashamūla tea. For pitta, gudūchī tea is the best uttara basti, while for kapha one can use yashthi madhu (licorice) basti. However, in cases of vaginitis and cervicitis, shatāvarī tea with ghee would be used as an uttara basti. In dryness of the cervix and vaginal wall and dysmenorrhea, use a dashamūla tea uttara basti with added nirgundī oil. In fungal or yeast infections, a shardunikā and neem tea uttara basti is used. When there is kapha dusthi with leucorrhea and fibroids, a punarnavā and yashthi madhu tea uttara basti is recommended. It is also said that if a woman takes a simple triphalā tea uttara basti with plain ghee once a week on a Saturday, good female health will be maintained.

In cases of PMS, uttara basti is done every day for one or two weeks, until the person is symptom free. Uttara basti should not be done during menstruation, the bleeding phase of rakta pitta conditions, vaginal prolapse, pregnancy, or when malignant lesions are present, especially during chemotherapy or active cancer.

To make an uttara basti tea, two tablespoons of the herb or herbs are added to one pint of water and boiled for two minutes. Once this has cooled down, half a cup of any recommended medicated oil or ghee can be added.

# Chapter 27

# Irritable Bowel Syndrome
## Pakvāshaya Kūpita Dosha

Winter 2008, Volume 21, Number 3

IRRITABLE BOWEL SYNDROME (*pakvāshaya kūpita dosha*) is the continuous inflammation of the intestinal mucous lining, anus, rectum, and distal part of colon. In some seriously ill patients, the entire large intestine is affected. This disorder usually becomes apparent during the second and third decades of life.

According to Ayurveda, irritable bowel syndrome (IBS) is a collection of symptoms that is a dual-dosha samprāpti. It is due to vāta pushing pitta or pitta pushing kapha in the colon. The moment the third dosha gets involved, it can lead to colon cancer. If that happens, it will usually occur about 20 to 30 years after the onset of IBS.

## Samprāpti of IBS

Typically, IBS begins with pāchaka pitta undergoing sañchaya and prakopa in the small intestine, at the same time that apāna vāyu is undergoing sañchaya and prakopa in the large intestine. Then, during the prasara stage, either vāta pushes pitta or pitta pushes kapha in the colon.

Symptoms are caused by intestinal irritability and irregularity in the bowel movements, with the symptoms occurring in both the small and large intestines. These symptoms are usually also influenced by emotional factors. Nervousness, anxiety, fear, and insecurity can trigger symptoms in a person with vāta prakruti or vikruti. On the other hand, anger, hate, and envy may bring on or aggravate symptoms in someone with pitta prakruti or vikruti. Less commonly, attachment, greed, and depression can produce symptoms in an individual with kapha prakruti or vikruti.

Some specific pathogens are also associated with IBS. Amoebic dysentery and amoebic colitis are examples of illnesses that can result in IBS symptoms.

Antibiotic-associated diarrhea is a third etiological factor. Prolonged antibiotic therapy can disturb the normal bowel flora, leading to either IBS or colitis.

A fourth factor that can lead to IBS is a chronic debilitating illness caused by exotoxins or environmental pollutants such as heavy metals.

Number five in this list is pseudo-membranous colitis. Exotoxins or prolonged exposure to radiation can damage the colon mucous membrane and produce inflammation and IBS symptoms.

Sixth, there are commonly dietetic factors involved. Excessive consumption of coffee, chocolate, raw fruits or raw vegetables can lead to irritable bowel, as well as consumption of hormones or toxins in the diet. Lactose intolerance is also associated with IBS, due to an inability of the body to digest lactose milk sugar, and so is wheat intolerance.

Seventh, an overuse of laxatives is a causative factor. In fact, many drugs can be involved in the formation of irritable bowel syndrome.

Finally, genetic predisposition is an important etiological factor that should always be kept in mind.

IBS is a syndrome, which means the presence of several clinically recognizable signs, symptoms or other characteristics that usually occur together. Predominant symptoms can include alternating diarrhea and constipation, accompanied by abdominal cramps and straining during elimination. The stools may be loose, or they may be compacted. At times, the patient can pass mucous with the stools, produced by irritation of the bowel lining. There is often gas, bloating, occipital headache, and fatigue, which are vāta symptoms. Pitta symptoms include diarrhea, nausea, temporal headache, and burning of the anal canal.

### Categories of IBS

Clinically, there are two main types of IBS. The first is vāta type, called spastic colon. It is marked by cramps, bloating and dull, aching pain in the lower abdomen. There is discomfort, and the pain often begins immediately after eating. Symptoms usually disappear after a bowel movement.

The second category is pitta type of IBS, characterized by loose stools without pain and an urgent need to have a bowel movement upon awakening or immediately following a meal.

Many diseases are similar to IBS, such as sprue syndrome, amoebic dysentery, and bacillary dysentery. So, when a person comes to you with IBS symptoms, one has to rule out all those other diseases that have similar signs and symptoms. A stool examination is helpful in that regard, and possibly a barium enema to assess the colon. In certain cases, a doctor needs to examine the lower colon using a procto-sigmoidoscope, to rule out ulcerative colitis and other diseases.

*Chikitsā (Treatment).* If there is no organic disease found, the Ayurveda practitioner has to recommend a suitable diet and lifestyle, and help the patient with any emotional factors. The first principle is to avoid the cause. That often includes reducing the amount of raw food that is eaten as well as the person's consumption of cigarettes and alcohol.

There are some useful yoga āsanas that can be practiced, which should be chosen according to the person's prakruti and particularly their vikruti:

Vāta vikruti: camel and cow āsanas; alternate nostril breathing and ujjāyi prāṇāyāma

Pitta vikruti: boat, bow and bridge āsanas; shītalī and shītkāri prānāyāma

Kapha vikruti: locust, lotus and lion āsanas; gentle bhastrikā and kapāla bhāti prānāyāma

So'hum meditation is good for all body types.

Exercise is an important part of the therapy for a person with IBS. Long walks, bike rides, swimming and underwater exercise can all help the person to relax, thereby promoting better bowel movements.

Even though IBS is not a serious disease, it can continue to be a problem despite having treatment. Therefore, regular medical checkups should be scheduled to be on the safe side. This is especially true for people over the age of 40.

## Herbal Remedies

For vāta (and kapha) type of IBS, one can use:

| | |
|---|---|
| Jātī phaladi guti | 200 mg |
| Kutaja vati | 200 mg (or kutaja churna) |
| Bhallataka guti | 200 mg |

These three tablets are given TID.

> T.I.D. = from the Latin means *ter in diem*, three times a day

Other remedies for vāta IBS include:

Roasted cumin, fennel, vidanga, and nutmeg powder (1 part cumin, 1 part fennel, ¼ part vidanga, pinch of nutmeg) with a teaspoon of ghee.

Tagara 200 mg is a tranquilizer that helps with anxiety or insomnia.

Vidārī 300 mg is a mild analgesic and sedative that is good for vāta IBS symptoms.

Ashvagandhā 500 mg is a mild analgesic, sedative, and muscle relaxant that is also good for vāta IBS symptoms.

Lasunadi vati 200 mg is a common remedy for gas and bloating.

Shanka vati 200 mg is useful for abdominal cramps.

Chitrakadi vati 200 mg can be given for nausea, low appetite, and poor digestion.

An anti-inflammatory herbal formula that helps with pitta-type IBS is:

| | |
|---|---|
| Shatāvarī | 500 mg |
| Gudūchī | 300 mg |
| Kāma dudhā | 200 mg |

This mixture is given TID.

Another good formula for pitta type of IBS is:

| | |
|---|---|
| Shatāvarī | 500 mg |
| Kāma Dudhā | 200 mg |
| Pravāl Pañchāmrit | 200 mg |
| Bilva | 200 mg |

Take ½ teaspoon TID, with pomegranate juice or cranberry juice, if pomegranate juice is not available.

Other pitta-pacifying remedies that can help include:

Mahā tikta ghrita (or tikta ghrita)

Bilva avaleha (or bilva churna)

Cumin, coriander, and fennel tea (equal parts of the whole seeds boiled in water)

A specific remedy for all types of IBS is kutaja arishta.

A second line of treatment is used to manage depression and emotional factors. The following tranquilizing and antidepressant herbs can be useful:

Brahmī              300 mg
Jatamāmsi          400 mg
Shankha Pushpī   200 mg .
This mixture may be taken TID.

## Diet

Reduce the person's dependence on laxatives by giving a dosha-pacifying diet. If there is constipation, recommend the use of prunes, raisins, and milk. Prune juice is particularly effective to manage constipation. The person can also try sat isabgol, oat bran, or wheat bran, and/or eat two bananas between meals.

For diarrhea, stop the intake of those foods. During the diarrhea stage of IBS, one can use kutaja, bilva, arrowroot, and nutmeg.

If there is a problem with gas or bloating, the person should not eat cabbage, beans, and uncooked vegetables. Many IBS patients do not digest milk properly, so those people should avoid milk in the diet.

Helpful foods for most people with irritable bowel syndrome include basmati rice, mung dal, and kitchari. Banana, pomegranate, and cranberry are the best fruits for IBS patients. Ghee is good for most people with IBS, because there is no lactose in the clarified butter. Buttermilk (takra), which can be made from one part of plain yogurt with two parts of water, is another helpful form of dairy for most IBS sufferers.

In general, people with IBS should eat a diet that pacifies the doshas and see an experienced Ayurvedic practitioner who can give them appropriate lifestyle and herbal remedies.

# Chapter 28

# The Art of Parenting Hyperactive Children
## Chanchalatā

Fall 2009, Volume 22, Number 2

THERE ARE INNUMERABLE srotāmsi in the human body, but we use thirteen main channels in Ayurveda. These include the seven *dhātu-srotamsi* and majjā vaha srotas (the nerve channel) is one of those important channels. Even though the mind functions throughout the body, the mental functions are intimately connected to majjā dhātu (nerve tissue and bone marrow) and thus to majjā vaha srotas. Hence, any nervous disorder is bound to affect the mind.

Attention Deficit Hyperactivity Disorder (ADHD) is known in Ayurveda as *chanchalatā*. It is a nervous disorder that usually affects children. Though ADHD is a relatively new term in Western medicine, this disorder has been known to Ayurveda for many centuries and can be understood by ancient Ayurvedic principles.

In chanchalatā (ADHD), high systemic vāta undergoes accumulation (sañchaya), then provocation (prakopa), and then spreads into majjā dhātu, affecting majjā vaha srotas and mano vaha srotas (the mind channel) simultaneously. The qualities of vāta that are most aggravated determine the types of symptoms that occur.

Due to increased mobile (chala) quality, the child is hyperactive. Increased mobile and light qualities of vāta make the affected child consistently impulsive and create an extremely short attention span. Owing to an imbalance of erratic (vishama) attribute, he or she cannot concentrate well or stay focused on a task. Vāta's cold, dry and rough attributes may be responsible for immature behavior, just as a cold, dry, refrigerated fruit will never ripen and become fully mature. The clear and empty attributes mean that these children live in their own world and don't respond to other people in a normal way. Vāta is also subtle, so when it is aggravated, there is an increase of subtle thoughts, feelings and emotions. According to modern classifications, there are different types of ADHD: hyperactive impulsive, hyperactive inattentive and hyperactive combined. From an Ayurvedic perspective the hyperactive impulsive has excess vāta qualities, the hyperactive inattentive has both kapha and tamasic qualities and the hyperactive combined has more pitta qualities and is due to the fluctuations of drava guna (the liquid quality).

ADHD may physically damage the body and it can trigger long-lasting social, emotional and educational problems. Teachers may complain about the child. The child is often not able to sit still and concentrate for long periods of time, which can lead to trouble in schooling, as the child appears immature, uncoordinated and boisterous. He or she usually has trouble getting along with other classmates, and with teachers and parents, and invariably suffers from a poor self-image. This is a book picture of disturbed vāta dosha.

The behavioral patterns depend upon the severity of the vāta disorder. If there is a lower intensity of vāta aggravation, the child proba-bly won't be a disturbance in the classroom, nor show all the above signs. However, he or she may still have difficulty in paying atten-tion and will appear unusually active.

### Causes (Nidāna)

- Vāta-provoking diet or malnourish-ment during pregnancy, especially stimulants such as caffeine, tobacco, sugar and chocolate, can disturb the central nervous system of the fetus, which may cause central nervous sys-tem malfunctioning. Watching movies excessively or visiting busy locations such as shopping malls may also disturb vāta dosha in the fetus.
- Mother drinking alcohol or taking drugs during pregnancy
- Food additives – chemical colors and preservatives that are added to food that the child eats, or those eaten by the mother when she is pregnant or breastfeeding
- Exposure of pregnant mother to radiation, such as repeated X-rays or radiation therapy
- Chemical toxicity, such as exposure to dyes, formaldehyde and so forth
- Damage during pregnancy, e.g., induced delivery, obstructed labor, premature rupture of amniotic fluid bag, forceps delivery, administration of drugs during delivery
- Premature delivery – this gives rise to congenital vāta disorders that may affect majjā dhātu, rendering the child hyperactive
- Complications of child birth that can cause neurological defects, e.g., CPD (ceph-alopelvic disproportion), face presentation, hand presentation, cord presentation or hip presentation
- Gender – boys are more prone to ADHD than girls

There are two systems of the brain that respond to situations. One results in prompt action, and in Ayurveda this is known as prāna vāta. The other encourages hesitation (tarpaka kapha) and consideration (sādhaka pitta). If prompt action is stimulated, hesitation is diminished, and that can be the mechanism that causes impulsive behavior.

For instance, a hyperactive child may see a flower in a pot on a table above and will jump to catch it, no matter how high, without considering the consequences of grabbing the flower. For a normal child, the prompt action is controlled by consideration and hesitation. The neurotransmitters that control the hesitation response are malfunctioning in the case of a child with ADHD. One factor may be vaccination shots, which can be hugely stressful to the immunological system. Mercury was previously used as a preservative, and one school of thought says that this mercury resulted in toxins affecting the brain. Consuming food preservatives, canned food, or frozen food may also be an important factor in disturbing the functional integrity between prāna vāta, sādhaka pitta and tarpaka kapha.

- Hereditary traits – genetic predisposition to ADHD; pitta or vāta predominant individuals are more likely to get ADHD—specifically those with $V_3 P_3$, $V_3 P_2$, or $V_2 P_3$
- Deficiency of tarpaka kapha; malfunctioning neurotransmitters that control the hesitation response

## Signs and Symptoms (Lakshana)

A child affected by ADHD can display the following signs and symptoms:

- Overactive
- Fidgety
- Restlessness
- Overly talkative
- Boisterous
- Overly excited
- Impulsive
- Poor coordination
- Short attention span (especially noticeable at school)
- Creates disturbances in the classroom
- Skips words when reading
- Laughs loudly
- Prefers to play with younger children

## Diagnosis (Roga Nidāna)

There is no specific laboratory test to diagnose ADHD. Diagnosis is done by consideration of the signs and symptoms that the child presents. Vāta vikruti children are hyperactive in behavior, so ADHD can seem like a rather vaguely defined term for these children. The quantity, intensity, and duration of symptoms should be carefully observed before diagnosing ADHD. Only then should one say that a particular child has attention deficit and hyperactive disorder.

Many times, ADHD is wrongly diagnosed and the child is put on medication that really affects the growth of that 'flower.' Don't label a child by the word 'hyperactive' simply because the parents or teachers may have a low level of tolerance for the child's activity level. They may not tolerate the normal intense activity of a child with vāta prakruti or vāta vikruti. That in itself does not mean that the child has ADHD.

## Treatment (Chikitsā)

In the standard medical treatment protocol, several stimulant medications may be given to treat ADHD since these stimulants affect the hesitation response thereby having a calming effect. This is an example of *tadarthakāri* (protagonistic) *chikitsā*. Methylphenidate and amphetamines are two common drugs of choice. After taking the drug, the child ends up being exhausted and does not have much energy left to act hyperactively. The drug makes the child's nervous system exhausted and the child appears calm. However, the child is made quiet, rather than being quiet.

These stimulant drugs have some hazardous side effects, such as stomachaches, muscle cramps, runny nose, colds, congestion, and stunted growth. In extreme cases, it is okay to use these drugs for a short period of time. However, it is better to bring the child back into balance by nature's way, through Ayurveda.

The Ayurvedic protocol for hyperactive children is to calm down vāta dosha. First, do oil massage (abhyanga) with a mixture of balā, dashamūla, and mahānārāyana oils. This can be followed by sweating therapy with nirgundī svedana, because nirgundī helps to relax the muscles. Anuvāsana basti is then given, with plain sesame oil. Also, rub bhringarāja oil onto the soles of the feet and scalp at bedtime.

Internally, give an herbal formula made of some or all of the following herbs:

| | |
|---|---|
| Dashamūla | 500 mg |
| Ashvagandhā | 400 mg |
| Vidārī | 300 mg |
| Yogarāja guggulu | 300 mg |
| Jatamāmsi | 200 mg (or Mustā 200 mg if jatamāmsi is unavailable) |
| Shankha Pushpī | 200 mg |
| Licorice | 200 mg |
| Tagara | 200 mg |

Children can be given ¼ teaspoon of this mixture three times daily (TID), and it is best taken with a teaspoon of honey and a teaspoon of ghee, all mixed together. One can also keep the doshas flowing well (anuloma) by using ¼ teaspoon of nishottara or triphalā before bedtime.

The child should be put on a vāta pacifying diet. Good foods are basmati rice and mung dal kitchari, with mustard seeds, cumin, and cilantro. Soaked almonds or almond milk are good, as are walnuts and cashews. A quarter teaspoon each of holy basil (tulsi) and turmeric can be boiled in a cup of milk and given to the child to drink at bedtime.

Brahmī-almond-date-cashew milk is a rich nervine tonic that can really help a child with ADHD. To make this, boil a cup of milk with a few dates, almonds, and cashews, and ½ teaspoon each of date sugar and brahmī (gotu kola) powder.

One special Ayurvedic treatment is to rub some pure gold on a rough stone, along with the fresh juice of brahmī, anantā mūla, and vacha and a teaspoon of honey. Give this mixture regularly for a month or two and it will really calm down a hyperactive child.

Ayurveda also recommends a number of rejuvenative therapies (rasāyana) for ADHD. Jatamāmsi, sarasvatī, and brahmī are three herbs that help to improve the attention span. One can give a child with ADHD 200 mg of each of these herbs TID. Shankha pushpī syrup is another beneficial remedy, and it enhances the ability to focus. Brahmī prash, brahmī ghee, and sarāvat arishta are good nervine tonics that enhance the attention span. One teaspoon of sarasvatī ghee can be given twice a day to calm the child down.

Suvarna vacha (calamus root in gold water) is another specific rejuvenative remedy for ADHD children. One can also boil a quarter ounce of pure gold in two cups of water, until the liquid evaporates down to one cup. Then remove the gold and give five to ten drops of this 'gold water' to the child, twice a day.

### Conclusion

Children with ADHD need tender, loving care. Don't order around a child with ADHD. Be gentle and polite and make everything go step-by-step. Activities such as getting up, eating meals, watching TV, and doing homework should all be done calmly and skillfully. Don't say, "Hurry up and get ready for school!" Instead, say, "Hi honey, time to get up and go to the kitchen to eat."

Chart a daily schedule for the affected child and help the family to follow that *dinācharya* (daily routine). Sweetly remind the child of things they forget, like a parrot. Get the child involved in sports and other activities that can keep them involved and relax their muscles at the same time.

Have a family rap session, where everyone meets and discusses their feelings. Then the affected child will start to discuss his or her feelings. The response to the child should be kind and appreciative.

Please don't be in a panic if your child is labeled 'hyperactive.' Ayurveda has some simple, direct, and practical remedies, and provides a great protocol for childcare through diet and herbs that will allow your precious flower to grow beautifully and bloom. Should the ADHD condition affect the education or family stability, medical intervention may be required.[36]

---

**AUTISM**

ADHD is a disorder of increased vāta, whereas autism is caused by kapha blocking vāta. In that disorder, tarpaka kapha blocks prāna vāyu and causes mental introversion. The person's attention is focused mainly on himself or herself. There is withdrawal from communication with other people and repetitive, childish behavior. This means that the child is self-absorbed and there is inaccessibility, aloneness, an inability to relate, and highly repetitive play. There can be strong resistance if this play is interrupted. The child also has language disturbances, as he or she is too introverted to learn what others are trying to communicate. Autism is more passive and introverted, whereas ADHD is more active and extroverted.

---

36. Helpful diagnostic information for ADHD is contained in the Diagnostic and Statistical Manual of Mental Disorders, Fourth Edition by American Psychiatric Publishing, 2000. You can find a good summary of this information here: http://en.wikipedia.org/wiki/ADHD#DSM-IV_criteria. Or put ADHD in the Search box at http://en.wikipedia.org then click on DSM in the Diagnosis section of the table of contents for that page.

## Chapter 29

# Sleep and Dreams

Summer 2011, Volume 24, Number 1

ACCORDING TO SANKHYA'S PHILOSOPHY of the creation of man and the universe, the whole universe is a creation of Purusha and Prakruti. Purusha is choiceless, passive awareness, while Prakruti is creative potential and primordial matter. Purusha doesn't need any sleep, because it is the full awakening of awareness. In that pure awareness, we are not aware that we are aware. The moment you become aware that you are aware, that is the beginning of the dream.

I have decided to write an article, which is also a dream. This whole world is the dream of Purusha. Prakruti is the beautiful creative bed, and on that bed of Prakruti, Purusha is lying and dreaming. An ancient sūtra from *Vishnu Sahasranāma* states, '*Vasudeva shavasanat vasati akhilam vishvam:*' "It is the dream of Vasudeva (Purusha) that creates this whole world."

Within ahamkāra (self-identity), the three *mahā gunas* (qualities) are present in an unmanifested form. When sattva, rajas, and tamas are equal and balanced, it is pure mahat (intelligence). Then, for the purpose of experience, sattva creates the concept of an observer, rajas creates the concept of observation, and tamas creates the objective world. Our mind is the pure essence of sattva, split from ahamkāra. This mind has three states: *jagrat, svapna,* and *sushupti.* The wakeful state (jagrat) is associated with sattva, the dream state (svapna) is related to rajas, and deep sleep (sushupti) to tamas.

Jagrat, the wakeful state, functions with more of a sattva quality, which is clarity and purity. Sattva creates individual consciousness and the concept of an observer. The moment we become conscious of consciousness, it creates a center—this is the observer. This observer projects outside of itself because of the rajasic quality. The movement of observation is rajas, and it relates to the dream state. When awareness flows from one point to another, it becomes attention, and that flow of attention is perception. Perception is the process of rajas carrying awareness through the doors of

> One sūtra says:
> Nidrāh shleshma tamah prayah.
>
> This means:
> We sleep because of increased kapha dosha and tamas quality.

215

perception (the senses) to meet with the objective world, which is tamas. The visible world is an expression of tamas, which is inertia, matter. Tamas relates to the state of deep sleep.

## Table 5: The Three States of the Mind

| State (Sanskit) | Guna | Consciousness | Mind | Senses |
|---|---|---|---|---|
| Waking (Jagrat) | Sattva | Conscious | Active mind | Sensory impressions |
| Dream (Svapna) | Rajas | Subconscious | Active mind | Sensory impressions |
| Deep Sleep (Sushupti) | Tamas | Unconscious | Inactive mind | No sensory impressions |

Sattva is the observer, rajas is observation, and tamas is the thing to be observed. The moment the observer (sattva) touches the thing to be observed (tamas) via observation (the medium of rajas), that gives us experience. In that experience, our awareness becomes materialized or crystallized. Experience is the precipitation or residue of awareness, so it is always of the past. Every experience nourishes ahamkāra. The bigger the experience, the bigger the experiencer; the smaller the experience, the smaller the experiencer. If ahamkāra does not identify with the experience, then awareness can remain in the present moment, becoming bliss.

You cannot experience the truth. You can only experience reality. Truth is universal, timeless, causeless, boundless, pure Purusha. Reality is sattva meeting tamas via rajas. The meeting point of these three gunas gives shape to the truth in the form of reality. Reality is a personal affair. It is a product of time and space, of cause and effect. Reality in Albuquerque is different from the reality in New York or New Zealand. Reality now is different from yesterday's reality.

*Yadā tu manasi klānte karmātmānah klamān vitāh*
*Vishayebhyo nirvartante tadā svapiti mānavah*

*Charaka Samhita, Sūtrasthana,* ch. 21, vs. 25

This beautiful sūtra states that our body, mind, and senses become tired of being consciously active because of our daily activities, thoughts, feelings, and emotions. Then the mind withdraws from the sensory world and enters the sushumnā nādī, which is the central canal of the spinal cord.

Passing through several lighter stages of sleep, we enter into a dark timeless zone called deep sleep, where the mind becomes relatively unconscious and inactive. We are cut off from the sensory world. In deep, dreamless sleep, there is no color, no light, and no form. Tarpaka kapha, prāna vāta, and sādhaka pitta are active, but the mind doesn't think about or feel anything. In deep sleep, the person is close to his own being–there is only being, no becoming. Deep sleep is not possible with dreams. Dreams are due to rajas, which is movement.

All sensory faculties are affected in deep sleep. For example, smell, taste, and sight are suppressed and the person cannot smell, taste, or see anything in the external world. However, touch and hearing are least affected, which is why touching a person or calling his or her name can easily arouse someone who is sleeping.

In between jagrat and shushupti, there is a transitional period, in which we are neither awake nor asleep. We enter into a subjective world. This junction between wakefulness and deep sleep is dreaming. Sleep is not a constant process, rather it fluctuates from wakeful to deep sleep to dreaming, to light sleep, back to dreaming and then to deep sleep, and so forth.

Sleep and wakefulness occur alternately within the daily sleep cycle during the whole life of the individual. During sleep, the brain is still active and the body still performs most of its functions. Externally sleep can appear to be a very passive state, but internally it is active. The heart rate, respiration, kidneys, gastrointestinal tract (GI), and other organs are still active in deep sleep. The kidneys are still performing filtration, and the GI tract may still be digesting the previous meal. Similarly, the brain is also active during sleep. The brain undergoes rejuvenation and reorganization rather than inhibition.

> **WHAT IS SLEEP?**
>
> At Stanford University, I visited William Dement, the retired dean of sleep studies, a co-discoverer of REM sleep, and co-founder of the Stanford Sleep Medicine Center. I asked him to tell me what he knew, after 50 years of research, about the reason we sleep.
>
> "As far as I know," he answered, "the only reason we need to sleep that is really, really solid is because we get sleepy."
>
> *Secrets of Sleep* by D. T. Max, National Geographic Magazine, May 2010

Sleep can be defined as a state of consciousness that moves from alert wakefulness to a loss of critical activity and response to the events in the environment, accompanied by profound alteration in the function of the brain. Sleep is not a continuous uniform phenomenon. There are ups and downs, fluctuations, and variations in the nature and depth of sleep. Even in the same person, the depth and nature of sleep will vary.

The nature of sleep varies according to a person's prakruti and vikruti doshas. For a vāta person, sleep is light and interrupted. Pitta people find it difficult to go to sleep, but once they fall sleep, they have relatively sound sleep. They are intermediate sleepers. Kapha people have deep prolonged sleep.

Vāta is mobile, light, and cold and if there is cold weather or a cold room, a vāta person cannot get to sleep. The same is true about noise coming into the bedroom. The light quality of vāta creates light sleep. The dryness of vāta leads to constipation and drowsiness with insufficient sleep. Pitta is hot, sharp, penetrating, and liquid. If the room is too hot or there is a light on, a pitta person will not sleep well. A pitta person needs a dark, quiet room and comfortable temperature, not too hot or cold. Kapha is heavy, dull, and slow or static. Kapha people can sleep comfortably in almost any room, cool or warm and with or without a bed. Sleep can vary in these ways.

## The Rhythm of Sleep

The rhythm of sleep varies according to an individual's age and his or her prakruti and vikruti. One's diet and habits, the environment, the season, work responsibilities, stress, and daytime sleep can also change it. Sleep requirements vary according to age as well.

In adults, the maximum depth of sleep comes at the end of the first hour or two. In children, there are two periods of deep sleep: one period is between the first and second hours, while the second period is between 8–9 hours after going to sleep. So children often go to sleep right away for one and two hours, then they start tossing and turning and have phases of rapid eye movement, and then they go into deep sleep for the remaining hours.

The Ayurvedic understanding of sleep is that older people usually need less sleep than younger adults. Elderly people sometimes feel they don't sleep enough, as they may only sleep for 4-5 hours per night. However, because of physical weakness or fatigue that may accompany aging, they often feel they need more sleep than this.

| Age and condition | Average amount of sleep per day[a] |
|---|---|
| Newborn | up to 18 hours |
| 1-12 months | 14-18 hours |
| 1-3 years | 12-15 hours |
| 3-5 years | 11-13 hours |
| 5-12 years | 9-11 hours |
| Adolescents | 9-10 hours |
| Adults, including elderly | 7-8 hours |
| Pregnant women | 8(+) hours |

a http://en.wikipedia.org/wiki/Sleep#Optimal_amount_in_humans

## Stages of Sleep

*Stage 1, light sleep.* It is the beginning of the sleep cycle, the junction between the jagrat and sushupti stages. This stage lasts for about 5-10 minutes. Theta waves (4-7 Hz) are present, producing a slow brain wave pattern. By comparison, when still awake, there is a predominance of alpha waves, which range from about 8-13 Hz. Stage 1 sleep is governed by prāna vāta and sees the calming down of prāna.

*Stage 2, the junction between light sleep and deep sleep.* There is a predominance of sigma waves, also known as sleep spindles (11-16 Hz). This second stage accounts for about 50% of the time a typical adult spends asleep. Body temperature drops, heart rate slows, and breathing deepens and becomes parasympathetic. Stage 2 sleep is governed by sādhaka pitta.

*Stage 3, deeper sleep.* There are an increased number of delta waves (0.5-4 Hz). There is still a deep, slow breathing pattern. This is the inhibition of sādhaka pitta and a predominance of tarpaka kapha. This third stage generally lasts for about 20-30 minutes per sleep cycle.

*Stage 4, deepest sleep, with more than 50% delta waves.* The whole brain becomes slow, as this stage is governed by tarpaka kapha. It typically lasts for about 20-30 minutes per cycle. During this stage, tarpaka kapha and prāna vāta can stimulate each other, which is why bedwetting or sleep walking can occur during this fourth stage.[37]

*Stage 5, rapid eye movement (REM) sleep phase, in which there is an increase in respiration and brain activity.* This is the svapna state of mind. While voluntary muscles are paralyzed, dreaming occurs at this stage. Vascular engorgement of the genitals in this stage can result in dreams of sex. REM sleep can comprise 20% to 25% of total sleep time.[38]

37. These first 4 stages are all non-REM sleep. Stages 3 and 4 have recently been combined into stage N3, under the 2007 American Academy of Sleep medicine (AASM) Guidelines, with the first two stages now referred to as stages N1 and N2.

There is more deep sleep earlier in the night, whereas there is a greater amount of REM sleep later in the night. A sleeper constantly transitions between stages of sleep. Sleep begins in stage 1 and progresses into stages 2, 3 and 4. After stage 4 sleep (deep sleep), stage 3 and then stage 2 sleep are repeated before entering REM sleep, stage 5. Once REM sleep is over, the body usually returns to stage 2 sleep. Sleep cycles through these stages approximately 4 or 5 times throughout the night. Most dreaming occurs in REM sleep. Although dreams also occur in stages 3 and 4, most people do not recall those dreams.

## Table 6: Three Stages of Sleep

| 1 | 5-10 minutes | Theta waves. Gradual cessation of prāna vāta |
|---|---|---|
| 2 | 10-25 minutes | Sleep spindle brain activity. Rapid, rhythmic brain waves. Temperature drops, breathing, and heart rate slow down. Cessation of sādhaka pitta. |
| 3 | 20-30 minutes | Delta waves. Slow brain activity. Deep sleep induced by tarpaka kapha |
| 4 | 20-30 minutes | Delta waves. Governed by tarpaka kapha. However prāna may become active, causing bedwetting or sleepwalking. |
| 5 | Initial occurrence can be very short but each cycle becomes longer, lasting up to an hour as sleep progresses | Rapid eye movement (REM) stage of sleep, which indicates activation of prāna. It is the dream stage, respiration becomes faster, and repressed emotions activate, causing some to have dreams of sex in this stage. |

# The Physiology of Sleep

In normal sleep, the eyes are closed, the jaw is relaxed, and muscles are relaxed; there is a deep parasympathetic breathing. The person breathes into their belly. During the wakeful state, most people breathe into their chest, called sympathetic breathing. Ayurveda says that sleep is due to excess tarpaka kapha secretion in the majjā dhātu, and that slows down the activity of prāna vāta and sādhaka pitta. Logical intellectual activities slow down and physical motor activities slow down as well.

During sleep, the srotāmsi are still active, but some srotāmsi are much less active than when awake, while others remain in a similar state of activity. Many reflexes are elevated, whereas responsiveness is lessened. People cannot remember any physiological events during their sleep. For example, rasa and rakta vaha srotas are somewhat inactive, as pulse rate, cardiac output, blood pressure, and heart rate are all reduced. In prāna vaha srotas, there is slow breathing, which sometimes becomes shallow. This diminished rate of respiration indicates that prāna vaha srotas also slows down.

In deep sleep, the activity of agni is reduced by 10-15%. Thus, one's basal metabolic rate, which is governed by jathāra agni and dhātu agni, becomes slower.

---

38. There are two main types of sleep: non-rapid eye movement (NREM) sleep (also known as quiet sleep) and rapid eye movement (REM) sleep (also known as active sleep).

Māmsa vaha srotas is completely relaxed, as all voluntary muscles are relaxed during sleep, and meda vaha srotas also slows down. Mūtra vaha srotas activity is reduced, so the volume of urine is less than during the day. The specific gravity and concentration of urine is raised because globular filtration diminishes. Bodhaka kapha and thus salivary secretions are diminished, as is lacrimation.

Majjā vaha srotas is intermittently relaxed and active. The eyeball, a part of majjā, is rolled up outwardly, eye lids are closed, and pupils are contracted when a person is in a deep sleep. However, there are periods of rapid eye movement when dreaming occurs.

### Historical Theories of Sleep

We discussed the Ayurvedic theory of sleep earlier in this article. Even today, we have not yet found the exact cause of sleep. Historically there have been many theories that try to explain sleep. From the late 1800s to the mid-1900s, one prevalent theory was that of cerebral ischemia or lack of blood supply to the cerebral cortex. In the 1950s, Mangold and Sokoloff did studies on cerebral metabolism that showed an increase of blood flow during sleep, putting to rest the cerebral ischemia theory. I. P. Pavlov believed that sleep is conditioned inhibition.

These were followed by biochemical theories such as the accumulation of acetylcholine creating sound sleep or the accumulation of lactic acid in the tissues causing fatigue. Other theories include studies of reserpine, serotonin, and the amino acid precursors of serotonin, 5-hydroxytryptophan (5-HTP) and L-tryptophan, and their role in sleep. Others focused on the reduction in muscle tone experienced during sleep, positing that the afferent impulse to the cerebral cortex creates sleep. This theory is interesting because oil massage does cause the muscles to relax and reduce their tone and transmission of the afferent impulse, which can lead to sleep. In Ayurvedic terms, this relaxes vyāna vāyu and prāna vāyu, creating sleep. Today, most sleep researchers agree that sleep has restorative, memory processing, and preservative functions.

## Dreams

Sleep is a biological need and a psychological requirement because of these rejuvenating, relaxing, and revitalizing functions. Sleep creates a total reorganization of the brain structure. Our brain cells' neurons undergo changes in deep sleep. Dream sleep has a different function.

What happens in our day-to-day activities? There are a lot of incomplete or unresolved thoughts, feelings, and emotions. These are all stuck in our brain tissue and, during second and fifth stages of sleep, the brain cells create a dream state so that these incomplete actions and unresolved emotions can be completed.

A dream is a discharge of an incomplete action. After a dream, the brain becomes orderly. Ayurveda says that the dream state (svapna) is rajasic. Wakefulness (jagrat) is sattvic, whereas dreamless deep sleep (shushupti) is tamasic. However, in a deep sleep, we are close to our being, close to our pure Purusha or soul.

Yogis practice *yoga nidrā,* which is psychic sleep, according to Vedic science. Because deep sleep is a way of being close to the inner source of being, when you sleep with awareness and maintain that awareness in the deep sleep state, you will become enlightened; that kind of sleep becomes a form of samādhi. Sleep is not samādhi, but samādhi is like sleep when it occurs with total awareness. In that awareness, there is no judgment, no criticism, no likes, or dislikes. In this awareness, there is a complete cessation of ego, because to some extent we forget our ego or identity in a deep sleep. Hence, the Ayurvedic approach to sleep is one of the gateways to becoming enlightened. In deep sleep, even a king and a beggar are the same. The moment they wake up, they become king and beggar again. This is due to identification.

There are different dream states. In these dreaming states, systemic vāta dosha may activate prāna vāyu, systemic pitta dosha may stimulate prāna vāyu, or systemic kapha dosha may disturb prāna vāyu, leading to three different categories of dreams.

## Vāta Dreams

Dreams of falling, being attacked, being pushed, or of always doing something in the dream as well as being frozen with fright, seeing the death of a loved one, or being locked up or flying are vāta dreams. Certain animals such as snakes, camels, and flying birds are related to vāta. Dreams about the autumn season are about vāta. In vāta dreams, the person is trying to fulfill a desire.

These dreams are about a person falling or being attacked. In some cases, kapha or pitta may attack vāta dosha and prāna vāta may receive the dream. It is a successful or unsuccessful effort of the dosha or higher consciousness to convey the message to the lower consciousness.

## Pitta Dreams

From the hot and sharp qualities, pitta people will teach or will be learning, even in the dream state. They will also release their anger through sex, killing someone, being inappropriately dressed, being nude in public, by arriving too late, or by eating in dreams. They will dream of summer, fires such as burning buildings, problem solving, or failing in some way because of their desires for success. They tend to see frogs and cats in their dream as well as wild animals like tigers.

## Kapha Dreams

Kapha dreams are very romantic. They dream about swimming, finding money, enjoying romantic sex, or being in the snow. They also dream about eating candy, doing the same thing repeatedly, or arriving too late, satisfying unconscious needs. They can also see themselves as dead. Kapha dreams will be about the spring or winter season, seeing the ocean or a lake, and animals like elephants, swans, or lions.

Ayurveda classifies dreams according to the doshas. Other dreams are spiritual dreams. An example may be a dream in which you see a teacher or deity whom you worship. Devotion can come in the form of a dream. In a dream, the mind goes beyond the past and present, seeing into the future. Suggestions about the future are given in some dreams. In this way, we can classify dreams.

One can meditate upon a dream; make your own dream diary. That way, by studying the patterns of your dreams, you can understand underlying etiological factors, such as your khavaigunya or weakness. I had a patient who told me, "Dr. Lad, for three days I have had a repeated dream about the back of my house, where there is a lake that is on fire." I could see that the lake represented the bladder, the fire is pitta, and the three days were her vāta pushing pitta in the bladder. Her bladder was giving her the message she has high pitta in the bladder and is likely to get cystitis or a bladder infection.

Other dreams can indicate death. To dream of teeth falling out means someone near you will die. Or seeing a cremation in your dream can mean that someone is going to die. There are also cultural dreams. In the Indian tradition, if someone dreams that people are rubbing sindhu on his forehead and flour over the body, it indicates that person will die. If a person dreams of a hole in the wall, that individual is likely to get tuberculosis in the lung cavity. If someone sees holes in a pole or pillar, it means that the person has osteoporosis or will likely get a medical fracture.

## Categories of Sleep Disorders

There are many environmental factors that induce insomnia. Insomnia may be due to noise (vāta), too much movement or travel (vāta), changing time zones or a change of altitude (vāta), cold weather or a cold room (vāta), too much heat in the room (pitta), or eating hot, spicy food (pitta).

There are different categories of sleeplessness. Dissomnias are sleep disturbances or excessive sleepiness and include types of insomnia, hypersomnia, narcolepsy, sleep apnea, brief limb jerks, and restless leg syndrome. Parasomnias include night terrors, nightmares, sleepwalking, and disorders related to mental illness. There is also sleep pattern disruption associated with medical illness such as endocrine disorders or pulmonary disease.[39]

There are various causes of insomnia and other sleeping disorders:

- Dietary factors – foods that the person finds hard to digest can cause indigestion and result in insomnia
- Lack of exercise
- Strenuous exercises before bed
- A bath immediately before bed
- Daytime sleep, such as an afternoon nap or siesta
- Sleep apnea
- Narcolepsy
- Restless leg syndrome
- Illnesses that cause pain, such as rheumatoid arthritis
- Mental illness
- Psychological factors such as anxiety, worry, and stress
- Drinking coffee, tea, and other caffeinated beverages

Drugs can cause drug-induced insomnia from consumption of alcohol, recreational drugs, or pharmaceuticals. For instance, if people drink whiskey, they will likely wake up at 2 o'clock in the morning as the liver tries to metabolize the alcohol. Certain medications can also cause insomnia.

---

39. *Taber's Cyclopedic Medical Dictionary*, 20th Ed., 2005, Venes, Donald, editor; page 2013.

## Doshic Types of Insomnia

Vāta insomnia is more likely with cold temperatures, excess travel, noise, excessive exercise, and consumption of vāta-aggravating foods such as raw foods, pinto, adzuki, or black beans. It is typically worse in the fall season. In vāta type of insomnia, the person often wakens every hour or two and usually has many dreams or nightmares. As a result, the person wakes up fatigued and feels drowsy during the day. This often results in constipation and difficulty in concentrating. Vāta tendencies towards constipation, bloating, arthritis, and rheumatism can create vāta insomnia. Excessive sexual activity can also cause insomnia.

Pitta insomnia is often caused by hyperacidity, staying up late at night, a bedroom that is too hot or exposed to light, or excessive consumption of foods such as citrus, sour fruits, chili pepper, coffee and other caffeinated beverages, red wine, or hard liquor. It is worse in summer season. In pitta type of insomnia, it is difficult for the person to get to sleep and they often waken during 'liver time,' which is around 2 AM. If the person doesn't get to bed by 10 PM or so, they get a burst of energy and tend to burn the midnight oil. They are often night owls who like to read, work, or watch TV at midnight. Pitta types like to read one or two chapters before bed. They generally need a completely dark and silent room to go to sleep.

Kapha insomnia is mild. The person goes to sleep right away but may wake up at dawn and have early morning insomnia. Kapha insomnia is usually related to overeating, which can cause breathlessness, snoring, sleep apnea, restless leg syndrome, seasonal affective disorder, mild depression, and/or kapha-type emotional dreams.

## Management of Sleep Disorders

To have naturally healthy sleep, we should receive periodic massage. Abhyanga is Ayurvedic oil massage and it will help to induce sound sleep. For better sleep, rub bhringarāja oil onto the scalp and soles of the feet before going to bed.

Milk is a good source of tryptophan, which can increase sound sleep. Drink a cup of warm milk about an hour before bedtime. Alternatively, vāta types can have garlic milk, pitta types can choose shatāvarī milk, and kapha people will benefit from turmeric milk. These medicated milks are made by boiling the herb in the milk for a few minutes and then allow the milk to cool a little.

The layout of your bedroom is another important factor. Don't sleep under ceiling beams or dividers. Your feet should not point towards a doorway. There should not be much of a gap between the headboard of the bed and the wall—a few inches distance is okay, but a larger gap can create insomnia.

Your sleeping position is also important to consider. Lying on your right side is calming, but lying on your back or left side can be okay. If you lie on your back or side, do So'hum meditation, inhaling with "so" and exhaling with "hum." With a peaceful mind watching the breath, you can go straight to sleep.

### Herbal Protocol for Sleep

"Herbal Formulas for Sleep" has some helpful herbal formulas for sound sleep, according to one's prakruti and vikruti.

Each of these remedies can be taken an hour before bedtime along with a cup of warm milk or the medicated milks listed above. These are simple but effective remedies to help induce sound sleep. Additionally, put an ounce of the Ayurvedic herb jatamāmsi in a little silk bag and place it under your pillow to create sound sleep.

If you take melatonin, there should be complete darkness. If there is a little light, it will create more drowsiness. It is a 2 multi-functional hormone that has many usages, but side effects include headaches, an altered sleep pattern, mood swings, itching skin, tachycardia, and depression. One should be careful not to take more than a 10 mg dose of melatonin. Melatonin side effects are usually temporary, so if you stop the medicine, within a week these can clear up.

### Table 7: Herbal Formulas for Sleep

| Vāta | Pitta | Kapha |
|---|---|---|
| Dashamūla 5 parts<br>Ashvagandhā 4 parts<br>Tagara 3 parts<br>Jatamāmsi 3 parts<br>½ teaspoon of this mixture nightly | Shatāvarī 5 parts<br>Gudūchī 3 parts<br>Jatamāmsi 3 parts<br>Shankha Pushpī 2 parts<br>½ teaspoon of this mixture nightly | Punarnavā 5 parts<br>Sarasvatī 3 parts<br>Chitrak 2 parts<br>Tagara 2 parts<br>½ teaspoon of this mixture nightly |

# Chapter 30

# Sleep Disorders

Fall 2011, Volume 24, Number 2

In this article, we will examine the following conditions as they relate to sleep disorders:

* Chronic Fatigue Syndrome (CFS)
* Depression
* Migraine
* Sleep Apnea
* Snoring
* Bedwetting
* Restless Legs Syndrome
* Sleepwalking

Any dosha can disturb sleep if it becomes high in majjā dhātu and mano vaho srotas. Sādhaka pitta is present in the cerebral-cortical area, tarpaka kapha in the medulla area of the brain, and prāna vāta governs sensory stimuli and motor responses. If any of these are increased, the individual's sleep pattern can become disturbed.

## Chronic Fatigue Syndrome

Chronic fatigue syndrome (CFS) is an uncommonly common condition these days in clinical practice. In CFS, an infectious mononucleosis virus can disturb rasa dhātu and particularly the lymph nodes in the neck area, which can become inflamed and swollen. Sthāyi and asthāyi rasa are affected, which causes āma and in turn results in sroto rodha (clogging of the channels). There are inflamed and swollen lymph nodes with low-grade fever, sore throat, and aches and pains. The person feels as if he is "dead on his feet," with extreme fatigue, and is often confined to bed for long periods. Ojas can become severely depleted.

CFS and sleep disorders can go together, as poor sleep depletes ojas. Sound sleep is necessary to restore and even build ojas. Hence, those with constitutionally low ojas can become susceptible to diseases if they get insufficient sleep.

To heal, the person should follow the following guidelines:

* Don't over-exert oneself
* Have enough restful sleep
* Eat home-cooked meals
* Don't eat foods with additives or preservatives, or canned food
* Take multi-vitamins
* Take care of allergies: food intolerances and *prāna sroto dushti* are particularly common in CFS
* Take this herbal formula TID (TID) with warm water: dashamūla 500 mg, ashvagandhā 400 mg, vidārī 300 mg, and jatamāmsi 200 mg[40]
* If there is fever, sore throat, or upper respiratory congestion, take sitopalādi 500 mg and mahāsudarshan 300 mg
* Good Night Sleep Tea[41] contains chamomile, skullcap, and tagara. It is particularly beneficial for this condition.
* If there are more pitta symptoms, one can take the following formula TID: shatāvarī 500 mg, gudūchi 300 mg, sarasvatī 200 mg

## Depression

If a person doesn't get proper sleep, it can lead to depression. In this condition, the individual keeps anxious and sad feelings inside.

In our daily life, we can see two types of depression. 'Healthy depression' comes from realistic feelings of pain, sadness, disappointment, guilt, anger, anxiety, or physical or psychological trauma. Suppression of these feelings or keeping one's feelings inside will create depression. This can lead to sleeplessness and insomnia and, in turn, the sleeplessness and insomnia can lead to depression. Effect becomes cause and cause becomes effect.

All healthy people feel this type of depression in their life. It comes and goes. The person is capable of functioning normally in relationships and in life in general. However, prolonged 'healthy depression' can produce chemical changes in the brain, leading to chronic depression. Therefore, don't take any depression lightly.

'Unhealthy depression' comes about when the individual is unable to function in one or more areas of life—relationship, work or so forth. Prolonged, persistent bad feelings will produce chemical changes in the brain, leading to unhealthy depression. The person can suffer from insomnia, or can become more passive and less active, sleeping for greater amounts of time than normal. Sleeping during the day and insomnia at night is one common scenario.

---

40. This amount of herbs, combined together, is a single serving. Most often, herbs are taken for a period of time, such as a week or a month. Then your herbalist would formulate a larger amount using these proportions and give you enough of the mixture for the recommended time period and number of servings per day.
41. Vasant Lad's tea formula, sold at the Institute. The traditional formula is made with jatamāmsi, shankha pushpī, and tagara. Jatamāmsi and shankha pushpī are endangered and/or threatened species. See cites.com for more information. Our current formula is quite effective.

Depression

Lifestyle changes can help in cases of 'healthy depression' and short-term 'unhealthy depression:'

- Regularize the lifestyle by sticking to a daily routine
- Wake up early and watch the sunrise
- Go for a morning walk
- Increased periods of activity are better than prolonged periods of passivity
- Cultivate friendships and enjoy a social life
- Try not to take things personally
- Watch your life objectively and know yourself as you are
- Eat fresh food (steamed vegetables, basmati rice, mung dal, fruit, etc.)
- Don't eat leftovers, or canned and frozen food
- Do daily yoga, prāṇāyāma, and meditation or relaxation

One can easily handle short-term depression by adopting these lifestyle changes. The most important thing for someone suffering from depression is to love their life and not engage in comparison.

People who are depressed live in the past or future. They do not live in the eternal present. Meditation means to bring awareness to this moment, without comparison or judgement. It means to be here now. Now is peace and bliss. Meditation is not hollow; it is whole, complete. Therefore, meditation can be of great benefit for someone with depression.

## Treatments of Doshic Types of Depression

Vāta-type depression with fear, anxiety, and insomnia:
- Abhyanga (sesame oil massage of the whole body) followed by a hot shower
- Gentle yoga āsana followed by calming prāṇāyāma
- Dashamūla 500 mg, ashvagandhā 400 mg, vidārī 300 mg, jatamāmsi 200 mg, TID
- Triphalā ½ teaspoon (tsp.) nightly
- Basti made from a tea containing 1 tablespoon (Tbs.) each of dashamūla, gudūchi, and brahmī
- Vacha oil nasya

Pitta-type depression with competitiveness, failure, anger, hate, envy, or jealousy (someone with this condition can become suicidal and need medical help):

- Abhyanga (sunflower oil massage of the whole body) followed by hot shower
- Yoga āsana followed by cooling prāṇāyāma
- Shatāvarī 500 mg, gulvel sattva 300 mg, kāma dudhā 200 mg, shankha pushpī 200 mg, TID
- Bhumi āmalakī ½ tsp. nightly
- Basti made from a tea containing 1 Tbs. each of gudūchi, shankha pushpī, and jatamānsi
- Brahmī ghee nasya

T.I.D. = from the Latin means *ter in diem*, three times a day

Kapha-type depression with attachment, greed, possessiveness, hypersomnia, and emotional eating:

- Abhyanga (sesame oil massage of the whole body) followed by hot shower
- Vigorous yoga āsana followed by heating prānāyāma
- Punarnavā 500 mg, chitrak 200 mg, kutki 200 mg, sarasvatī 200 mg, TID
- Bibhītakī ½ tsp. nightly
- Basti made from tea containing 1 Tbs. each of punarnavā and brahmī
- Anu tailam nasya or vacha powder nasya

Note that vāta and kapha types of depression are relatively easy to handle, but the pitta type of depression can become serious and may need medical help.

## Migraines

Migraine headaches are a vāta-pitta type of disorder. They are more common in women and in people with pitta constitutions, especially perfectionists, compulsive types, or type A personalities who are success-oriented and who live more in the head than the heart.

There are two main theories about the causes of migraine:

1. The blood vessels (rakta) expand due to the hot quality of pitta, exerting pressure on the nerve fibers (majjā), causing pain. This is the cause of pitta type of migraines.
2. The blood vessels (rakta) contract, due to the cold attribute of vāta, blocking flow to part of the brain (majjā). This causes pain and is the cause of vāta type of migraines.

One of the main causes of sleep disorders is aggravated vāta pushing pitta in rasa-rakta and majjā dhātus. People with disturbed sleep patterns are prone to migraine.

Migraines can cause visual impairment, because the eyeballs are an important part of majjā dhātu. The aura of the migraine begins in the eyes.

### Causative Factors of Migraines

- Disturbed sleep
- Emotional factors
- Food allergies and intolerances
- Coffee
- Chocolate
- Cola drinks
- Citrus fruits
- Sour foods

### Symptoms of Vāta-type Migraines

- Throbbing pulsating pain
- Cluster headaches
- Constipation
- Gas and bloating

## Symptoms of Pitta-type Migraines

◆ Sharp pain
◆ Excessive sweating
◆ Nausea
◆ Photosensitivity
◆ Flashes of light (ophthalmic migraine)

## Healthy Lifestyle Tips for Acute or Sub-Acute Migraines

◆ Sufficient sound sleep
◆ Avoid artificial sweeteners and MSG
◆ Avoid prolonged exposure to sunlight, or wear a hat and sunglasses
◆ No smoking or drinking alcohol
◆ Avoid excessive sexual activity
◆ Take time to relax
◆ Munch on magnesium, which means green leafy vegetables, pumpkin seeds, oats, barley, and soy beans
◆ Ensure you drink enough water
◆ Avoid foods to which you are allergic
◆ Cool the scalp by applying coconut oil medicated with brahmī oil
◆ Take a brisk walk or do other aerobic exercise in the early morning (kapha time)
◆ Rest, read, and relax during the middle of the day (pitta time)

## Management of Chronic Migraine Headaches

The following herbal formula TID: dashamūla 500 mg, shatāvarī 300 mg, kāma dudhā 200 mg, tagara 200 mg, and jatamāmsi 200 mg

One-half tsp. of bhumi āmalakī nightly with warm water

Take Good Night Sleep Tea herbal mixture

Do nasya daily: 1) vacha oil nasya for vāta types or 2) brahmī ghee nasya for pitta types

Super Nasya Oil® is suitable for all constitutions

Rub bhringarāja oil and brahmī oil on the scalp and soles of feet before bedtime

## Sleep Apnea

Sleep apnea is another important sleep disorder. It is characterized by abnormal pauses in breathing (apnea) or periods of unusually shallow breathing (hypopnea) during sleep.

One in ten Americans suffer from abnormal snoring. The person can stop breathing for between ten seconds to two minutes, typically for ten to fifteen times per hour. In my hospital clinical practice, I have observed patients stopping breathing for 30-40 seconds. The patient doesn't know that he is snoring or that he has stopping breathing.

Loud snoring, noisy breathing, gurgling, and harrumphing during sleep can all be associated with sleep apnea. Such snoring sounds can be terrifying to the person's partner. Those suffering from sleep apnea are usually obese. The patient may have nasal congestion, a snuffly nose, deviated nasal septum, or other such condition.

There are various factors that can cause these symptoms. For instance, noisy breathing can be due to food intolerances or food allergies. Sleep apnea can also be induced by cold medicines and other drugs.

### Lifestyle Recommendations
* Nasya with Super Nasya Oil® or vacha oil before going to bed
* Use nasal spray that relieves nasal congestion
* If overweight, reduce weight
* Don't drink alcohol (as it can increase sleep apnea)
* No smoking
* Avoid allergic foods
* Don't eat late in the evening and no late-night snacks
* Āsana and prāṇāyāma can be particularly beneficial, especially anuloma-viloma and kapāla bhāti prāṇāyāma
* Punarnavā 500 mg, sitopalādi 400 mg, tālīsādi 300 mg, abhrak bhasma 200 mg, trikatu 100 mg TID
* Before going to bed, inhale steam with 2 drops of eucalyptus oil

Sleep apnea is potentially a serious condition. It can induce a heart attack in some patients as well as cause other complications, so it needs to be properly managed. In particularly serious cases, this treatment may not be sufficient, so it will be necessary to see a medical doctor and have a sleep evaluation.

## Snoring
When a person sleeps on his or her back, gravity acts on the loose tissue in the upper respiratory passage and the tongue falls backwards into the throat. This can create snoring.

Snoring is particularly common in men, because they have a more oval vocal cord, due to the physiology of the Adam's apple, as opposed to women's more round vocal cords. It also frequently occurs in obese people and those with upper respiratory congestion.

### Causative Factors
* Sleeping on your back
* Obesity
* Upper respiratory congestion
* Heavy consumption of alcohol in the evening prior to sleep
* Sleeping pills and tranquilizers
* Insufficient sleep
* Stress
* A soft, saggy mattress
* A pillow that is too low or too high can exacerbate snoring

### Management
* Sleep on one side, especially the left side (as this promotes better digestion)
* Ensure sufficient sound sleep
* Sleep on a firm mattress

- Use an appropriate-sized pillow
- Elevate the head-end of the bed by placing a brick under it, raising it by about 2 or 3 inches
- Nasya with Super Nasya Oil® or other nasya appropriate for the constitution
- Inhale steam with eucalyptus oil
- No smoking
- Avoid drinking alcohol in the late evenings
- The following herbal formula is to be taken TID: sitopalādi 500 mg, tālīsādi 400 mg, mahāsudarshan 300 mg, and abhrak bhasma 200 mg
- One tsp. of bhumi āmalakī before bedtime will also help this condition.

# Bedwetting

This is a common condition for children. A family history of bedwetting is frequently present for those who wet their bed.

The main causes of bedwetting are:

- A small bladder
- Overactive prāna vāyu
- Respiratory allergies, which can cause insufficient sleep
- Psychological factors, such as stress, fear, or anxiety

Dealing with bedwetting is a delicate situation, as it can strongly affect the child's self-esteem. Do not humiliate or punish a child for wetting the bed, as this can increase his or her stress levels and thereby worsen the problem. It is important not to tell other people that your child wets the bed, as this can undermine self-esteem.

## Management

- No beverages just before bedtime
- No carbonated drinks
- Encourage the child to urinate before going to bed
- Before the child goes to bed, gently massage the lumbosacral area of the back, the hypogastric region on the front, and the scalp and soles of the feet. Use oil or cream, or just do dry massage if that is more practical
- Check out if there are allergies and get those managed
- Check if the child snores and, if so, treat the cause of the snoring
- Train the child to hold onto his or her urine as long as possible

Nowadays, there are wireless moisture sensors with an alarm attached, and the sensor can be placed in the child's underwear. This can be shocking, so I do not think this is suitable for children under age five. It may help older children who have this condition.

Externally, apply vacha paste to the belly button. Internally, give sesame-jaggery candy, made from one tsp. of ground sesame seeds and ½ tsp. of raw sugar or jaggery mixed together. This is called *tila-guda rasāyana*.

Also, boil one cup of milk and ½ cup water with 5 whole pippalī in it. Keep it cooking until the water evaporates and the mixture reduces to one cup in total. Then give this mixture to the child to drink an hour or so before bed. Alternatively, give the child a cup of warm licorice milk to drink a few hours before bedtime.

Gulpha marma is a set of marma points that can be gently massaged with vacha oil before bed. Connected to the kidneys, ureter, and bladder, gentle massage will calm down undue stimulation of apāna vāyu.

Scary stories and horror movies can aggravate bedwetting by increasing vāta dosha, so these things should be strictly avoided. Scary dreams can cause the child to pass urine in his or her sleep. Giving 200 mg each of brahmī, jatamānsi, and shankha pushpī can have a helpful tranquilizing effect and thereby minimize bedwetting.

I have observed that children who have worms can suffer from bedwetting. Therefore, it can be beneficial to de-worm the child by giving 200 mg each of vidanga, palash, kamilla, and krumi kathar. Also clean the perineal area before bed with a cotton swab dabbed in neem oil.

## Restless Foot / Leg Syndrome

This chronic disorder may be due to the increased mobile (chala) and irregular (vishama) qualities of vāta dosha. The feet and legs are the lower extremities, so they come under the physiological functioning of apāna vāyu.

Chronic constipation, diverticulosis, irritable bowel syndrome (IBS), kidney stones or stones in the bladder or ureter, renal colic, pregnancy, iron-deficiency anemia, and intake of stimulants such as caffeine or tobacco are all etiological factors that may activate the mobile and irregular attributes of vāta in māmsa and majjā dhātus, thereby contributing to restless foot/leg syndrome.

Many times, restless foot/leg syndrome may be due to an internal itching sensation or intolerable creeping sensation in the lower extremity. This sensation can be so strong that there is an irresistible urge to move the leg. It can also be drug-induced.

This syndrome occurs mainly at vāta times (dawn and dusk) or at the end of the day when the patient goes to bed tired or fatigued. The condition is worse in cold climates. Modern medicine still does not know an exact etiology for this condition. One has to thoroughly investigate the patient's history and family health history, and rule out other conditions such as thyroid disorders, renal colic, anemia, and so forth.

One may be able to discern a relationship between restless foot/leg syndrome and coffee intake or other factors. Then one can treat the cause of the condition.

### Management
- Snehana – massage with sesame oil

- Svedana – soak feet for five to ten minutes in a bucket of warm water with a mustard seed tea bag; 2 Tbs. of slightly crushed mustard seeds in a piece of cheese cloth.
- The following mixture TID before food: ashvagandhā 500 mg, vidara 300 mg, jatamāmsi 200 mg, and yogarāja guggulu 200 mg
- One half tsp. of gandharva harītakī at bedtime, to maintain the normal movement of vāta dosha (anuloma)
- Rub a mixture of 50:50 mustard oil and vacha oil on the soles of the feet before going to bed
- For pregnant woman with this condition, give one cup of warm milk with a tsp. of ghee (clarified butter)
- If the condition is due to the side-effects of a psychotropic drug, use an antidote such as nutmeg. A good mixture is jatamānsi, nutmeg, and mustā.
- If due to anemia: 200 mg each of loha bhasma and abhrak bhasma, or 4 tsp. of loha āsava after food. Also, take natural sourced iron, such as Floradix®, currants, raisins, beets, or carrots.
- If due to caffeine, eliminate coffee or other caffeinated drinks and increase protein and grain drinks, such as kefir and soups made with barley, quinoa and so forth
- Tranquility Tea is a natural alternative to valium, a frequently prescribed drug that has many undesirable side effects
- Beneficial yoga āsana include palm tree pose, standing on one leg, eagle pose, leg lifting, plough pose, and locust pose. These poses should be maintained for at least one minute each. Lotus pose (*padmāsana*), easy cross-legged pose (*swastikāsana*), and accomplished pose (*siddhāsana*) are also helpful for restless foot/leg syndrome.

# Sleepwalking

This condition is called somnambulism, which translates as sleeping ambulance. It is an autonomic action performed during sleep due to high vāta in majjā dhātu. The person has little or no recollection of any sleepwalking the following day.

Sleep is induced by tarpaka kapha, sādhaka pitta, and prāna vāta. When tarpaka suppresses prāna, prāna vāyu can get disturbed and stimulate the autonomic nervous system. The person appears to awaken partially, with open eyes but a blank facial expression. The patient is not fully aware. He or she may sit up, sit on the edge of the bed, walk in the bedroom, or even leave the room. Some can even get in their car and drive off! There is a real danger of physical trauma to the patient or to others.

Sleepwalking is surprisingly common in children, but rare in adults. It is more common in male children and female adults. The exact cause is not known. However, women can suffer from this condition during the menarche age, as hormonal changes may trigger the hypothalamus, which governs autonomic actions.

Psychic children who are also oversensitive can have an overactive autonomic nervous system. Thus, they can experience sleepwalking or other sleep disorders. Night terrors may accompany sleepwalking, so scary stories and horror movies should be avoided.

**Management**

- The first thing is to prevent injury by removing sharp or dangerous objects from the bedroom
- Lock the door and windows in the room
- Place a safety gate at the top of any staircase
- Don't keep any fire or water hazards
- Hide the car keys
- Keep the patient under observation
- Avoid horror movies or scary stories before bedtime
- Where appropriate, another person should sleep on the side of the room closest to the door
- Rub bhringarāja oil on the scalp and soles of feet at bedtime
- The following herbal mixture can be given TID: ashvagandhā 500 mg, brahmī 400 mg, shankha pushpī 300 mg, and jatamāmsi 300 mg
- Nasya with brahmī ghee or vacha oil
- Place a silk bag (4 inches by 4 inches) of jatamāmsi root under the pillow
- Massage *Mūrdhni, Sthapanī, Oshtha,* Jatru, and Hasta/Pāda Kshipra marma points[42] with nutmeg oil
- Mantra, yantra, homa, and havana therapy can be beneficial if done under expert guidance

---

42. Illustrations are shown in the appendix on page 237.

# Appendix

## Marma Chikitsā Protocols

*From chapter 20, Backache and Sciatica, page 160.* Trik, Ūrū, Sakthi Ūrvī, Jānu, Gulpha, and Pārshni are marma points that are specific for treatment of this syndrome. Pārshni marma is a point at the central part of the heel that will relieve sciatica pain when it is pressed.

**Pārshni Marma**

Press this point with the blunt end of a pencil to relieve the pain of sciatica and lower back pain.

*From chapter 22, Headache, page 168.* Apply the appropriate doshic oil to the marma points shown in the illustration below. Other points for headache include Ūrdhva Skandha (mid-point along top of shoulders, between neck and arm) and Hasta Kshipra and Pāda Kshipra.

*From chapter 26, Female Health Issues, page 197.* Marma chikitsā is also helpful and the best marmas for PMS are Nābhi, Bhaga, Sakthi Ūrvī, Jānu, Gulpha, and Trik. Nutmeg essential oil can be applied to these energy points.

*From chapter 30, Sleep Disorders, page 234.* Massage Mūrdhni, Sthapanī, Oshtha, Jatru, and Hasta/Pāda Kshipra marma points with nutmeg oil.

# Herbs and Other Substances Mentioned in This Book
## Table 8: Types of Preparations for Herbs and other Substances

| Type | Method |
| --- | --- |
| Āsava | a medicinal herbal wine[a] |
| Arishta | a fermented herbal concoction |
| Arka | a distillation of herbs suspended in water |
| Avaleha or leha | a semi-solid preparation made with jaggery, herbs and ghee or oil and honey |
| Vati | medicinal pills or tablets, also called gutikā |
| Bhasma | medicinal ash |
| Churna | a fine powder of herbs |
| Ghrita | preparations of ghee infused with a decoction and a fine paste of the herb |
| Guggulus | preparations having the exudate as the main effective ingredient |
| Kalka | crushed herbs made into a pulp or paste; a wet bolus |
| Kshira pāka | herbal preparations that are boiled in milk |
| Kvātha | a combination of coarsely powdered herbs; a decoction |
| Lepa | medicinal paste |
| Mandūra | preparations containing purified mandūra (Ferroso-ferric oxide) along with other herbs |
| Parpati | a rasa preparation using purified mercury and sulphur |
| Prash | an herbal preparation cooked with ghee that results in a jam or jelly-like substance |
| Rasa | preparations containing minerals as the main ingredients |
| Taila | oil is boiled with a decoction and a fine paste of the herb(s) |

a. Herbal preparations, as used in this table, can include other substances such as minerals, foods, etc.

In this book, Dr. Lad has mentioned many herbs, herbal preparations, oils, ghees, and other healing substances. The table that follows is a compilation of these substances. It has the name of the substance as mentioned in the text but it does not include every variation of that substance.

For example, punarnavā can be used variously as punarnavāsava, punarnavā lepa, punarnavā guggulu, punarnavā rasāyana, etc. The table lists the name of the substance as mentioned in the text, the Sanskrit name, its Common name, and its Botanical name. While the Sanskrit names often offer alternative names, the selection is by no means comprehensive, and is only included if it differs from the name used in the book. In many cases, the substance mentioned is a compound or mineral and there is no botanical name or possibly no common name. Occasionally, the name of the substance is known more commonly in a language other than its Sanskrit, Common, or Botanical names. The Name in Book is usually Sanskrit. When it is not, we have added a parenthetical designation: B for Bengali, C for Canarese (also known as Kanarese), E for English, G for Gujarathi, H for Hindi, K for Kashmiri, M for Mahrathi, and P for Punjabi.

## Table 9: List of Herbs and Other Substances in this Book

| Name in Book | Sanskrit Name | Common Name | Botanical Name |
|---|---|---|---|
| Āma pachak vati | | | *Compound* |
| Āmalakī | Āmalaka | Indian Gooseberry | *Emblica officinalis* |
| Ārogya vardhini | | | *Compound* |
| Ātmaguptā | Kapikacchū | Cowitch Plant | *Mucuna pruriens* |
| Abhrak | Abhraka | Mica | *Talcum purification*[a] |
| Abhrak bhasma | | Mica Ash | *Compound* |
| Agaru | Agar (H) | Eaglewood, Agarwood | *Aquilaria agallocha* |
| Agni mantha | Jayā | | *Clerodendrum phlomidis* |
| Agni tundi rasa | | Agnitundi Rasa | *Compound* |
| Ahiphenam (resin) | | Opium, White Poppy | *Papaver somniferum* |
| Ajagandha | Pasugandha | Wild Mustard | *Cleome viscosa* |
| Ajvain (H) | Ajamoda, Yavānī | Ajwain | *Carum roxburghianum, Trachyspermum ammi, Carum copticum* |
| Aloe Vera (see kumārī) | | | |
| Alum (E) | | | *Alumen* |
| Amber (E) | | | *oil from multiple tree resins, primarily Liquidamber orientalis* |
| Amrita (see guduchi) | | | |
| Anantā mūlā | | Indian Sarsparilla | *Hemidesmus indicus* |
| Arjuna | Kakubha | Arjuna Myrobalan | *Terminalia arjuna* |
| Arka | Ravi | | *Calotropis procera* |
| Arka patra (see arka) | | | |
| Arka pushpa (see arka) | | | |
| Asafoetida | Hingu | | *Ferula foetida* |
| Ashoka | Kankeli | | *Saraca indica* |
| Ashvagandhā | | Winter Cherry | *Withania somnifera* |
| Asthi poshaka vati | | | *Compound* |
| Avipattikar | | | *Compound* |
| Bachan | Bacha nāga, Vatsanaba | Monkshood | *Aconitum ferox* |
| Balā | | Indian Country Mallow | *Sida cordifolia* |
| Basil (see tulsi) | | | |
| Bhallataka | Arushkara, Bhallatā | Marking Nut | *Semecarpus anacardium* |

## Table 9: List of Herbs and Other Substances in this Book

| Name in Book | Sanskrit Name | Common Name | Botanical Name |
|---|---|---|---|
| Bhangā (see vijayā) | | | |
| Bhringarāja | Kesharāja | False Daisy | *Eclipta alba* |
| Bhumi āmalakī | | Feather-foil Plant | *Phyllanthus amarus*[b] |
| Bibhītakī | Vibhīta, Aksha | Beleric Myrobalan | *Terminalia belerica* |
| Bilva | Shrīphala | Bael Fruit | *Aegle marmelos* |
| Bitter Gourd (E) (see karela) | | | |
| Black Pepper | Maricha, Vellaja, Ushana | | *Piper nigrum* |
| Borax (E) (see tankana) | | | |
| Brahmī | Mandūka Parnī | Gotu Kola | *Centella Asiatica is most common* |
| Brahmī | | Water Hyssop | *Bacopa monnieri* |
| Calamus (E) (see vacha) | | | |
| Camphor (E) | Karpūra | Camphor | *Cinnamomum camphora* |
| Cardamom | Elā | Cardamom | *Elettaria cardamomum* |
| Castor | Eranda Mūla, Gandharva-hasta | Castor-oil Plant | *Ricinus communis* |
| Catechu (see khadira) | | | |
| Chamomile (E) | | German Chamomile, Camphor Plant | *Matricaria recutita, used internally in teas, etc.* |
| Chandana | Shveta Chandana | Sandalwood | *Santalum album* |
| Chandrakalaras | | | *Compound* |
| Chandraprabhā | | | *Compound* |
| Chitrak | Agni, Vahni, Jvalanājhya | Ceylon/white Leadwort | *Plumbago zeylanica* |
| Chitrakadi tailam (see chitrak) | | | *Compound* |
| Chyavānaprāsh | | | *Compound* |
| Cilantro (E) (see dhānyaka) | | | |
| Cinnamon (E) | Tvak, Dārusitā | Cinnamon | *Cinnamomum cassia* |
| Coriander (E) (see dhānyaka) | | | |
| Cumin (E) | Shvetajīraka, Jīraka | | *Cuminum cyminum* |
| Dāruharidrā | Dārvī, Katamkateri | Indian Barberry | *Berberis aristata* |
| Dūrvā | Shatavīrya, Doorwa | Bermuda Grass | *Cynodon dactylon* |

Table 9: List of Herbs and Other Substances in this Book

| Name in Book | Sanskrit Name | Common Name | Botanical Name |
|---|---|---|---|
| Dashānga paste | | Ten Herbs Paste | Compound |
| Dashamūla | | Ten Roots | Compound |
| Deer Horn Ash (E) (see shringa bhasma) | | | Compound |
| Deer Musk (E) | Kasturi, Mushkaha | | Moschus chrysogaster |
| Deodara (see devadāru) | | | |
| Devadāru | | Deodara | Cedrus deodara |
| Dhānyaka | Dhanika, Dhānya, Dhānyakam | Coriander, Cilantro Leaf | Coriandrum sativum |
| Dhattūra | Krishna-dhatura | Thornapple | Datura alba |
| Dhattūra | Kanaka,Dhustūra, Ummatta, | Angel's Trumpet, Devil's Trumpet | Datura metel f. fastuosa |
| Drākshā | Mridvīkā, Gostanī | Grapes | Vitis vinifera |
| Echinacea (E) | | American Cone Flower | Echinacea purpurea |
| Eucalyptus (E) | | Fever Tree, Blue Gum Tree | Eucalyptus globulus |
| Evening Primrose (E) | | | Oenothera biennis |
| Fennel (E) | Shatapushpa, Mishi, Madhurikā | Fennel | Foeniculum vulgare |
| Flax seed (E) | Uma, Atasī | Flax Seed, Linseed | Linum usitatissimum |
| Gandhak rasayana | | | Compound |
| Gandharva harītakī | | Haritaki & Castor Oil | Compound |
| Ghee or Ghī (H) | Ghrita | Clarified Unsalted Butter | |
| Ghrita madhu | | Ghee and Honey | |
| Ginger Root (E) | Ārdrakam (fresh), Shunthi (powdered) | | Zingiber officinale |
| Gokshurādi guggulu | | | Compound |
| Gokshura | Gokshuraka, Trikantha | Puncture Vine | Tribulus terrestris |
| Goldenseal (E) | | Yellow Root | Hydrastis canadensis |
| Gudūchī | Amritā, Amritvallī, Madhuparnī | Heartleaf Moonseed | Tinospora cordifolia |
| Guggulu | Purā, Mahishāksha | Indian Bedellium | Commiphora mukul, Balsamodendron mukul |
| Gulvel sattva | | Special Preparation of Gudūchī | |

# Appendix

## Table 9: List of Herbs and Other Substances in this Book

| Name in Book | Sanskrit Name | Common Name | Botanical Name |
|---|---|---|---|
| Guñjā | Raktikā, Kākanantī | Wild Licorice | *Abrus precatorius* |
| Harītakī | Abhayā, Pathyā, Kāyasthā, Shivā | Chebulic Myrobalan | *Terminalia chebula* |
| Haridrā | Rajanī, Nishā, Rātri | Turmeric | *Curcuma longa* |
| Hawthorn (E) | | | *Crataegus laevigata*[c] |
| Hema garbha | | | *Compound* |
| Hibiscus (E) | | | *Hibiscus rosa-sinensis* |
| Hing | Rāmantha, Sahasravedhi | Asofoetida | *Ferula foetida/narthex* |
| Hingvastak chūrna | | | *Compound* |
| Indra | Vāruṇī | Bitter Apple | *Citrullus colocynthis* |
| Jātīphalā | Jātishasya | Nutmeg | *Myristica fragrans* |
| Jaipāla | Jayapāla, Mukula | Croton or Kroton | *Croton tiglium* |
| Jambul | | Indian Beech, Java Plum | *Syzygium cumini* |
| Jatamāmsi | Māmsī, Jathā, Jathilā | Indian Spikenard | *Nardostachys jatamamsi* |
| Jyotishmatī | Malkungi (H) | Staff Tree | *Celastrus paniculatus* |
| Kākolī | Kshirakākolī, Vāyasolī | | *Lilium polyphyllum* |
| Kāma dudhā | | | *Compound* |
| Kāñcanāra (H) | Kāñcanāraka | | *Bauhinia variegata* |
| Kaishore guggulu | | | *Compound* |
| Kapikacchū | Ātmaguptā | Cowitch Plant | *Mucuna pruriens* |
| Kapittha | Danta shatha | Wood Apple | *Feronia elephantum* |
| Karanja | Naktamala | Pongam Tree | *Pangamia glabra* |
| Karaskara | Kupīlu | Nux-Vomica Tree | *Strychnos nux-vomica* |
| Kasturi | | Musk-deer, Musk | *Moschus moschiferus* |
| Katukā (see kutki) | | | |
| Karela (H) | Kāravella, Kāravallaka | Bitter Gourd / Melon | *Momordica charantia* |
| Khadira | | Catechu | *Acacia catechu* |
| Khurasani ova | Pārasīka Yavānī, Yāvanī | | *Hyoscyamus niger* |
| Khus (G) | Ushīra, Vīrana, Ādhaya | Khus-khus Grass | *Andropogon muricatus* |
| Kumārī | | Aloe Vera | *Aloe barbadensis* |
| Kushtha (M) | Āmaya, Puskara | Costus | *Saussurea lappa* |

Table 9: List of Herbs and Other Substances in this Book

| Name in Book | Sanskrit Name | Common Name | Botanical Name |
|---|---|---|---|
| Kutaja | Kalinga, Shakra, Vatsaka | Conessi Bark | *Holarrhena antidysenterica* |
| Kutki | Titkā, Tiktarohinī, Katukī, Kutukā | Hellbore | *Picrorrhiza kurroa* |
| Laghu mālinī vasanta | | | *Compound* |
| Laksha | Laksha (lac) | Resin | *Cateria lacca* |
| Lakshmī vilas | | | *Compound* |
| Lasunadi vati | | | |
| Latākaranja | Putikaranja | Molucca Bean, Fever Nut | *Ceasalpinia bonducella* |
| Lavanga | Devapushpa | Clove | *Syzygium aromaticum* |
| Lodhra | Rodhra, Paththīkā | Lodh Tree | *Symplocos racemosa* |
| Loha (H) | Lauha | Iron | *Ferrum* |
| Loha bhasma | | Iron Bhasma | |
| Lotus (see padma) | | | |
| Mākaradvāja | | Insoluble Sulfide of Mercury-Gold | *Compound* |
| Mūtrala | | | *Compound* |
| Madana phala (M) | | Emetic Nut | *Randia dumetorum* |
| Madhu | | Honey | *Mel* |
| Mahā vāta vidvamsa | | | *Compound* |
| Mahānārāyana | | | *Compound* |
| Mahārasnādi kvath | | | *Compound* |
| Mahāsudarshan | | | *Compound* |
| Mahāyogarāja guggulu | | | *Compound* |
| Mandhūra bhasma | | Ferric Iron Oxide Calcination | *Compound* |
| Manjishthā | Vastraranjinī, Rakta | Madder Root | *Rubia cordifolia* |
| Mocharas/Mocha rasa | | | *Compound* |
| Moti bhasma | Muktā | Pearl Ash | *Mytilus margaritiferus* |
| Multani mitti or mati | | Fuller's Earth, Armenian Bole | *Silicate of alumina, magnesia, and oxide of iron* |
| Mustā | Mustaka, Nagar motha (M) | Nut-grass | *Cyperus rotundus* |
| Nāgakeshara (see also Saffron) | Keshara, Hemā, Nāgapushpa | Cobra's Saffron | *Mesua ferrea* |

## Table 9: List of Herbs and Other Substances in this Book

| Name in Book | Sanskrit Name | Common Name | Botanical Name |
|---|---|---|---|
| Neem (see nimba) (H, B, P) | | | |
| Nimba | Arishta, Picumarda | Neem, Indian Lilac | *Azadirachta indica* |
| Nimbu (H) | Jambha | Citric Acid | *Citrus bergamia* |
| Nirgundī | Sinduvāra, Nīla | Chinese Chaste Tree | *Vitex negundo* |
| Nishottara (M) | Trivrit, Nishota | Turpeth | *Ipomoea turpethum* |
| Nutmeg (E) (see jātīphalā) | | | |
| Osha (E) | | Colorado Cough Root | *Ligusticum porteri* |
| Pāshana bheda | | | *Compound* |
| Pātthā | | Velvet Leaf | *Cissampelos pareira* |
| Pachak vati | | | *Compound* |
| Padma | | Lotus | *Nelumbo nucifera* |
| Palash (M) | Palāsha, Kimshuka, Raktapushpaka | Bastard Teak | *Butea monosperma* |
| Parijata (see parijatak) | | | |
| Parijatak | | Night-flowering Jasmine | *Nyctanthes arbortristis* |
| Parpati | | | *Compound* |
| Passionflower (E) | | Maypop | *Passiflora incarnata* |
| Pippalī | Māgadhī, Granthikā | Indian Long Pepper | *Piper longum* |
| Pradarāntak vati | | | *Compound* |
| Pravāl pañchāmrit | | | *Compound* |
| Punarnavā | Kathhilla, Shothaghnī | Spreading Hogweed | *Boerhaavia diffusa* |
| Pushkaramūla | | Elecampane | *Inula racemosa* |
| Rāsnādi guggulu | | | *Compound* |
| Rāsna | Vandaka | | *Inula helenium* |
| Raktachandana | Raktānga | Heartwood, Red Sandalwood | *Pterocarpus santalinus* |
| Rasa | Pārada | Mercury | *Hydrargyrum* |
| Rasagandha | | | *Compound* |
| Raupya bhasma | | | *Compound* |
| Rose (E) | | | *Rosa damascena* |
| Sūkshma triphalā | | | *Compound* |

Table 9: List of Herbs and Other Substances in this Book

| Name in Book | Sanskrit Name | Common Name | Botanical Name |
|---|---|---|---|
| Saffron (E) | Kunkuma, Nāgakeshara | Kesar (H) | *Crocus sativus* |
| Saffron (E) | Nāgakeshara, Nāga | Cobra's Saffron, Indian Saffron | *Mesua ferrea* |
| Sandalwood (see raktachandana or chandana) | | | |
| Sanjīvanī | | | *Compound* |
| Saptaparnī | Sapthaparna | Dita Bark | *Alstonia scholaris* |
| Sarasvatī | | | *Compound* |
| Sarpagandha | Chandrika | | *Rawolfia serpentina* |
| Sat isabgol (H) | Ashvakarna | Psyllium Husks | *Plantago ovata* |
| Shanka vati | | | *Compound* |
| Shankha | | Conch | *Turbinella rapa, xanchus pyrum, or gastropoda* |
| Shankha bhasma | | Conch Ash | |
| Shankha pushpī | Shankhapushpā, Shankhinī | | *Evolvulus alsinoides* |
| Shardunikā | Meshasringī | Gurmar (H) | *Gymnema sylvestre* |
| Shatāvarī | | Asparagus Root | *Asparagus racemosus* |
| Shilājit | | Mineral Pitch, Asphalt | *Asphaltum* |
| Shringa bhasma | | Deer Horn Ash | *Compound* |
| Shuddha shilajit | | | *Compound* |
| Shulah vati | | | *Compound* |
| Shunthi (see ginger) | | | |
| Sitopalādi | | | *Compound* |
| Sudarshan | | Poison Bulb | *Crinum asiaticum* |
| Sudarshan gana vati | | | *Compound* |
| Sutshekhar | | | *Compound* |
| Suvarna | Svarna | Gold | *Aurum* |
| Suvarna malini vasant | | | *Compound* |
| Suvarna sutshekhar mātrā | | | *Compound* |
| Swayambhu guggulu | | | *Compound* |
| Tālīsādi | | | *Compound* |
| Tagara | Kālānusārī | Indian Valerian | *Valeriana wallichii* |
| Tankana | | Borax | *Sodii biboras* |
| Tikta churna | | | *Compound* |

## Appendix

### Table 9: List of Herbs and Other Substances in this Book

| Name in Book | Sanskrit Name | Common Name | Botanical Name |
|---|---|---|---|
| Tikta ghrita | | Bitter Ghee | *Compound* |
| Tobacco (E) | Tamakhu | | *Nicotiana tabacum* |
| Tribhuvan kirti (ras/ rasa) | Tribhuvana kirti | Traditional Formula | *Compound* |
| Trikatu | | | *Compound* |
| Triphalā | | | *Compound* |
| Tulsi | Tulasī, Surasā, Krishnatulasī | Holy Basil | *Ocimum sanctum* |
| Tumbī | Tumbinā | Bottle Gourd | *Lagenaria siceraria* |
| Turmeric (E) (see haridrā) | | | |
| Ushīra | Vīrana, Ādhaya | Vetiver | *Vetiveria zizanioides* |
| Ushīra (see khus) | | | |
| Vāsaka | Vāsā, Vrisha, Ātharūsha | Malabar Nut | *Adhatoda vasica* |
| Vacha | Vācā, Ugragandha | Sweet Flag | *Acorus calamus* |
| Vanga bhasma | | | *Compound* |
| Vangeshvara | | | *Compound* |
| Varuna (B) | Varana (S), Vayavarna (M) | Three-leaved Caper, Sacred Garlic Pear | *Crateva religiosa* |
| Vasant kusumakar ras (H, M) | | | *Compound* |
| Vetiver (see ushīra) | | | |
| Vidārī | Bhumikushmānda, Vidārikā | Indian Ginseng | *Ipomoea digitata*[d] |
| Vidanga | Jantughna, Vella, Krimighna | Embelia | *Embelia ribes* |
| Vijayā | Bhangā, Bhang (M) | Marijuana | *Cannabis sativa* |
| Visha garbha tailam | | | *Compound* |
| Wild Caraway (E) (see ajvain, yavānī) | | | *Carum copticum* |
| Yashthi madhu | Yashthikā, Madhūka | Licorice Root | *Glycyrrhiza glabra* |
| Yavānī | Ajamoda | Bishop's Weed | *Trachyspermum ammi, Carum roxburghianum, Carum copticum* |
| Yogarāja guggulu | | | *Compound* |

a. Black form is used in medicine.
b. Often erroneously known as Phyllanthus niruri, according to *Ayurvedic Medicine* by Sebastian Pole
c. Also known as Crataegus oxyacantha.
d. Used interchangeably with Pueraria tuberosa, according to *Ayurvedic Medicine* by Sebastian Pole.

## Table 10: Yogāsana Used in this Book

| | |
|---|---|
| Accomplished Pose | Siddhāsana |
| Boat Pose*a | Paripūrna Nāvāsana |
| Bow Pose* | Dhanurāsana |
| Bridge Pose* | Setu Bandha Sarvāngāsana |
| Camel Pose* | Ustrāsana |
| Cobra Pose* | Bhujangāsana |
| Corpse Pose | Shavāsana |
| Cow Pose* | Gomukhāsana |
| Eagle Pose | Garudāsana |
| Full Boat Pose | Paripūrna Nāvāsana |
| Head Stand | Shīrshāsana |
| Lion Pose | Simhāsana |
| Locust Pose | Salabhāsana |
| Lotus Pose | Padmāsana |
| Moon Salutation | Chandra Namaskār |
| Palm Tree Pose | Tālāsana |
| Peacock Pose | Mayūrāsana |
| Plow Pose | Halāsana |
| Cock or Rooster Pose | Kukkutāsana |
| Shoulder Stand | Sarvāngāsana |
| Half Spinal Twist | Ardha Matsyendrāsana |
| Sun Salutation | Sūrya Namaskār |
| Easy Cross-Legged Pose | Swastikāsana |
| Triangle Pose | Trikonāsana |
| Thunderbolt Pose | Vajrāsana |
| Tree Pose | Vriksāsana |

a. Photos of the poses with asterisks are on page 181.

## About The Ayurvedic Institute

The Ayurvedic Institute was established to promote the traditional knowledge of Ayurveda. In support of this, the Institute also offers programs in the sister disciplines of Ayurveda—Sanskrit, Yoga and Jyotisha (Vedic astrology.)

The Ayurvedic programs reflect the style of sitting with a traditional Indian teacher. The Vedic educational model is quite different from the "western" experience with which most of us are familiar. The knowledge is taught with the body, mind and spiritual components intact, along with practical examples, ceremonies and stories.

Vasant Lad, *Ayurvedic Physician*, founded the Ayurvedic Institute in 1984 and is its principal instructor. He graduated with a Bachelor of Ayurvedic Medicine and Surgery (B.A.M.&S.) from the University of Pune, India in 1968 and received a Master of Ayurvedic Science (M.A.Sc.) in 1980 from Tilak Ayurved Mahavidyalaya, also in Pune.

- **The Educational Department,** offers the Ayurvedic Studies Programs, Level One and Two, the Pune Gurukula Program, Yoga, and the Jyotish courses. Also available are the Ayurvedic correspondence course *Lessons & Lectures on Ayurveda* by Dr. Robert E. Svoboda and various weekend and intensive seminars with Vasant Lad and others.

- **The Herb Department** offers custom formulas made from Ayurvedic and Western herbs, CDs, DVDs, books, incense, and a variety of Ayurvedic and other products.

- **The Panchakarma Department** offers traditional Ayurvedic procedures for purification and rejuvenation that include oil massage, herbal steam treatment, shirodhara, cleansing diet, herbal therapy, and other treatments.

- **The Publishing Department**—The Ayurvedic Press—primarily publishes Vasant Lad's new books and articles, but also publishes other traditional Ayurvedic and Vedic works.

- **Membership** in the Ayurvedic Institute supports the aims and objectives of the Institute. Members receive the quarterly journal, *Ayurveda Today*, and a 10% discount on products and seminars.

---

## Contact us for more information:

**The Ayurvedic Institute**

PO Box 23445 • Albuquerque, New Mexico 87192-1445

(505) 291-9698 • Fax 505.294.7572

www.ayurveda.com